PHARMACY CLINICAL COORDINATOR'S HANDBOOK

Lynn Eschenbacher, PharmD, MBA, FASHP

National Director of Pharmacy Operations
The Resource Group, LLC
An Ascension Subsidiary
St. Louis, Missouri

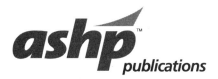

Any correspondence regarding this publication should be sent to the publisher, American Society of Health-System Pharmacists, 7272 Wisconsin Avenue, Bethesda, MD 20814, attention: Special Publishing.

The information presented herein reflects the opinions of the contributors and advisors. It should not be interpreted as an official policy of ASHP or as an endorsement of any product.

Because of ongoing research and improvements in technology, the information and its applications contained in this text are constantly evolving and are subject to the professional judgment and interpretation of the practitioner due to the uniqueness of a clinical situation. The editors and ASHP have made reasonable efforts to ensure the accuracy and appropriateness of the information presented in this document. However, any user of this information is advised that the editors and ASHP are not responsible for the continued currency of the information, for any errors or omissions, and/or for any consequences arising from the use of the information in the document in any and all practice settings. Any reader of this document is cautioned that ASHP makes no representation, guarantee, or warranty, express or implied, as to the accuracy and appropriateness of the information contained in this document and specifically disclaims any liability to any party for the accuracy and/or completeness of the material or for any damages arising out of the use or non-use of any of the information contained in this document.

Director, Special Publishing: Jack Bruggeman
Acquisitions Editor: Beth Campbell
Editorial Project Manager: Ruth Bloom
Production Manager: Kristin Eckles
Cover Design: Carol Barrer
Page Design: David Wade

Library of Congress Cataloging-in-Publication Data
Pharmacy clinical coordinator's handbook / [edited by] Lynn Eschenbacher.
    p. ; cm.
Includes bibliographical references and index.
ISBN 978-1-58528-478-8
    I. Eschenbacher, Lynn, editor. II. American Society of Health-System Pharmacists, issuing body. [DNLM: 1. Pharmacy Administration. 2. Administrative Personnel. 3. Pharmacy Service, Hospital--organization & administration. QV 737.1]
RS100
615.1068ʾ3--dc23
                    2015033759

ISBN: 978-1-58528478-8

10 9 8 7 6 5 4 3 2 1

Dedication

This book is dedicated to all of the pharmacy clinical coordinators who have worked tirelessly to develop and provide high-quality pharmacy services. Keep up the great work and strive for your best.

Thank you to my extremely supportive husband, Stephen, and my caring and loving children, Audrey, Madison, and Sloane. You encourage me and inspire me to be the best that I can.

Thank you to ASHP for providing so many opportunities for leadership and to advance our profession to provide the best care possible for our patients. All patients deserve a pharmacist as part of their care, and we need to continue to demonstrate our ability to impact patient care and advocate for our involvement.

Lynn Eschenbacher

Table of Contents

Contributors

Carrie A. Berge, PharmD, MS
Director of Pharmacy
Parkland Health & Hospital System
Dallas, Texas

Jennifer Burnette, PharmD, BCPS
Medication Safety Officer
Manager, Medication Policy, Quality
  & Investigational Drug Services
Jackson Memorial Hospital
Miami, Florida

Samuel V. Calabrese, BS Pharm, MBA, FASHP
Associate Chief Pharmacy Officer
Cleveland Clinic
Cleveland, Ohio

Steven S. Carlisle, PharmD, BCPS
Residency Program Director
Parkland Health & Hospital System
Dallas, Texas

Noelle R. M. Chapman, PharmD, BCPS, FASHP
Pharmacy Manager/PGY1 Residency Program
  Director
Northwestern Memorial Hospital
Chicago, Illinois

Jean B. Douglas, PharmD, FASHP
(Former) Clinical Pharmacy Coordinator
The Moses H. Cone Memorial Hospital
Cone Health
Greensboro, North Carolina

Lynn Eschenbacher, PharmD, MBA, FASHP
National Director of Pharmacy Operations
The Resource Group, LLC
An Ascension Subsidiary
St. Louis, Missouri

Robert P. Granko, PharmD, MBA
Director of Pharmacy
The Moses H. Cone Memorial Hospital
Cone Health
Greensboro, North Carolina

David Hager, PharmD, BCPS
Manager, Patient Care Services and
  Professional Development
Department of Pharmacy, UW Health
University of Wisconsin–Madison
Madison, Wisconsin

Jenna M. Huggins, PharmD, MBA, BCPS-AQ Cardiology
Senior Vice President, Retail Business
  Development
Mutual Drug
Durham, North Carolina

Scott Knoer, PharmD, MS, FASHP
Chief Pharmacy Officer
Cleveland Clinic
Cleveland, Ohio

Laurimay L. Laroco, PharmD
Pharmacy Clinical Coordinator–Adult
Emergency Department and Clinical Evaluation
  Areas
WakeMed Health & Hospitals
Raleigh, North Carolina

Bob Lobo, PharmD
Director, Clinical Programs
Department of Pharmaceutical Services
Vanderbilt University Medical Center
Nashville, Tennessee

Trista Pfeiffenberger, PharmD, MS
Director, Network Pharmacy Programs
  & Pharmacy Operations
Community Care of North Carolina
Raleigh, North Carolina

Kate M. Schaafsma, PharmD, MBA, MS, BCPS

Manager, Department of Pharmacy
Froedtert & the Medical College of Wisconsin
Milwaukee, Wisconsin

Jennifer M. Schultz, PharmD, FASHP

Clinical Pharmacy Supervisor/Residency
    Program Director
Bozeman Health Deaconess Hospital
Bozeman, Montana

Mark Sullivan, PharmD, MBA, BCPS

Executive Director, Pharmacy Operations,
    Vanderbilt University Hospital and Clinics
Vanderbilt Hospital Pharmacy
Nashville, Tennessee

Antonia Zapantis, PharmD, MS, BCPS

Associate Professor
Director of Experiential Education
Nova Southeastern University
Fort Lauderdale, Florida

Rhonda Zillmer, PharmD

Pharmacy Manager
WakeMed Health & Hospitals
Raleigh, North Carolina

Preface

The pharmacy clinical coordinator is a valuable member of the healthcare team. If you are an experienced clinical coordinator, this book will help enhance your practice. If you are just starting on your journey as a pharmacy clinical coordinator, this book can be your step-by-step guide to succeeding in this essential and demanding position. There is much to learn and master to be an effective and high-performing pharmacy clinical coordinator. First, *clinical* is just the start. You have discovered, or soon will discover, that you are also a coach, mentor, innovator, and visionary as well as an expert in human resources, operations, logistics, finance, safety, and risk management. Use this book to help you generate the ideas you will need as a pharmacy leader to impact your staff in a positive way and ensure optimal patient care outcomes.

The *Pharmacy Clinical Coordinator's Handbook* will be your guide for practical tools and tips on just about everything related to being a pharmacy clinical coordinator or clinical manager. We have brought together top experts from our profession to provide you with real-life, practical information. The tone of the book is conversational, as if you had one of these experts sitting right with you all the time providing knowledge and expertise just for you. We hope this book will be the go-to resource for coordinators or managers who want to take their practice to the next level and make a difference in healthcare and patient care.

Have you ever asked these questions as a clinical coordinator?

- How does pharmacy provide value to the healthcare team?
- Who should I get to know in my organization so that if I need something I have already developed that relationship?
- How do I build my team and inspire them to achieve high-quality outcomes for patient care?
- What can I do to advance practice?
- There is so much to do. Where do I start, and how do I even know what to do?
- I have been a coordinator for many years. Is there more that I can do?

We have provided answers to all of these questions and many more. The book includes many charts, checklists, protocols, processes, diagrams, references, and websites for you to generate ideas on how you can improve what you are doing and how you can impact your team.

You should enjoy what you do as a clinical coordinator or manager. You are in a position in which you can positively impact the lives of your staff as well as the patients that you serve. Being in middle management can be tough, but if you have a clear vision and strategy and set clear expectations for your team members and hold them accountable, you can achieve anything!

If your actions inspire others to dream more, learn more, do more and become more,
you are a leader.

—*John Quincy Adams*

I shall pass this way but once; any good that I can do or any kindness I can show to any human being; let me do it now. Let me not defer nor neglect it, for I shall not pass this way again.

—*Stephen Grellet, Quaker Missionary*

These two quotes will help you remember the great power that you have as a clinical coordinator to do your best and to lead others to do their best. Our patients count on us as pharmacists to touch their lives in such a way that they either stay healthy or get better as a result of our involvement.

Go forward, and do great things for yourself, your employees, and your patients.

Lynn Eschenbacher

List of Figures, Tables, and Appendixes

Chapter 15. Incorporating Students and Residents into It All

Chapter 16. Putting It All Together: The Effective Clinical Coordinator

n/a

CHAPTER 1

Getting Started

Noelle R. M. Chapman

KEY TERMS

Credentialing—Credentialing is used by organizations to validate professional license, clinical experience, and other preparation for a specialized practice; qualifications documentation expected and/or required for a healthcare provider to practice in a specific setting.

Delegation—Delegation is entrusting a task or responsibility to another person, typically one who is less senior than oneself.

Practice Model—A practice model describes how pharmacy department resources are deployed to provide patient care.

Privileging—Privileging is a process to define specific services provided by a pharmacist practitioner; ensures the individuals that are granted privileges to perform said activities can demonstrate competency and have ample experience providing services.

Introduction

Congratulations on your decision to become a clinical coordinator! The first feeling you may be experiencing after the initial excitement is fear. If you experience a crisis of confidence when taking on new challenges, be assured it is a normal feeling. I have two pieces of advice to help you fight your way through it:

1. *Trust yourself and those around you.* If you have been offered a position as a clinical coordinator, chances are you have already proven you can be successful doing a portion of what will be required of you. This means you know more than you think you do! Additionally, positions are not typically offered unilaterally, so there were likely several people that made the decision to choose you. Trust your own experiences and their knowledge and wisdom to put you in a coordinator position. Your success is directly tied to theirs, so do not be afraid to consult them or other experts for advice, and follow your instincts.

2. *Learn from your mistakes, and let them make you better.* Remember when you first got your pharmacist license? You were really excited to be a "real" pharmacist, but then somewhere along the line you made your first error. You were terrified because the reality of your responsibility and power hit home in a very real way. Hopefully, we all take the errors we make and use them to transform ourselves into better pharmacists. Having a coordinator position is no different. You have a new level of authority and power that is exciting! You are actually going to make changes that improve the overall care of patients in a more wide-reaching way than before; however, like everything else in life, you should consult manuals, handbooks, and experts to help you through common issues and prepare you for circumstances that lie ahead. As humans, we are prone to error; we may communicate ineffectively or miss a deadline. Take your misstep, handle it graciously, and learn from it.

In this chapter, we will explore transitioning into the clinical coordinator role, evolving into an effective leader, and maintaining balance. This chapter is meant to provide you with a road map for success by introducing you to some of the concepts developed throughout the book. Buckle your seatbelt!

The First 90 Days (5-point vehicle check)

Before you go on a road trip it is important to make sure your oil has been changed, the tires are aligned and at the right pressure, your lights and windshield wipers are in working order, and your gas tank is full. The last thing you want is to get partially through your trip and need a tow truck because your tires blew out. Starting out as a clinical coordinator is similar; all of the pieces must be in working condition to get you to your destination.

Vehicle Walkaround

When you rent or purchase a new vehicle, you are usually required to walk around the car to make sure every dent or scratch is taken into account. Until this point, I have assumed you have done the appropriate preparatory work to be an effective clinical coordinator. Make sure you have the information you need to start the journey and have assessed your new situation appropriately. Write down the answers to the following questions to ensure you have all the information you need to set personal goals.

Know your institution. Have you taken the time to familiarize yourself with your environment and its culture? What is your patient population? Does your institution serve a wide variety of patients with various clinical services, or does it have a narrower focus? For example, if you work at a large academic medical center, your clinical scope is going to differ from a mid-sized institution that primarily treats cancer or cardiac patients. Additionally, what is important to your institution? What is the vision and mission and specific goal(s) the institution is trying to achieve? This will become important as you set your personal goals to help to create a common language.

Know your department and staff. As a clinical coordinator you will be leading the clinical charge of the department. This is a key element for success. What is the **practice model** of the pharmacy? How does the department work with physicians, nurses, and other healthcare professionals to positively impact patient care? How does the staff view professional development and experiential education? What are the demographics of the department? Working with a large group of recent graduates with specialized residency training will present very different challenges than working with a small staff of seasoned pharmacists. How integrated is technician practice? What is the departmental leadership like, and how do you integrate into that?

Know your job requirements. Where a clinical coordinator fits into the organization chart varies greatly from institution to institution. Some clinical coordinator roles are at a staff pharmacist level (preparing materials and guiding decisions of the pharmacy and therapeutics committee), whereas others are at a manager or assistant director level. Knowing how and where you fit in the department will drive the responsibilities of your job. What percentage of your time will be on the front line taking care of patients? What percentage is off-line office work? What are you expected to *do* versus whom are you expected to *lead*? What are required tasks and their frequency (e.g., are you responsible for preparing quarterly quality reports or running monthly clinical team meetings)? Are the expectations of the job realistic? Do you have an affiliation with a college of pharmacy and/or teaching requirements? Are your teaching requirements didactic or experiential? It is easy to get excited about the direction you want to move in or the changes you want to implement, but you will never make progress on those things unless you know and fulfill the tasks and responsibilities that are required of you.

Know yourself. It is important to have a firm grasp of your skills, abilities, and opportunities for improvement. This continual analysis will be discussed in more depth later in this chapter; however, if you cannot easily state what you are good at, what you are passionate about, and what your weaknesses are, spend some time identifying those pieces of information before you dive into the rest of this journey.

Oil Change

One of the crucial elements to vehicle maintenance is checking the oil. Before beginning any long trip, it is wise to make sure your vehicle has had an oil change based on the manufacturer's recommended distance (e.g., every 3,000 miles). Likewise, when you are starting off as a clinical coordinator it is very important to assess your team. What is their attitude toward clinical programs? What about growth of those programs and themselves? How comfortable are they interacting with physicians, nurses, and patients? You need to have a clear understanding of the culture of the team, but more importantly you need to spend time getting to know the individual team members and assessing them as well. Who is motivated? Who is complacent? What are they comfortable doing, and how much do they "own" medication management? If your team is highly motivated and very clinically involved and you start off talking about adjusting medications for renal function, you will lose credibility. Listening to and assessing your team are essential.

How do you go about assessing a team? Initially, take the time to work alongside team members performing various duties and learn how they round, document, teach, and dispense. Work with technicians who perform clinical duties, such as taking medication histories, and with pharmacists from outside your department (e.g., transplant and medication safety pharmacists) to learn their responsibilities and how they integrate into your department. This knowledge will become invaluable because you will empathize rather than sympathize with staff members. Initially, you should focus on information gathering and not on introducing change. It takes time to know what your team does, but the initial investment will make work easier and more effective down the road. An added benefit to knowing what people do is getting to know them personally in the process.

Knowing people and developing a meaningful relationship with them is the cornerstone to accomplishing anything. It is perhaps the most time-consuming part of what you will do, but it is essential to being an effective and relevant coordinator. Not all of us are vocal, transparent, or communicate easily, and we do not all have the same values or motivations. How can you know the members of your team well enough within the first few months to start doing the things you want to do? Be systematic. Schedule one-on-one time with each team member and emphasize that this is a two-way learning process. One technique that has been successful for me is to ask everyone the following series of questions:

1. What are your strengths?
2. What are your opportunities for improvement?
3. What are your interests?
4. What would you like to see changed?
5. What are your future career goals?

Although these five questions seem simple enough, you can learn a lot about a person from the responses you receive. Do they only answer in a pharmacy-related manner or as a whole person? Are they critical thinkers? What is their passion, or have they not yet determined that? If you get to know the people you are working with, you should be able to align their strengths and interests with your department/institution's goals to create a highly satisfying and productive environment for both of you. As with changing your vehicle's oil, it is important to ensure that this process occurs at a predetermined time interval. That interval will depend on the size and scope of your responsibilities and the role the clinician plays; however, having these conversations at least every 6 months keeps the engine running smoothly. As you continue past the initial few months in your role, your questions may morph or become less systematic. Ideally, you will not need to routinely ask question 4 because you will have built up such strong relationships with your team members that they will openly come to you with ideas or issues.

Tire Check

At some point the "rubber needs to hit the road," meaning you have work to do and you need to make sure your tires are appropriately rotated, have enough tread, and have adequate air pressure. Knowing your requirements requires a balance among tactile responsibilities—doing and leading.

If you hope to make a positive impact on patient care, you need to know what is expected of you. What meetings must you attend, or lead? What reports need to get out and on what time frame? What metrics are you expected to work on? Hopefully at this point in your career you have mastered time management skills. Moving into a new level of

responsibility requires you to re-evaluate your skills. You may have to step back, assess your time commitments, and put everything back together in a way that is more effective. If you are starting at a new institution, this can be an easier process because you have left all your old job responsibilities behind. If you accepted a clinical coordinator position at the same institution, it can be a difficult process to let go of duties and make the transition. **Delegation** is often the most difficult skill to master at any level. You do not want to delegate tasks and responsibilities inappropriately because you may then be viewed negatively; however, it is necessary to delegate some duties otherwise you may be viewed as either a micromanager or someone who does not trust others. As a general rule of thumb, the questions you should ask yourself are listed in **Figure 1-1**. Thinking through and aligning your requirements and priorities will go a long way toward being an effective coordinator.

Having your tires rotated and aligned is only part of the process. Without the appropriate amount of tread (i.e., clinical coordinator's knowledge or skill), you can slip and slide all over the place. If you continue to self-evaluate, you will be one step ahead because you will know your opportunities for improvement before anyone else. (This applies to personal qualities as well as skills.) However, if you want to do the best job you possibly can, you must know where your gaps are and make a concerted effort to hone your skills. You have already started personal assessment by taking stock of your requirements and expectations. Use this list to identify what abilities are needed to meet expectations. A common way to think of your skills is to divide them into the following three categories: tactile (technical or clinical skills), professional, and leadership. When making your list of necessary skills, do not overlook the obvious such as baseline clinical knowledge in a particular subject or knowing how to operate the pharmacy computer system. Clinicians can become ineffective simply because they were trying to make clinical recommendations that computer systems or formularies do not support. Once you have a completed list, be honest with yourself about your abilities in each area. **Figure 1-2** contains examples of potential skills necessary for a clinical coordinator role. These are just a few examples to get you started (the table is not intended to

FIGURE 1-1. Delegation Flow Chart

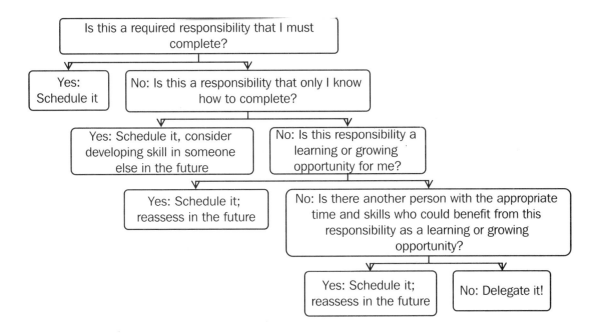

be all-inclusive). Evaluate your level of comfort or knowledge for each skill. In addition to self-assessment, it is beneficial to have a mentor or coworker fill out the table so you have a more accurate view of where you need to exert your energies to get desired traction. Once you have identified your personal gaps, there are various ways to address filling in those gaps, such as developing a personal action plan. Almost always, this plan will include consulting your mentor, education, and reassessment.

Taking a look at the air pressure in your tires helps you to avoid serious issues. It is the same with analyzing your team's skill gaps. Once you have completed your self-assessment, do the same with your clinicians. Often coming up with the list of abilities your team members need is easier than coming up with your own, but validating their abilities is more difficult, especially when it comes to abstract qualities like communication and decision-making. As with gauging tire pressure, you will need a tool to assess whether their assessment of their comfort and knowledge is under- or overinflated. The tool's effectiveness relies on defining what high, moderate, and low comfort/knowledge means. There is no need to reinvent the wheel as it is likely your institution already

has some of this defined as part of its annual evaluation process. For the areas that are not defined, consult with your leaders and team to set definitions for the group. For example, how do you assess another pharmacist's communication skills regarding clinical decisions? One way may be to have them submit three or four examples of notes they have written in patients' charts. Another way would be to survey nurses, physicians, and other team members as you surveyed your mentors and colleagues when doing your own skill assessment.

Once you are further along in your position, surveying and assessment will become less formal because you have built relationships; however, it is important to have a process for reassessment (perhaps through the annual evaluation process) as the intention of identifying gaps is to eventually fill them. What was once an opportunity for improvement could potentially become a strength, so you want to guard against pigeonholing your team members or yourself.

Headlights, Tail Lights, and Brake Lights

Lights are an important safety feature on any vehicle. They help you to see where you are

FIGURE 1-2. Skill Assessment Chart

	Necessary Skill or Ability	Level of Comfort or Knowledge		
		High	Moderate	Low
Tactile	Medication order review			
	Patient discharge education			
	Knowledge base: cardiology			
	Communicating with team on rounds			
Professional	Effective meeting management			
	Implementing plans			
	Communicating with other departments			
	Making patient-focused decisions			
Leadership	Direction setting			
	Role modeling			
	Team building			
	Organizational involvement			

going and work to communicate your actions with those around you. In this way, your headlights, tail lights, and brake lights are your institutional leaders. You need them to see where you are going and direct your vision and plans. Anticipate working with some leaders more than others; identify these leaders and set up interviews with them. Be thoughtful about your list as everyone's time is valuable, and you want to be considerate and effective. For example, having a relationship with the chief executive officer could be beneficial, but unless you are at a director level or above it is not likely an appropriate use of his or her time or your own. Your list should include pharmacy leaders (which you will already know from your walkaround and assessment of your team); appropriate senior management; nursing managers; key medical staff; safety and quality members; and information technology personnel. During your meetings, ascertain their opinion of current clinical pharmacy services and their future expectations for scope and quality. The primary goals of these interviews are to listen and develop relationships. Come prepared with questions, but make sure to be conversational to facilitate your goals. Because you will meet with or talk to these people frequently, do not feel you need

to discuss everything in this initial interview. Write down ideas mentioned during these interviews as they may help you generate alignment and quick wins when you start working toward development.

Depending on how progressive your institution is regarding pharmacy practice, you may be disappointed by some of the opinions or the information you receive. Do not be discouraged! Elevating pharmacy practice and affecting positive change in your institution may be part of the reason you were hired. It is far more important for you to get an accurate idea of how clinical pharmacy practice is viewed during these interviews than to start pushing an agenda immediately. This will help you see down the road to create common goals and set the tone for future practice.

Making Sure the Wipers Work

Have you ever been in a vehicle and the windshield wipers do not completely clear off the windshield? Fortunately this problem has a simple remedy, but you have to think ahead and check the wipers before you are on the road in a rainstorm. As you start your journey as a clinical coordinator, do not wait to have issues before identifying a mentor. A mentor is an experienced and trusted advisor and is commonly referred to in business, leadership, and educational literature as a key component to success. If you do not have an established mentor, there are resources available to find a mentor; however, the best place to look for a mentor is right within your organization. Some key questions to consider when choosing a mentor have been described in the pharmacy literature[1]:

- Do you have a sincere willingness to grow?
- Do you admire this person professionally?
- Do you feel comfortable with this person and trust your conversations will be held in confidence?
- Is this person positive, optimistic, encouraging, and enthusiastic?
- Are you okay with having this person be candid with you and challenge you to reach your career potential?
- Are you willing to share your fears, failures, and concerns?

Like checking your windshield wipers routinely, maintaining a mentor–mentee relationship requires frequent contact. Once you have established a mentor, make sure to routinely schedule meetings. This is especially important during the first 90 days as you get to know each other.

Filling the Gas Tank

Now that you have assessed your team, figured out what you need to do, built a personal network, and established a mentor relationship, you have the required pieces to start planning what you would like to accomplish. Having a firm but flexible plan is like having gas in your tank—you will not get far without it! Strategic planning will be discussed in more detail later in this handbook, but there are several key components you will need in the first 90 days.

- **Issues.** Your list may be lengthy at first and should contain information gathered from your team, your own observations, and interviews with institutional leaders.

- **Resources.** You need to know what you are working with and what is working well. This list should include both tangible resources like computer systems and intangible resources like motivated personnel, which show leadership potential.
- **Metrics.** What measures does your institution aim to hit? Which ones are looming that you could potentially impact? Think outside the box, and take into consideration the views of those you interviewed.
- **Needs.** It is unlikely you began this position with everything you need at your fingertips. Define what you need to get the job done (note that this is different than the list of issues). Again, the items may be tangible (e.g., a reliable pharmacy documentation system) or intangible (e.g., preceptor development).
- **Priorities.** Determining the issues of highest importance will help you define your short-term and long-term focus.

Every trip has its unavoidable developments. You may get into a fender-bender or get a flat tire; however, if you prepare adequately you can minimize your risks and increase your chance of a successful journey.

Evolving into a Leader

It is essential to see ourselves as leaders so we need to devote time toward developing leadership skills. The levels at which we lead may be different. Some people lead entire departments, and some lead clinical initiatives. On the most basic level, we all should be leading medication management for our patients. As a clinical coordinator, you are expected to lead *something*, so starting off with a plan to develop or enhance your leadership skills will increase the likelihood of your success.

Leading You

One of the most inherent yet overlooked leadership principles is that to lead you need someone to follow. Why would someone follow you? Do you have great ideas or natural charisma? Do you stand for something? There is not just one type of leader. Obviously, everyone cannot lead all of the time. What and when you lead will emerge through your personal style.

Your leadership style is a compilation of many things such as your inherent qualities and abilities, your conflict resolution abilities, your views on change, etc. To be an effective leader, you need to really know yourself. The famous psychologist Viktor Frankl once said, "Between stimulus and response there is a space. In that space is our power to choose our response. In our response lies our growth and freedom."[2] Having a good sense of self can move you from

Stimulus→Response

to

Stimulus→**Choice**→Response

Becoming less reactionary will likely lead you to make choices that can result in happiness and success. Earlier in the chapter you were asked to think about what you are good at, what you are passionate about, and what your weaknesses are. This is just the tip of the iceberg. Below are some activities that are used with departmental leaders and trainees to increase self-awareness. By no means is this an exclusive list, but it can help you get started. The important part of any of these activities is honesty. View yourself as you really are, not as you think you should be. It is helpful to validate results with someone who will keep you accountable, such as your mentor.

Personality Assessments

There are several types of personality assessments available (see Chapter 8: Staff Development—10 Factors to Guide Performance and Chapter 14: Leadership from the Clinical Coordinator's Perspective). One of the most widely used assessments is the Myers-Briggs Type Indicator (MBTI) based on the psychological typology identified by Carl Gustav Jung and further developed by Katharine Cook Briggs and her daughter Isabel Briggs Myers. The assessment identifies your natural preferences in a series of four dichotomies: extraversion (E)/introversion (I), sensing (S)/intuition (N), thinking (T)/feeling (F), and judging (J)/perceiving (P). Another common personality assessment is the DiSC assessment that focuses on four different personality traits: dominance, influence, steadiness, and conscientiousness.

A certified administrator should perform the assessments, and many institutions have it available; however, if not available, uncertified assessments are available on the Internet.

The purpose of a personality assessment is not to typecast you but to bring insight to your preferences and how you direct your energy and efforts. If you know your natural tendencies, then you have the opportunity to make cognitive decisions and interactions to either enhance or modify your natural tendencies. For example, my natural preference is to be introverted. I decided that to do the things I wanted to do, I needed to be more comfortable in social settings. I pushed myself out of my comfort zone and, over the course of time, adapted my tendencies to become more extroverted. Please note that there is nothing wrong with being an introvert. Personality testing is not intended to state that one preference is better than another. I share this example because I made the conscious choice to shift my tendencies; knowing yourself and your preferences is what allows you to do that. To know which direction you need to go, you need to know where you are.

Conflict Management

As with personality testing, there are many different options for determining your conflict style. Most of the conflict style inventory tests were designed on the basis that there are five main conflict styles, most commonly referred to as directing, harmonizing, compromising, avoiding, and cooperating. Similarly, there is no right and wrong conflict style, but there are advantages and disadvantages to each. As you shift into the new role of clinical coordinator, you will find that there will be times when you have to play peace keeper between conflicting parties. You may need to make a hard call on a patient's therapy, or there may be battles you simply want to avoid. Knowing your conflict style will allow you to move along the continuum to be most effective. Sometimes to stay true to who we are, we need to change tactics.

Mission Statement

In my opinion, the most important thing you can do to develop yourself is to have a personal mission statement. We all have a visionary self: the person that we want to be. I have yet to meet a person who says "I want to make bad decisions," yet we all do from time to time. Your personal vision takes into account all the various pieces of you (deciphered from the above assessments) and leads you to your visionary self. Your mission should be based on your unique personal values and principles. It should focus on what you want to be and do, so it can serve as a guiding light through your future decisions. If you have never written a personal mission statement, make it a priority to do so right away. It is a difficult endeavor you likely will modify over time, but without one you cannot have a solid professional or leadership mission, and your goals are just tasks without context in a bigger picture.

Goal Setting

Although many people cringe at the thought of New Year's resolutions, I love the concept. What a perfect time to think about your personal mission and determine what you will do to reach it. The steps toward reaching that mission are your goals. If you have never set personal goals, there are many tools available to walk you through the process. Regardless which process you decide on, make sure to write your goals down and to make them SMARTER.[3,4]

Specific—Who, what, where, when, which, and why

Measurable—Determine if you have met the goal

Achievable—Attainable but not too easy

Relevant—Consistent with mission and other goals

Timebound—Set a due date

Evaluated—Bring out the yard stick

Reviewed—Consistent reminder of what you want to achieve

Personal Development

If you read any leadership or personal development books and articles, you will find that everyone has a set of principles on which they build their theories. Below are five leadership principles from my readings and experiences that are applicable to my practice in the clinical pharmacy arena.

1. **Team building is essential to success.** You are not alone in your quest for better

patient care. Think about the information you have gathered from your team, discuss with your mentor, and start building.

2. **Surround yourself with people better than you.** This is not intended to suit the self-deprecating. The reality is that we cannot be the best at everything. In your personality and conflict assessments you should have learned the value of people who think and act differently than you do. Find those with amazing talent and those that complement your gaps, and get them on your team to make your concerted effort stronger.

3. **Align and empower.** You can have an amazing team and the best people surrounding you, but if you are all moving in different directions, you will accomplish very little. Have a plan and communicate it clearly and often. Set and communicate clear expectations, and hold yourself and others accountable to those expectations. If you have done a good job surrounding yourself with talent, empower those people to use their talents to execute the plan. You want to create an open environment where people are free to be creative within their limits. As a generalization, pharmacists tend to be a little meticulous. Do not let your own meticulousness get in the way of what you want to accomplish. For example, if you are implementing an antimicrobial stewardship team, have your team train all of your staff to recognize and be able to make recommendations for the most common antimicrobial scenarios in your institution. You do not need an infectious diseases specialist to dose vancomycin or treat community-acquired pneumonia. Save their expertise for the situations that really need them.

4. **Have a system for accountability.** As with your own personal or professional goals, write down what you are working toward as a team. Check in with your team members to ensure that they are hitting deadlines and maintaining service standards.

5. **Inspire.** Your role as a clinical coordinator means people are looking to you for direction. If you do not give positive feedback, those people will eventually lose interest

and become callous. Inspire them to work toward your common goal. Communicate quick wins, and reward participation and hard work. You do not need to break the bank to do this. Simple thank-you cards and a positive attitude goes a long way (so does pizza or chocolate—people love food).

Although these five principles are what I have found to be the pillars in my leadership success, find ones you are comfortable with and that work for you.

Lifelong Learning Plan

Maybe you are reading this thinking, "I already know this. I know myself, and I'm not new to leadership, but I'm looking to sharpen my skills." Terrific! There is always something new to learn or a skill to improve. To know what those are in ourselves, we need a lifelong learning plan. As you master certain skills or your path leads you in new directions, your learning plan may morph, but there are some fundamentals to help you stay on your game.

Reading. It is exceptionally difficult to stay on top of medical literature! It is so overwhelming to see so many new articles come out and not be able to scratch the surface. Establishing a reading plan leads to many benefits. First, determine what journals, subject areas, or professional social media sites you are either interested in or need to stay on top of for your job. Now that you are in a leadership role, consider some journals outside of pharmacy that have a business focus, such as *Modern Healthcare*, *Becker's Hospital Review*, and *The Wall Street Journal*. Then set up an electronic CliffsNotes version of those items. Many journals, websites, and libraries will compile a list of new postings or articles and a brief description so you can quickly scan to pull out those you want to further explore. Be discerning. First, review the abstract to get the gist of what you need to know. By doing this, you create your own mental card catalog that enables you to review that reference when you need the details. Have a similar process for listservs and professional social media sites. To organize your information, create email folders for the compiled lists you receive. Periodically go through those folders and, if you have not used any of the information in there, edit your

initial list. If something new catches your attention or your focus moves in a new direction, you may need to add to your initial list. In addition to periodic literature, read books or magazines for pleasure. Not only is it a great way to relax, but it also gives insight to generate creative solutions to problems or helps you to see situations in a different light.

Professional organizational involvement. There are many benefits to being actively involved in professional organizations, and education is one of them. Education through professional organizations comes in many formats: live CE sessions, roundtable discussions, webinars, online resources, journals, etc. However, I have found that the most useful educational points I gain are through networking with people who are facing similar issues. To reap these benefits, you need to be engaged. Chose an organization that speaks to you—whether it is local or national, focuses on a specialty practice area, or has a more general approach—and explore various ways to get involved. Sometimes information on how to become involved is detailed on a website, such as the ASHP Section of Inpatient Care Practitioners.[5] Most organizations have many opportunities to get involved that do not require a large time commitment. One of the easiest ways to find out more is to attend the organization's networking events, which are typically smaller in size than a meeting with the opportunity to meet people face-to-face. There are usually sign-in sheets where you can leave your email address and request more information. However you choose to get involved, professional organizations provide you with an opportunity to stay up-to-date with issues and receive current educational information.

Building your portfolio. Reading and educational sessions only take you so far. Sometimes we need opportunities to sharpen our skills or explore things on a deeper and formal level. Fortunately there are several established voluntary postresidency educational opportunities including certificate programs, certifications, and degree programs within the profession. These opportunities are very important not just to keep you abreast of knowledge, but to keep you informed on the significant changes of pharmacists' roles on the healthcare team. In your role as clinical coordinator, you may be expected to expand services to include more direct patient care opportunities or develop specialized teams. **Credentialing** helps to demonstrate competency in advanced practice areas, helps in the pursuit of compensation for services, and helps to elevate our accountability to our patients. ASHP has a useful resource center that outlines resources and the importance of credentialing and **privileging**.[6]

Certificate programs (also called *practice-based continuing pharmacy education activities*) are typically awarded by educational institutions or pharmacy organizations and include didactic instruction, demonstration of professional competency, and/or simulations. They are shorter in duration than other programs listed but longer than a standard continuing education session. Some examples of certificate programs include immunization delivery, medication therapy management, and diabetes management programs. Traineeships are similar to certificate programs but tend to be of a longer duration (e.g., 5 days) and have a more intense individualized focus.[7] There are traineeships available for specific clinical areas (e.g., pain and palliative care) as well as in leadership training (e.g., Pharmacy Leadership Institute).

Certifications are granted to pharmacists who have demonstrated a level of competency beyond that needed for licensure in a focused area of practice. Pharmacist certification programs are primarily undertaken by the Board of Pharmacy Specialties (BPS). To achieve certification, a pharmacist must successfully pass a written examination. Some specialties also include an experiential component. Specific continuing education modules or re-examination are required for recertification. Some certification specialties include pharmacotherapy, oncology, and ambulatory care pharmacy; however, BPS is consistently reviewing petitions for new specialties.

Degree programs are available at any higher education institution and are not necessarily pharmacy specific (e.g., master's in business administration); however, the ASHP Foundation offers the Pharmacy Leadership Academy (PLA), which takes general business and leadership principles and ties them in with pharmacy practice. The program consists of various modules on a range of critical topics, incorporating self-learning and reading, presentations, and case based interactive components. The PLA is recognized by colleges and universities as a graduate-level program, and participants are eligible for consideration of waiver of graduate credit hours toward a master's degree (e.g., master's in healthcare administration).

Depending on whether you are looking to hone a particular clinical skill or have a more broad-based approach to your growth, building up your portfolio can have long-lasting personal and professional benefits.

Leading Others

There are too many leadership concepts to adequately cover in this chapter (see suggested readings); however, there are a few concepts to be thoughtful of at the beginning of your tenure as a clinical coordinator to avoid pitfalls along the way.

Leading "Friends"

A natural part of working alongside people is forming friendships. One of the most challenging aspects of becoming a clinical coordinator is guiding those you are currently working beside or have recently been your peers or friends even if you do not have people reporting directly to you. Although there is no magic formula to follow, and peer leadership is fraught with peril, some basic building blocks can help you avoid disasters along the way.

Deidentify. Leading peers can be difficult because you know them on another level. The pitfall is that sometimes this can lead either to favoritism or reverse favoritism (being harder on those you know). A helpful technique when determining how to approach a situation is to do what we do in clinical education: deidentify. Personalize after you have decided on a course of action. For example, when you treat someone with heart failure you look at their symptoms and test results to determine what treatments they need. After you determine the course, you adjust the angiotensin-converting-enzyme inhibitor to ensure that it is covered by insurance or change the timing to be compatible with the patient's lifestyle. Gather the facts, respect the rules, and be consistent. If you can adopt this approach, you will avoid bending the rules or having different expectations for friends.

Privacy. Being a clinical coordinator is a position of authority. Like it or not, that means that there is a larger target on your back than there was before. Consistency in upholding your values has become more important. As a general rule, we need to be cautious of what we allow people to see on social media. Although people like to have fun and let their hair down, do not advertise your escapades with your friends. Being accepted and being respected are of equal importance as they directly relate to your professionalism. In addition, your coworkers may bring forward items of sensitive nature. Confidentiality is important as well as knowing when to elevate something of a critical nature.

It is not about you. As much as we have focused on getting started, knowing yourself, and developing your skills, the bottom line is that this is all for a bigger purpose and not for your own benefit. By keeping the spotlight on what you want to accomplish, you will show you are working toward the good of the whole and not just for yourself or a certain select few.

Breed competence. Earlier we discussed surrounding yourself with people who are better than you. If your peers are objectively practicing at the top of their game, it becomes more about them getting what they deserve and less about you handing out favors. I have found that people I chose to surround myself with are hardworking, intelligent, and self-driven. These are qualities that I respect and admire regardless if they are coworkers, friends, or both. Surrounding myself with greatness has not only made me better, but also has made peer leadership much easier.

Be aware of distrust. There is always someone wanting to fight "the man." No matter what you do, there will be people who automatically distrust you because of what you stand for instead of whom you really are or what you are working toward. Stay true to core values and you will not have to waste your time trying to fight other people's issues.

Use what you know. There is one advantage to leading peers. You know firsthand what they want to accomplish and the frustrations that are holding them back. Use that knowledge to make things better. It may not be on upper management's radar that it takes 47 clicks to write a pharmacokinetic note in a patient's chart, but it might be a huge annoyance to the staff. Help to resolve some of these smaller issues and you will gain support from your peers.

Accountability. Whether you are interacting with your friends, peers, or people who refer to you as their supervisor, accountability is essential. Additionally, you need to be accountable for the expectations of your position. Accountability can be viewed either as a support group or a stick depending on your approach and the situation. In theory, it should be much easier to hold those you are friendly with accountable, but that is not always the case.

Authentic Leadership

The skills required for leadership—motivation, clear communication, influence, and organization—are not a secret. Some ways to develop or acquire these traits are described above. How to use these traits in practice is much more difficult. Think back to some of the most effective and influential people in your career. Did they appear to use the above skills as tools, or were the skills seamless with their personality? Did they behave differently in front of peers than in front of people they were leading? Or were they consistently genuine in every interaction? As you start out on your journey, you will acquire skills and knowledge that make you a stronger and better practitioner and leader. Do not wield those skills as weapons in an arena. Incorporate them into who you are and how you react so you are genuine in your approach. There is no one clear profile for a great leader. Because you have taken the time to know yourself, use your natural strengths to enhance who you are as a clinical coordinator. Use your head, but lead with your heart. Be *authentic*. This is a true challenge, however, as you are starting out. If you begin with this as your target, you will be less likely to get caught up in the work, stress, or power of your position.

Balancing It All

If you have more than one interest or responsibility, you have probably faced the challenges of trying to balance it all. It can be difficult to find your new normal especially after transitioning into a new role. The quest for sublime balance is like searching for the Holy Grail, and, generally speaking, we put too much value in having equal attention to the yin and yang portions. We all have finite abilities and time and have to identify where to allocate those at any moment. We are shooting for a time balance chart in **Figure 1-3** to feel balanced. The reality is that there will always be peaks and valleys as in **Figure 1-4**.

The amount of time we allocate to each interest is based on many variables. What do you *need* to do? What do you *want* to do? What requires more concerted effort? What is more self-sustainable? What acute events are occurring in each domain? How motivated are you? To devote time to something, it automatically takes time away from something else, so

FIGURE 1-3. Idealized Time Balance Chart

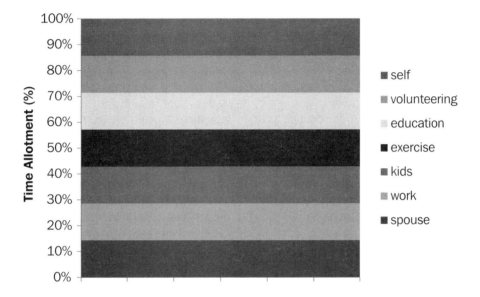

FIGURE 1-4. Realistic Time Balance Chart

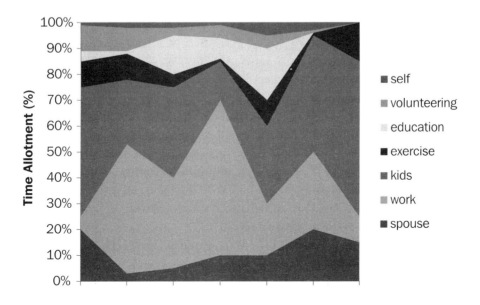

the pressure we put on ourselves to do it all becomes a mathematical equation.

Another way to think about balance is to look at life like a dinner plate. What you choose to put on the plate and the portion sizes are up to you, but you only have one plate and only so much can fit on it. Do you eat the same items in the same portions for every meal? Whether you are referring to managerial–clinical balance, job–professional involvement balance, or work–life balance, many of the same principles apply. Let's look at some ways to have a successful and balanced approach.

Pearl #1: Make healthy choices

An essential component to balancing it all is making choices that are in line with what you are trying to accomplish. It is very easy to feel overwhelmed or get caught up in saying yes to every opportunity if you have not defined your personal goals. Setting personal goals helps you to see your life as a whole and *why* you are doing things when you may not particularly want to be doing them. Your goals guide what you choose to put on your plate and help define your priorities.

Pearl #2: You took it, you eat it

One of the most difficult positions I have ever had required a 50/50 split between front-line responsibilities as a clinical pharmacist and managerial oversight of five clinical specialties. It was not difficult because the expectations or the scope were unreasonable, but because I had to balance time between leading and doing. I quickly came to realize that when I was fulfilling my role as a clinician, the responsibilities of being a department leader did not dissipate. I could manage my schedule to have meetings on my off-line days or split patient coverage with my partners in any number of ways, but I had to face that you cannot plan crises or change the way that people view you from one day to the next. I had taken a slice of the leadership pie, and although the size of my slice would change from day to day, I would always have at least a little bit on my plate. (Incidentally the same concept can be applied to parenting.) Accepting that who I am and what I do are entwined, and that I chose the piece of pie to begin with allowed me to come to terms with the fact that I took it and now I had to eat it. Once you accept that there are certain foods that will be on your plate daily, it becomes much easier to shift the foods around those items.

Pearl #3: Control portion size

Of equal importance to acceptance is empowerment. Regardless of the items you have on your plate, you can moderate how much or how little you take on a daily basis. When attempting to balance clinical versus managerial responsibilities, it is acceptable to focus your time and put your best effort forward. If you are responsible for direct patient care, spend the time taking care of your patients. Trying to work on your other responsibilities while you are rounding only will distract you from your priority and decrease your efficiency. Likewise, if you are working on a project and keep getting interrupted to take care of clinical issues, your project will suffer. This concept is incredibly difficult to execute in the current age of instant electronic gratification, so it is especially important to set boundaries. Designate a time (or times) for these maintenance activities so you can devote 100% of your effort to what you are doing. Depending on your clinical model and capacities, changing your physical location can also help. Staying on the nursing unit when fulfilling clinical responsibilities keeps you closer to the patients you are serving and also decreases office distractions. Compartmentalizing will not always work as there are emergencies or high-priority situations that will arise on both sides, but if you can set up this type of framework then your work will be completed with 100% effort 100% of the time instead of 50% effort all of the time.

Similar to controlling your focus, become comfortable setting limits for yourself. Some work will never be done. There is always more we can do for our patients, final touches we can add to make projects better, or emails to be answered. Control how much time you allow yourself to devote to individual activities. Both these tactics will allow you to shift your attention to another portion of your plate and allow you to feel a sense of empowerment that often gets lost when we try to do too much for too long.

Pearl #4: Find your motivation

No matter how good you are at setting goals, accepting your choices, and empowering yourself, motivation is a necessity. Finding motivation and keeping it in front of you, like hanging a picture of yourself on your refrigerator when you are dieting, will help you through any number of situations. Internal motivation is likely what brought you to where you are in many sectors of your life including this role as clinical coordinator. Internal motivation is a key factor to success, but supporting that motivation externally is a key factor to balance. Surround yourself with people who will keep you accountable to your goals and lift you up through the process, such as friends, family members, and mentors as well as professional organizations. Active involvement in professional organizations allows you to learn from people who are facing similar issues while giving back what you know. It does add another item to your plate; however, it is like gravy on your mashed potatoes: it enhances many of the other things you are eating.

Pearl #5: Nutrient timing

A key principle to healthy eating is nutrient timing. This is the concept behind increasing the number of frequent, smaller meals or not eating after 7 p.m. You want to consume most of your calories when you most need them. In the same way, time management is key to maintaining balance, especially with positions of split responsibility. If you have struggled with time management in the past, now is a good time to hone your skills and establish new habits. There is a lot of literature on how to best manage time, and we all need to figure out the things that work for us, but here are a few universal principles to help get you started:

- **Identify your goals.** Everything comes back to clearly defining your goals. If you know where you are heading, then you will make choices that help get you there.
- **Develop your sense of time.** Have you ever worked on something and wondered why it took so long to complete, or felt exhausted at the end of the day, but when you thought back you had no idea what you spent your time on? Take a few days and record every activity you are involved in and how long it takes you to complete it. This will give you an idea of where you

are wasting time and also help you to better estimate how long the tasks actually take.

- **Be structured, yet flexible.** You need to have a plan of attack to execute well; however, do not get so attached to your plan that you cannot adapt to the unexpected. At any moment you could have a patient that is crashing, a personnel emergency, or a sick family member. You have to be flexible, but not having a plan will make you less efficient.
- **Actually manage your time.** Some people feel that time management is simply managing their calendar or making lists. Time management also includes delegating responsibilities, managing meetings, helping people to stay on task, and following a routine.
- **Have a daily to-do list.** Writing down what you need to accomplish is helpful, but make sure you are prioritizing your list on a daily basis. I have a general rule of thumb to have a maximum of three tasks on my daily to-do list so that I can actually accomplish what I need to accomplish.
- **Outline clear expectations.** Learn to communicate clearly regarding time frames and requirements. This is particularly helpful when working in groups. At the end of conversations or meetings, recap tasks, the people responsible for completing them, and corresponding deadlines to make sure everyone is on the same page.
- **Learn to graciously decline.** You will never stay in balance if you blindly agree to every opportunity that presents itself. Ask for time so you can think about which of these opportunities fits into your goals on your own time. You should never have to make a large decision in haste. If you decide to turn down an opportunity, make sure to be respectful and thankful for the offer.
- **Be positive.** Just like you have choices about what you put on your plate, you have a choice about how you view your

responsibilities. If you can see your glass as half-full instead of half-empty, it will make it easier to cope when things get tough.

- **Manage yourself.** Everything you are involved in will fall apart if you do not take care of yourself both physically and mentally. Schedule time for exercise, alone time, sleep, or whatever you do that makes you feel you are investing in yourself.

Pearl #6: Forgive and ~~forget~~ learn

Balancing the various aspects of life is difficult. There are many demands on your time coming from various angles, and knowing where to put your energy is not always clear. (Even if it is clear, we do not always do what we know we should!) You might take too large of a helping or someone might reach in and eat off your plate. One skill we all need to master is forgiveness. If you are a person who harbors guilt, then learn to forgive yourself. If you are a grudge holder, learn to forgive others. One mistake I believe that people make is to forget once they forgive. Forgetting leaves room for repetition. Whatever the situation, remember to move forward and learn from your experiences.

These pearls should aid you in your quest for balance, but results will vary depending on the number of interests you are attempting to balance and the acuity of events occurring in each of those interests. Most importantly, it is up to you to edit your plate. Know you have choices every step of the way, and remember you have mentors and support networks to help you.

Summary

As you get started in your role as clinical coordinator, remember you are playing the long game. To make a positive impact and have influence, take the time to gather the information you need. Invest in those around you and in yourself in a productive way. Come back to the beginning occasionally to re-center as well as appreciate the progress you have made. Most of all...enjoy the ride!

PRACTICE TIPS

1. Do your homework and get to know your institution, team, requirements, and yourself.

2. Stand for something, and set a clear vision. Be authentic in your approach.

3. Edit your plate wisely. Making smart choices about how you spend your time will keep you effective and balanced.

References

1. White S, Tryon J. How to find and succeed as a mentor. *Am J Health-Syst Pharm.* 2007;64:1258-1259.

2. Frankl VE. http://www.brainyquote.com/quotes/quotes/v/viktorefr160380.html. Accessed November 5, 2014.

3. Doran GT. There's a S.M.A.R.T. way to write management's goals and objectives. *Management Review* (AMA FORUM). 1981;70(11):35-36.

4. Yemm G. *Essential Guide to Leading Your Team: How to Set Goals, Measure Performance and Reward Talent.* New York, NY: Pearson Education; 2012:37-39.

5. http://www.ashp.org/DocLibrary/MemberCenter/SICP/Get-Involved.pdf. Accessed November 5, 2014.

6. http://www.ashp.org/menu/PracticePolicy/ResourceCenters/Credentialing-and-Privileging-Resource-Center. Accessed November 5, 2014.

7. The Council on Credentialing in Pharmacy. *Credentialing in Pharmacy: A Resource Paper.* Washington DC: The Council on Credentialing in Pharmacy; 2010.

Suggested Reading

Covey SR. *7 Habits of Highly Effective People.* New York, NY: Free Press; 1989.

DiSC profile. www.onlineDiSCprofile.com.

George B. *Authentic Leadership.* San Francisco, CA: Jossey-Bass; 2003.

Maxwell J. *The 360° Leader: Developing Your Influence from Anywhere in the Organization.* Nashville, TN: Nelson Business; 2005.

Myers-Briggs. http://www.myersbriggs.org/my-mbti-personality-type/take-the-mbti-instrument/.

Wollenburg K. Leadership with conscience, compassion, and commitment. *Am J Health-Syst Pharm.* 2004: 61(17):1785-1791.

CHAPTER 2

Building and Leveraging Key Relationships

Scott Knoer and Samuel V. Calabrese

KEY TERMS

Communication—The exchange of thoughts, messages, or information, as by speech, signals, writing, or behavior.

Credibility—The quality of being believed or trusted.

Integrity—The quality of being honest and fair.

Relationship—A state of connection or association between people and how they behave or work with each other.

Introduction

When he is having a particularly difficult day, a good friend often says, "The problem with life is that there are people in it." What he means is that it can take a lot of time and energy to get things done in a complex organization. Just when you think something is finished, someone comes up with a new twist to which you must respond. Even things that seem relatively simple can be exhausting due to the extensive amount of **communication** (emails, texts, and informal and formal meetings) needed to put an initiative over the goal line.

The best thing about life is that there are people in it because there are very few things of significance you can achieve by yourself. The inherently complicated nature of patient care forces us to act collaboratively. To be effective and successful, we must nurture strong **relationships** up, down, and across our care teams, professions, and organizations. As you take on more responsibility at work, the importance of these relationships only increases. As a direct care practitioner, relationships are important, but being a clinical superstar can take you a long way. These dynamics dramatically change when you become a clinical coordinator. Now you are evaluated not as an individual performer but as a facilitator. You are only successful if your team is effective. You are judged by the achievements of those you lead and mentor rather than by what you have done by yourself.

Life is about relationships. Success through relationships transcends all that we do. The ideas and tools discussed are universal truths for interacting with your family and friends; social, civic, and faith-based institutions; work and professional organizations; and in any social situation. Although subjects are broadly translatable, this chapter will focus on *how* to build and leverage key relationships and the essential players to ensure your success.

Knowing Yourself

Developing successful relationships requires us to know people on a more personal and professional basis. We have to understand what drives them. What are their interests and goals? What are their strengths? Who are they outside of work? However, before you can successfully develop the meaningful relationships to improve patient care, you must first understand yourself. What drives you? What are your strengths? What are your opportunities for improvement?

Without understanding ourselves well, we are prone to repeat our mistakes leading to diminished professional growth and an inability to reach our full personal and team potential. Because everyone makes mistakes, people are generally forgiving of minor missteps if you acknowledge the error and follow up with a sincere apology. Although mistakes happen, repeatedly committing the same errors without changing your approach has the potential to seriously damage relationships. When our mistakes alienate others, we limit our ability to work effectively as a team. Albert Einstein is attributed with defining insanity as "Doing the same thing over and over again and expecting different results."[1] This definition of insanity is broadly applicable to our lives. It fits well into a successful philosophy of interacting with people by understanding yourself and how you connect to the world.

A sports medicine physician gave one of the most simple and yet profound pieces of advice. If you do something that causes a negative response or outcome, do not do it again. Instead, modify your behavior and generate a plan that facilitates the achievement of realistic goals without the undesired consequences. Although this is a simple concept, it is surprising how many people perpetuate bad behaviors despite the consistent results of undesirable outcomes. Repeating harmful behavior and expecting different results is, in fact, by definition, insane. The question is "How do we avoid the insanity—the damage to relationships caused by repeating bad behaviors derived from our unique personality traits?" Do you roll your eyes in meetings when a particular person speaks? Do you raise your voice when debating? These are examples of behaviors that impair relationships and limit your ability to work effectively in teams.

To build and leverage relationships, we must first mitigate our inherent faults and, more importantly, learn from mistakes. The alternative of simply making excuses or failing to acknowledge the issue and replicating mistakes is a path to certain failure. People often justify their personality quirks with "That's just who I am and people need to understand me" or "I am not going to play politics." Statements such as these are attempts to rationalize and justify bad behavior or simply deny its existence. Life is about understanding how to relate to people effectively. Adjusting behavior when we err is critical to success. The key to self-awareness and successful relationships is to truly understand yourself and your actions, modifying behaviors based on success and failure.

In the quest to better understand oneself and better relate to others, there are innumerable resources available. Below are two self-improvement tools that are useful in developing ourselves and our teams. These widely used tools are designed to help individuals understand not only themselves but also others. Using these instruments will give insights into how you and your teammates process information and interpret the world, and they allow for tailoring of messages to your specific audience for optimum effect and receptivity.

Myers-Briggs Type Indicator

One of the most commonly used individual and social understanding tools is the Myers-Briggs Type Indicator (MBTI, http://www.myersbriggs.org/).[2] It is designed to classify individuals into categories, providing insight into how they perceive and react to the world. MBTI translates Jung's theory of psychological types into an understandable and useful tool allowing individuals to grasp their own personalities including their likes, dislikes, strengths, weaknesses, possible career preferences, and compatibility with other people.

The assessment centers around four preferences:

1. *Extraversion (E) or introversion (I).* Do you prefer to focus on the outer world or on your own inner world?
2. *Sensing (S) or intuition (N).* Do you prefer to focus on the basic information you take in or do you prefer to interpret and add meaning?
3. *Thinking (T) or feeling (F).* When making decisions, do you prefer to first look at logic and consistency or first look at the people and special circumstances?
4. *Judging (J) or perceiving (P).* In dealing with the outside world, do you prefer to get things decided, or do you prefer to stay open to new information and options?

Depending on your responses, you will be categorized into one element of each preference. When you put these four letters together, you get your personality type code, which is one of 16 possible combinations. For example, INTJ indicates you prefer introversion, intuition, thinking, and judging (remember, this indicates *preferences* only—an INTJ also uses extraversion, sensing, feeling, and perception). No one personality type is best or better than any other one. It is not a tool designed to look for dysfunction or abnormality. Instead, its goal is simply to help you learn more about yourself so you will have a better idea on how to communicate and interact with others.

Insights Discovery

Insights Discovery is a similar personality assessment tool that we have found effective and use in our department.[3] It has only four components that are relatively easy to understand and visualize through a color wheel. Because this tool is intuitive and, as the name suggests, insightful, the terms and concepts have become a common part of our department's relational vocabulary. Although each person has all of these personality traits or color energies to some degree, everyone has a dominant trait that reflects predispositions in perspectives and actions. The Insights Discovery color energies are listed below[4]:

1. *Fiery red.* An individual who is extroverted, high energy, and action-oriented; uses a direct, authoritative manner; and radiates a desire for power and control.
2. *Sunshine yellow.* An individual who is strongly extroverted, friendly, usually positive, and concerned with good human relations; uses a persuasive but democratic manner; radiates a desire for sociability.
3. *Earth green.* An individual who focuses on values and relationships, reliability, and dependability; prefers relationships that value the individual; and radiates a desire for understanding.
4. *Cool blue.* An individual who is introverted and wants to understand the world around them; prefers written communication to maintain clarity and precision; radiates a desire for analysis.

We will come back to these color energies later as an aid in understanding interrelations with our coworkers of various disciplines. However, before dissecting collegial interactions, it is important to highlight several common themes we consider universal truths of relationship-building.

The value with all of these tools is found in reflecting on their results and understanding how inherent biases and filters impact actions and decisions. Moreover, these tools generate appreciation and understanding of how others view the world. Through this knowledge, we discern how to most effectively communicate with people based on their world perspectives. The final step to effective relationship building is to actually modify your behavior based on this newfound awareness so you are more effective in your role.

Universal Truths of Relationship Building

Establishing Credibility and Trust

Establishing **credibility** and trust is paramount to the building and maintenance of meaningful, productive relationships, and it is the first theme of successfully working with others. Trust is achieved through the demonstration of **integrity** and consistently meeting commitments. This basic relationship tenant is best demonstrated by simply doing what you said you were going to do when you said you were going to do it. If you commit to performing a patient medication review for a provider on the potential causes of pancreatitis, then get it done in a timely manner, and make sure he or she knows where to find your response if it is not delivered verbally. If you tell your resident you will provide feedback on a poster being presented at the ASHP Midyear Clinical Meeting, then give timely feedback so the resident can meet the deadlines. When you agree to provide nursing staff education on the newest antiplatelet inhibitor, follow through. When individuals and their leaders trust each other and are trusted by others, communication improves and productivity accelerates as attention is redirected toward team objectives. The book *The Speed of Trust* states that establishing trust ensures projects and initiatives are accelerated and implemented faster because

the bureaucracy and concerns for fraud or backstabbing are eliminated, and real work can be accomplished.[5]

Commitment and follow-through are the relational equivalent of amino acids in your DNA. They are the building blocks of personal bonds; they lay the foundation for a solid relationship. Like the old Nike commercial says, "Just do it." No excuses. The reality is that unexpected events will occasionally limit the ability to follow-through as promised. This could result in harming your credibility, but if you communicate the circumstances honestly and proactively and reset the deadline in a mutually respectful way, you will likely preserve the relationship. Maintaining credibility necessitates your providing a quality product by the new deadline. Consistently delivering produces good will and reciprocity with your peers, resulting in relationships where others want to help you. This sets the stage for leveraging these key relationships for the betterment of patient care.

Always Do the Right Thing

Another vital component of building and leveraging relationships is to consistently act with personal and professional integrity. The *Merriam-Webster* definition of *integrity* is "the quality of being honest and fair."[6] This can be further simplified to *always do the right thing.* Integrity consistently applied to all aspects of professional discourse builds trust.

In our profession, this is best displayed in terms of patient care. Placing the patient at the center of every decision will make it obvious to your medicine, nursing, information technology (IT), finance, and facilities teammates that your motives are true. This means not breaking the rules, setting up systems, and providing care in cost-effective ways. Having limited resources means you cannot meet everyone's needs. Prioritizing organizational capacity in a patient-focused manner facilitates effective resource allocation and stakeholder buy-in. Sometimes a decision is the right thing for the patient but not the best thing for your department. It may require you to change an ingrained process.

Meet the Personal Needs of Others

Have you ever gotten a request from your finance director or facilities manager to have a relative who is considering pharmacy school shadow you for a day? Perhaps a coworker has a parent hospitalized, and you have time to stop by and see if there is anything you can do (assuming HIPPA appropriate). Maybe a nurse has a personal drug information question that you can research without too much time investment. Assuming there is not a conflict of interest or confidentiality issue, helping your coworkers with personal matters demonstrates a commitment not just to patient care but also to your coworkers. Even better, offer to help them before they ask you. These small actions deepen personal relationships and will pay dividends later on.

Understand Others' Values and Perspectives

The next universal truth of relationship building is understanding the values and perspectives of others. This can be crudely conveyed as playing politics, but in essence it is about understanding your patient care partners. Can you put yourself in their shoes and see things from their perspective? What is important to them? What are their challenges? What is inhibiting them from providing optimal care for your patients?

Understanding the values and perspectives of those you work with and applying this knowledge is fundamental to developing positive interactions with all of your direct and indirect caregivers. When formulating a proposal for your initiative, consider the values and perspectives of key stakeholders and decision makers, and make sure it resonates with their personal value system. This mindset will help you create the win-win strategies, which are crucial to achieving common goals.

Leveraging Relationships

Bias for Yes

A veteran employee told a pharmacy intern not to do too good of a job because that would just lead to more work. Although this cynical view has truth to it, getting more work is not necessarily a bad thing. In fact, it can bring significant opportunity for those with a bias for saying yes. The fact is that leaders do give more work to their high performers because they

have proven that they deliver. Saying yes when your supervisor asks for a volunteer demonstrates a willingness to go above and beyond the minimum expectations. When you successfully complete extra tasks, you will generally be given more opportunity. Also, the more you do, the more you hone your skills and cultivate your expertise. Starting a new anticoagulation or antimicrobial stewardship service may result in an invitation to present your project at a meeting. If you say yes, it may turn into a publication. A publication generally turns into phone and email inquiries from peers. Optimizing your chance to share your learnings fosters the growth of your professional network.

Be a Strategic Opportunist

As a general rule, there are great advantages by saying yes to opportunities. The danger of a bias for yes is accumulating more commitments than you are able to fulfill. As with anything else, this philosophy if carried too far can be detrimental. It is important to identify when the demands of new opportunities exceed your time and resource capacity, which can result in an inability to deliver and cause negative relational outcomes.

Strategic opportunists quickly identify situations that further the patient care agenda; they never throw away a good proposal. Do you want to add a pharmacist to your team to do medication reconciliation? Perhaps you put together a splendid cost-benefit analysis on this subject only to have it rejected due to cost concerns. Do not discard that proposal. File it away, and be ready to dust if off when the timing is right. We all hope that a negative event such as a medication error never happens at our organization. For example, if an adverse event occurs that could have been prevented with a complete and accurate medication history, this misfortune is the opportunity to improve patient care. Crises can shine a spotlight on problems, creating opportunities for change that were previously nonexistent. Burnis Breland captured the essence of strategic opportunism, "Always look for the opportunity that adversity and crisis may create. Management excellence is turning tragedy into opportunity."[7]

The caveat to being a strategic opportunist is that opportunities should be leveraged only for the good of the system and for improvements that better patient care, not for those advancing a personal agenda. Only take advantage of situations when it affords the ability to improve society or patient care. A strategic opportunist who only looks out for themselves will be quickly marginalized and loses the credibility and trust that took so much time to build.

Success Breeds Success

How does this bias for yes and embracing opportunity help you build and leverage key relationships? It goes back to the initial comments on establishing credibility and trust. Every time you follow through, you add to your relationship "bank"; every time you exceed an expectation, you build trust. Your success will be rewarded with more opportunity. When opportunity knocks, be astute enough to recognize it as an opportunity rather than more work.

Align with Organizational Goals

To be successful at work, it is critical to effectively leverage relationships with leadership including your supervisor and even further up the chain into the C-Suite (referring to senior executives). Interpreting organizational goals and translating them into actionable strategies and tactics is a necessity for a clinical coordinator's success.

The values and goals of the C-Suite drive the organizational vision, creating a framework within where all initiatives must align. Speaking a common language and reflecting back to organizational goals will facilitate improved understanding of how the proposal fits into the overall mission and will aid in the plan's justification. Demonstrating quality is always a C-Suite priority; implementing services that reduce readmissions and increase HCAHPS (Hospital Consumer Assessment of Healthcare Providers and Systems) survey scores is an effective way to validate departmental and team value. Your team can show significant organizational impact while fulfilling the C-Suite goals.

It is critical to identify the services your team can provide that advance the agenda of the C-Suite and improve patient care. But how do you know if the next big thing coming down the pike in healthcare will impact the system's finances and reputation? In essence, how do you see the future? How do you develop a vision for yourself, your team, and ultimately for your profession? To some, vision seems to be a genetic trait like height. Over the years, however, the secret to creating vision has become clearer. Vision is a learned skill; to develop vision, you must associate with smart, optimistic people.

You now know the universal secret to success, and it only cost you the price of this clinical coordinator's handbook. Seriously though, when you interact with "thought" leaders at local, state, and national meetings; talk to peers about innovative projects; or read the professional literature, you consciously or subconsciously synthesize these tidbits, and direction becomes clearer. The more information you put together, the better you will be at seeing the big picture and having a vision to guide your team and the department's future efforts.

Can you help establish a bedside delivery program? Can you work with your local college of pharmacy faculty to take more Advanced Pharmacy Practice Experience students? If you do this, can you use these pharmacist extenders to complete medication histories for every patient on your units within 24 hours of admission? Can you leverage these resources to discharge counsel every patient? Can you work with your IT team to create a flag that will ensure patients are counseled on all new medications?

These individual thoughts, which were derived from multiple sources, have coalesced into our vision for practice that reduces readmissions and increases HCAHPS survey scores. By developing a vision from casting a wide professional net, you can align your team with wider organizational goals.

Vision is best carried out when there is understanding how individual actions contribute to the big picture. Take the time to explain quality metrics to your pharmacists, students, and residents. To achieve organizational goals and carry out the vision, your team has to know how what they do impacts the greater good.

The Credit Belongs to the Team

The best leaders are humble and give away the credit for team successes. Sharing the credit with those involved builds a strong sense of value, engagement, and belonging within the team. By praising your pharmacists, technicians, and unit nurses, you make them look good. When you praise a technician on your unit when turnaround times are good, you let the technician shine. At a meeting when the vice president of nursing recognizes a service your team has implemented, tell everyone you could not have achieved it if her nurse manager had not been such a valuable and collaborative partner. Sharing the credit acknowledges the valuable roles of team members. Although some people are uncomfortable receiving praise in front of a group, most are appreciative when publically acknowledged for their contributions to patient care.

Taking goal alignment a step further in the context of relationship building, one of the most important relationships is the one you establish with your supervisor. A good supervisor can remove barriers and advocate for your team. Although we will soon discuss the importance of managing up, down, and across, we believe that this key relationship is important enough to highlight here.

Make Your Supervisor Look Good

The best way to develop a mutually beneficial relationship with your direct supervisor is to make sure your work reflects positively on your supervisor. This should be a central tenant of how you operate at work. If your team is successful, then your supervisor looks good. If your supervisor looks good because you make life easier by being a stand-out employee, then the vast majority of supervisors will give you more latitude to make decisions, more autonomy, and more responsibility.

Develop Your Team

As a clinical coordinator, you are responsible for the development of your team. The number one way for your team to thrive is by selflessly sharing what you know and have. Introduce them to your colleagues. Help them submit a proposal for a poster or talk at a state or national meeting. If they are leading a great project for patients, give them credit for it. Tell your supervisor and your multidisciplinary team what a good job they did.

It is critical as a leader to overcome personal insecurities. The desire to prove oneself and the innate nature of competition can inhibit

the ability to build a strong and effective team. You shine when your team shines, but beyond that it is your role as clinical coordinator to foster growth. Insecurities make people much less effective at establishing and leveraging personal and professional relationships. The preoccupation over whether someone on your staff will diminish your power and reputation is a fundamental perception error, which has the potential to be a leadership character flaw. If you succumb to this thought process, you need to reassess your philosophy. Conversely, if you are unable to delegate for fear that it will not be perfect, you will restrict your team, which will inhibit them from reaching their potential. Establishing relationships with your team means giving them honest feedback and opportunities to flourish. Remember, as a clinical coordinator you are no longer evaluated by the success of your efforts but by the success of your entire team.

Communication 101

The cornerstone of building relationships is communication. Unfortunately, we find that miscommunications frequently occur. Maybe it was the way we stated the message, or it may have been the emotions we were feeling at the time. Perhaps it was the way our expressions said more than the actual words. Whatever the reason, we soon learn that effective communication is more complicated than just the words we use. Additional skills must be developed including selecting the method in which we send a message, controlling our emotions and nonverbal cues, and accounting for who is receiving the message. The need to continue to cultivate and refine these skills over our lifetime is imperative for building and fostering good relationships.

As a clinician you have used these skills to work with your team to ensure optimal patient care. When taking on the clinical coordinator role, you become involved in conversations and decisions not only of a clinical nature, but also of an administrative nature. Your audience will broaden to include a multigenerational, multidisciplinary team. It is vital for you to be cognizant of how your communication style impacts the receipt of the message and the recipients' perceptions.

Communication can be broken down into basic components: the sender, the message, and the receiver. Any factors that influence these basic elements will have a positive or negative effect on the communication. Staying attuned to some common factors impacting communication can assist in avoiding potential miscommunication.

Emails and Text Messages

The tools available to us today to assist in communicating a message are abundant. Technology including social media, smartphones, email, and text messaging has become a mainstay in our lives. These channels are widely utilized due to the ease of use and ability to communicate to groups of individuals simultaneously. However, these channels are impersonal, inhibit the sender and receiver from reacting to nonverbal cues, and do not allow for rapid feedback. Only messages considered routine and straightforward with minimal ambiguity, such as factual information, should be communicated through these methods.

When using email or other electronic communication, think about the following:

- **Recipients.** Are you sending this to the appropriate parties? Ensure that only the individuals in need of the information are included as recipients. Including someone's supervisor may convey you do not trust them to respond appropriately or that you are telling on them.
- **Subject.** The subject of your email should be clear and succinct. An email should consist of only one major topic. Often emails are stored by subject for easy retrieval at a later date.
- **Content.** The body of the message must be delivered in a clear manner with the correct tone and accurate information. Think about the construction of the message. It should get to the point without reading like a novel. It is important to note that 43% of people who receive long emails delete or ignore them.[8] Finally, remember that an email is a written communication and creates a written record. Ask yourself if you are comfortable

with the chief executive officer (CEO), human resource representative, or the local newspaper reading the content because emails can be forwarded to anyone.

- **Responses.** Responses to emails should follow the same guidelines above; however, there are a few other items to consider. We tend to react as soon as we finish reading an email feeling that we must answer immediately and often hit send without thinking. You should pause and ask yourself a few questions. First, to whom will you be responding? Too often, the sender will "reply all" without considering if all of the individuals on an email list need to be involved with the conversation. Remember to identify your recipients. Replying to all can be a professional pitfall when responses contain information to which all recipients should not be privy. Second, are you the correct person to be receiving the email and providing an answer? If not, refer the sender to the appropriate individual. Finally, will a reply cause a debate or generate additional questions to be answered? Do not use email as a mechanism to debate a point. Email conversations that go beyond two exchanges should be resolved in person or by phone.

Ineffective communication through these channels is common and generally leads to misunderstanding, misinterpretation, and often results in unnecessary back and forth.

Face-to-Face, Phone, and Conference/ Videoconference Calls

Communication channels that allow for direct dialogue are most useful when discussing complicated or controversial messages. These channels consist of face-to-face meetings, phone conversations, and video/audio conference calls. Using this channel, the participants can interact with each other in real time to provide clarification, if needed, and to ultimately reach mutual understanding. An effective face-to-face communication is critical in building relationships. As a clinical coordinator, you will use this channel continuously with members of the medical team, coworkers, and peers. Consider the following when using this method of communication:

- **Words.** The words you choose have a direct impact on the effectiveness of the communication. Simplify the content, and organize your thoughts to clearly convey your message. Using empowering words during the conversation will have a positive effect on the perception of the receiver. Refer to the table below for empowering words to use in place of disempowering words (**see Table 2-1**).[9]

- **SBAR.** Using the communication tool **s**ituational **b**ackground **a**ssessment **r**ecommendation (SBAR) is an effective way to organize and prepare for face-to-face communication. This method has been shown to improve overall communication while decreasing communication errors.[10] It was first developed by the United States Navy and is now considered a best practice for standard communication by The Joint Commission. The following is the SBAR structure:

  - **Situation.** Identify the problem or concern and provide a brief description.

  - **Background.** Provide clear, relevant background information relating to the situation.

  - **Assessment.** Provide your professional conclusions.

  - **Recommendation.** Identify what can be done to correct the problem.

- **Tone/voice.** It is not just what you say during a conversation but how you say it. The tone of your voice has been found to be responsible for 35% to 40% of the message being sent.[11] This becomes particularly important during phone conversations and conference calls. It is defined as the quality of a person's voice, including the pitch and volume.[12] To illustrate how tone changes the meaning of a sentence, read the following sentence below. Place an emphasis on the bolded word to see how the meaning of the statement changes.

  > **I** did not say the dose was wrong (blaming someone else)

  > I **did not** say the dose was wrong (defensive)

  > I did not say **the dose** was wrong (insinuating something else may be wrong)

Be sure to review the key points you want to make and ensure the inflections of your voice deliver the corresponding message. Also, pay attention to the volume of your voice. A loud voice may signify aggression or defensiveness, while a soft voice may give others a perception

Table 2-1. Empowering and Disempowering Words

EMPOWERING WORDS	DISEMPOWERING WORDS
Could (implies option, potential)	**Should** (affixes a single outcome through guilt and manipulation)
Prefer, desire, choose	**Need** (implies desperation)
And	**But** (blocks, used to dismiss, does not acknowledge the value of what another has said)
Opportunity	**Problem** (creates immediate defense)
Will, explore	**Try** (creates doubt, focuses effort on no decision)
Not at this time	**Maybe** (says no by avoiding making a decision)
Idea	**Issue** (suggests inherent opposition and places attention on discord)

you lack confidence or knowledge. Like any other skill, identifying the proper tone takes practice. Rehearsing conversations beforehand is a method that may be helpful in developing this skill. Utilize a mentor to provide feedback during a rehearsal or use a tape recorder to assist in your training.

- **Body language.** Over half of the messages we send when communicating are nonverbal.[11] Our nonverbal communication or body language can inhibit us from getting our intended message across. Nonverbal communication is usually derived from our subconscious and includes facial expressions, posture, gestures with your arms or hands, and eye contact. A way to develop an understanding of body language is through observation. Observing how others use nonverbal communication is an easy way to pick up on best and suboptimal practices. Observing yourself, however, is more challenging. Asking for feedback from a peer is a method to identify your nonverbal communications. Select someone you trust and ask for them to evaluate your nonverbal communication skills. Have them observe you in a few meetings to identify patterns and triggers. Prior to any meeting, reflect on what may trigger poor nonverbal communication. Triggers include being hungry, needing to visit a restroom, having issues with someone in the meeting, already being angry, or being unprepared. Addressing these triggers prior to a meeting will help avoid unintentional negative nonverbal communication. Once the meeting begins, make a conscious effort to pay attention to your nonverbal communication. How are you sitting? Do you have your arms folded? Are you tapping your pen? Are you watching the clock? Self-awareness controls your body language, but it takes time to develop, and even then our subconscious may override our conscious intentions.

- **Active listening.** Communication is not just about speaking. It is also about hearing and understanding what is being said. Active listening is receiving the message and making a conscious effort to understand the complete meaning that is being sent. To become a good active listener, consider the following[13]:

  - Make and maintain eye contact (provide undivided attention)
  - Acknowledge you are listening (e.g., head nods)
  - Eliminate distractions (smartphones, watching the clock)
  - Paraphrase periodically (ensure message is received correctly)
  - Do not interrupt
  - Respond accordingly

Communicating Change

You have heard it before, and here it is again: "The only constant is change." This statement is as true today as it was when Greek philosopher Heraclitus first said it thousands of years ago. Change is inevitable, and how we communicate during times of change is critical. Whether it is a process or procedure change, a formulary change, a new medication restriction, or a staffing change, communication needs to be effective and efficient. Your relationships and how you are viewed by others are vital to your ability to effectively communicate change.

- **Know what exactly is changing and why.** Avoid using jargon such as "do more with less" or "the organization must be more responsive." Be able to articulate what is changing, why, and how it will affect others.

- **Know the results needed.** Understand the goal to be achieved with the communication. Is it acceptance, support, or an alternative view? This will assist in identifying the appropriate tactic for starting the communication.

- **Share information as soon as possible.** Your team expects you to communicate changes to them. Timely communication will prevent them from finding out about changes from other sources or the grapevine.

- **Overcommunicate.** Provide quality and consistent information regarding changes through various channels. Face-to-face communication is the best method, and used in combination with clarifying emails, newsletters, and websites, it provides the redundancy and repetition essential to ensure effective communication.

- **Provide feedback opportunities.** Give people multiple opportunities to share concerns, ask questions, and offer ideas. Follow up with timely answers and updates. Change requires a grieving process as something must end before the new way begins. Support your team as they move through the process to improve acceptance of change.

For more information on implementing change, we strongly recommend Kotter's *Leading Change*, which examines the actions of people who transformed their organizations. He introduces an eight-step model for helping managers deal with transformational change and provides a roadmap to achieving organizational change. The eight-step model allows change to be achieved by a process building on each step (see Chapter 14: Leadership from the Clinical Coordinator's Perspective, and Figure 14-2: Kotter's Eight-Step Change Management Process).

Crucial Conversations

Inevitably, disagreements and misunderstandings arise in all relationships. This generally necessitates having an unpleasant conversation. Communicating as issues arise can be difficult and is often avoided. These conversations may be repeatedly postponed because they are filled with emotion and have the potential to elicit conflict regarding the topic. Stop for a minute and think about a conversation you may be avoiding. Ask yourself what you are avoiding and how this is impacting the relationship. By not having the conversation, we unconsciously place a strain on the relationship. When we choose to address the issue, how these conversations are conducted has a lasting effect on the relationship. To preserve the relationship, you should adequately prepare to facilitate the conversation. Refer to Patter-

son's *Crucial Conversations* for the best ways to approach these conversations (see Chapter 7: Human Resources and People Management for more on crucial conversations).

Communicating with the C-Suite

Communicating with the senior executives outside of pharmacy is different than presenting a monograph at the pharmacy and therapeutics (P&T) committee meeting or making a recommendation on patient rounds. For P&T and patient rounds, pharmacists are taught to share all supporting evidence, build the case, then make the final recommendation. The C-Suite or senior executives are different. They want the "ask" or final recommendation first and then the supporting evidence. If they want to read it, they will; however, most of the time they just review the "ask" or recommendation. Remember to start with the executive summary first, and then share the supporting evidence.

Identifying and Working with Key Stakeholders

Now that we have covered the basic communication techniques, the next step is to establish which key stakeholders are critical to your success. As a clinical coordinator, you will be the conduit between the medical team and the pharmacy department. Strong relationships will provide the foundation for communicating information, requests, and decisions. Establish these relationships before you need them; it is a lot easier to ask for support or direction when you already know the individuals than having to cold-call them to ask for their opinion or recommendation. For example, there is a drug shortage and you need support to restrict or substitute a medication. If you already know the key physicians, nurses, and/or P&T chair, you can determine the plan of action faster and more successfully because you already know the key stakeholders. Another example would be if a physician requests an extremely expensive medication that might not be evidence-based or part of the formulary. If you already know the physician who ordered the medication, you can have a more comfortable conversation about the alternatives and rationally discuss options.

Relationships to cultivate are the direct patient care positions within the medical team including physicians, pharmacists, students, and residents. We will also highlight relationships with team members that also play a critical role in a complex organization, such as those in quality, safety, accreditation, finance, facilities and operations, IT, and all other disciplines that do not directly touch our patients.

Physicians

By nature of their role, physicians have predominant leadership positions within any healthcare team. This has translated into promoting physicians into formal leadership positions.[14,15] For example, all of the hospital CEOs within the Cleveland Clinic health system are physicians. In fact, on the organizational chart the pharmacy department reports to a physician leader. Given the skills and attributes most often possessed by physicians, this can be seen as a positive trend. Physicians in formal leadership roles are the same as the physicians who round with the clinical coordinator and the physicians on the P&T committee we work with to provide cost-effective care. They are data-driven caregivers who understand the metrics that measure quality and that good clinical services improve patient outcomes. Many have additional master's degrees training in business, which augments their clinical skills.

What are the keys to building successful relationships with physicians? Demonstrating integrity, always following through, and understanding others' values and perspectives will ensure improved understanding and interactions with these leaders.

Physicians today fall into two categories: those employed by organizations and those in private practice. The move toward physician employment has expanded rapidly and is likely to be a permanent reality.[16-18] The main difference between these groups is that private practice physicians are not only healthcare providers but also small business owners. When working with private practice physicians, understanding the pressures of maintaining a sustainable business in times of increased regulation and payer demands is critical. These pressures will impact decisions on how they utilize time and interact with the health system.

Dramatic changes in healthcare reimbursement and the focus on quality and population health have changed the relationship with physicians. Several years ago, as healthcare reform of financial incentives shifted toward rewarding quality, terms such as *standardization* had to be used with care. Discussion with nonemployed medical staff about standardization had the potential to elicit a reflexive and emotionally laden response of "cookbook medicine." Many physicians were concerned about the loss of control, as well as the concern for the loss of the art of medicine. It is still important today to understand that perspective.

Quality metrics and pay for performance are more entrenched in healthcare. Physicians face inherent challenges in this new model. Although employed physicians are generally free from the complex distraction of running a business, they are impacted by pressures to meet productivity and quality metrics. As healthcare evolves, it is important to understand how these changes impact our physician colleagues. The conundrum is that the current healthcare system necessitates a highly complex, integrated, team-based approach to patient care, yet measures success by outcomes heavily influenced by patient choices and behaviors. However, this system's design holds physicians ultimately accountable for measures well beyond the sphere of their influence.

As pharmacists, we are accountable for the care we provide, but physicians are held responsible for the patients' overall health and care. Physicians are the quarterbacks, directing the multidisciplinary teams. Therefore, it is critical we establish an understanding of our role as competent, patient-focused caregivers. In this model, pharmacists become invaluable team members who assume responsibility for certain aspects of patient care and, as a result, lighten the physicians' burdens. By becoming the physicians' partners in care, pharmacists can drive improvements in quality and efficiency. The best physicians hold themselves accountable; when they delegate a task, they feel the responsibility for any error that impacts their patients. Once we, as pharmacists, earn physician respect and are entrusted with providing patient care, it is our professional obligation to recognize that this trust is a privilege. We must respect and protect this privilege by delivering clinical skills, integrity, reliability, and accountability to the team.

Another key concept to understanding the physicians' perspective is remembering that they are data-driven clinicians who understand the complexities of clinical care. They are persuaded by facts and evidence-based recommendations; they only change their opinions when presented with empirical data. All discussions with physicians must be patient-focused and logical. Understanding this fundamental rule will help build and leverage key relationships with our physician partners.

Case Example 1

Who are the right physicians to work with when building relationships? Of course, a clinician's quick response may be "all physicians." Although this is true, as a clinical coordinator you will need to focus on those relationships that you can leverage for success: the department chair, the attending physician, and those physicians who are committee leaders. They not only hold key positions within the organization, but they also have influence over their peers.

Let's take a challenging formulary decision. Intravenous acetaminophen has caused much debate within our organization. The cost of this medication has quite an impact on the pharmacy's budget despite minimal therapeutic advantages. This medication was first added to formulary with restrictions; however, after performing a drug-use evaluation, the pharmacy made a recommendation to the P&T committee to further restrict the medication to allow only staff physicians to order the medication. This type of restriction places the responsibility and the burden on the staff physician to ensure that it is prescribed appropriately. How could strong relationships help in this scenario? Your goal is to acquire the P&T committee's approval for the recommendation. A key relationship with the physician leader of the P&T subcommittee responsible for this category of medication will give you an opportunity to present the recommendation rationale to a colleague with which you have gained trust. Provided you have a solid case, the key physician will be your advocate. Having a physician champion for a controversial idea is ideal for acceptance. It is also an opportunity for you to identify which physicians may be resistant to the proposed recommendation. Contacting these individuals prior to a P&T meeting will allow for candid and transparent discussion. These early conversations or "socializing the change" may

not result in agreement; however, it prevents those opposed to this recommendation from being blind-sided. Building strong relationships with key physicians and being highly transparent with communication will position you for successful navigation of the political landscape.

The new realities of payment shifts toward population health, and risk-based contracts are very positive developments for pharmacy. We thrive in the world of cost-effective care. This is our bread and butter. Managing medications across the continuum of care improves quality and outcomes and reduces overall costs. Demonstrating our ability to collaboratively impact outcomes and our value in the multidisciplinary team supports physician leaders and is critical to our professional success.

Nursing

Pharmacy's relationship with nursing is critically important to a clinical coordinator's success. To effectively cooperate with this key constituency, it is vital to understand some basic concepts. You must appreciate the unique challenges that nurses face in caring for patients and recognize some fundamental differences between our mutually dependent professions. Understanding these divergent perspectives will help you successfully leverage relationships within this important community.

The most significant issue that can negatively impact nursing/pharmacy relationships is immediacy. Looking at the nursing and pharmacy perspectives regarding medication turnaround times demonstrates this paradigm differentiation. Imagine a pediatric patient in pain. What is the patient's nurse most concerned about with regard to pediatric pain medication? If you answered the nurse wants the medication "now," you are correct. Nurses assume the medication will be safe and accurate, but they want it now!

Looking at this situation from the pharmacy perspective, what is the pharmacist most concerned about with regard to pediatric pain medication? Pharmacists universally answer it has to be safe and accurate. The pharmacist's perspective is safety above all. The nurse's perspective is to meet the immediate needs of easing patient pain.

Our nursing and pharmacy professions are also different in another way as demonstrated from the Insights Discovery perspective. The University of Minnesota Medical Center—Fairview utilizes the Insights Discovery tool widely. Overwhelmingly, nurses who took this assessment were dominant in the *earth green* or the relationship quadrant. That seems intuitive. People who go into nursing want to care for others and strongly value relationships.

Although pharmacists were more varied in their dominant color, *cool blue* was the largest quadrant for our profession. This is also intuitive; people who go into pharmacy are good at math and are trained as data-driven scientists. Pharmacists like data. We live to quote the latest published study on drug efficacy as related to our specialty. If we are not careful, this may appear as cold and insensitive. When we speak to nurses, we need to use the word *patient* often. You should always tie your message back to the patient. Start the conversation on a personal note, and do not go directly to what we need from them. Connect in a way that demonstrates you value your relationship with them. Relationship-oriented people need to know you value them for who they are, and then they will reciprocate. Establishing this type of relationship involves more than barging in with a request. It involves taking time, making eye contact, and asking personal questions.

Life is complicated, and we should not oversimplify the traits of an entire profession. *Fiery red* nurses and *sunshine yellow* pharmacists do exist in the world. Although individuals cannot accurately be painted with such broad strokes, these examples are still useful for illustrating some fundamental differences in perspectives due to their training or self-selection of profession. We can then appreciate how this understanding facilitates the development of positive interprofessional relationships.

Case Example 2

As a clinical coordinator, a strong positive relationship with nurses is important to ensure safe patient care. It is critical to recognize that formulary decisions may not directly reach these individuals from the P&T committee. As a clinical coordinator, you are the liaison for new medications as well as crucial medication administration changes.

> *Let's explore a new medication that has unique impact on nursing administration. Clevidipine was recently added to your formulary. Due to its properties, the vial and tubing must be changed every 12 hours to prevent line infections. Prior to implementation, you have a responsibility to ensure your nursing colleagues are knowledgeable regarding the safe administration of this medication. Working with a key nurse, you can decide the best approach to communication, training, and education. You realize you can relate it to a similar administration technique that is used for propofol. Because the nursing team is already familiar with a similar procedure, it will not be viewed as additional burden. Partnering with your nursing colleagues will help identify strategies when implementing changes or new procedures.*

Other Caregivers

Toby Cosgrove is a physician-trained CEO at the Cleveland Clinic. His background drives his relentless pursuit of clinical excellence, patient safety, and outcomes. One of the most admirable things about his leadership is his insistence to recognize all employees as caregivers. Physicians, pharmacists, care coordinators, housekeepers, food service workers, accountants, security, and everyone else who is employed by or volunteers at the health system has a role in patient care. Our jobs exist for one reason—to take care of patients. When everyone can see their vital role in improving patient care, they change their way of thinking. They also look at each other differently, realizing that groups like finance and facilities also have a huge impact on patient care. Everyone is aware they are on the same team working toward a common goal.

Who are some of those other caregivers whose relationships can make or break the success of a clinical coordinator? A few examples below are highlighted, but relationships with key caregivers who are not on the front line are also critical to the team's success.

IT/Informatics

For most organizations, all records of today's care reside within the electronic health record (EHR). The entire medication-use process—from prescribing to documentation of administration and outcomes—lives within this world. Many safety, quality, and cost control initiatives, such as dosing guidelines, protocols, care paths, and formulary decisions, are implemented through the EHR. We must foster strong connections with our IT/informatics teams. Developing relationships of mutual trust and respect will guarantee that we are seen as the experts who clinically drive the operational changes necessary to improve care through the implementation and optimization of automation and technology. If you do not know your IT team, get to know them. This will help when you need to make changes to systems that will improve patient care. You are the middle person between the technology and the frontline user. As an advocate for making changes and improvements, it is essential to know the technology so you can speak knowledgably in meetings and on projects. It is necessary to think broadly across the hospital or health system to determine how the request will impact others. Sometimes you have to gain support from other disciplines, but your role is to understand what the pharmacy staff needs related to technology, analyze it to ensure the best solution, and then work with the correct teams to implement the change. Also, remember to double check the requests to ensure they have been implemented correctly. There are many different aspects to technology and informatics, so make sure you know all the different teams and how you can be involved.

Finance

We live in a world of finite resources. Almost every service provided has both a cost and a benefit. For example, adding a pharmacist to the emergency department for 8 hours a day, 7 days a week requires us to hire 1.4 full-time equivalents plus a factor for nonproductive (vacation/sick/holiday) time. This salary must then be multiplied by a factor that represents fringe benefit costs (insurance, retirement, etc.). Any service proposed must be justified with a cost-benefit analysis that demonstrates a return on investment. Having a friend in the finance department is extremely helpful. It is also important for you to educate your finance team on the economic benefit that good pharmacy services bring to the organization. The finance team can help you better understand the departmental administrative allocations of expenses and advocate for reallocation of expenses based on actual utilization of resources.

Facilities/Operations

The significant role facilities and operations play in patient care is taken for granted until something fails. When you have a leak in the pharmacy satellite or need the cleanup of a biohazard, the relationships with these essential departments is as evident as the mess they are needed to help resolve. Building and leveraging relationships with the facilities staff is crucial.

Quality/Safety/Accreditation

The staff members in these roles are vital to advancing safe, effective patient care. When convinced of your team's value, they will see you as a partner to help advance their objectives. Likewise, you can leverage their perspective and support when attempting to meet accreditation and quality metrics. Having someone in another discipline advocate for the value of a pharmacy service can have more impact than you advocating for that service. One effective way to build relationships with this group is to volunteer in validating quality metrics related to medications to ensure they are accurate. Another is to use your knowledge of the most recent clinical guidelines to help make informed system changes based on the latest evidence.

Pharmacy Operations Team Partner

As a clinical coordinator, you may think the title implies you will focus only on the clinical aspect of healthcare. However, to be an effective clinical manager and to ensure the best patient outcomes and staff satisfaction, it is essential to collaborate with the pharmacy operations team within your department. You must understand operational issues and bridge any clinical/operational issues. If a patient needs a medication that is not currently stocked, you must determine if there is truly a clinical need and then work with the pharmacy buyer to secure the medication. If a patient is crashing, you must make sure that the required medication gets to the patient in a timely manner. If there are several medications that are clinical equivalents, you should determine the preferred agent and then work with the operations team to contract for a great price and stock the preferred agent. You will work with the P&T committee on restrictions or a therapeutic interchange. It is critical you understand how to analyze the many processes and steps involved in the medication management process and either recommend or implement the improvements. Sometimes these are considered operational initiatives, but you need to be involved as a leader in this domain as well. A successful leader and patient advocate never allows silos to get between their team and patient care. The best way to eliminate silos within your department is to follow through and ensure resolution of every patient care issue, not just clinical ones. Modeling this behavior will rub off on your staff and will lead to better patient care. The ASHP Pharmacy Practice Model Initiative states there needs to be an equal focus on both clinical and operational, and that these should not be divided but should work together collaboratively.

Leading from the Middle: Managing Up, Down, and Across

Managing Up

Hierarchy is a reality in the workplace. In the expanded role of clinical coordinator, relationships with direct supervisors and those in higher positions become increasingly important. These individuals are instrumental in promoting the work you do, providing assistance in removing obstacles, and assisting in identifying solutions to problems. A conscious effort must be made to manage these relationships. It is critical to remember that the supervisory relationship involves mutual dependence. That is, both parties need each other to achieve ultimate success.

Kotter provides the following to assist in managing up[19]:

- Understand your supervisor's goals and objectives. How do they relate to your goals and objectives? Part of your job is to ensure your supervisor is seen in the best light possible. Alignment of goals is imperative for this to be successful.

- Understand your supervisor's pressures. Remember that he or she reports to someone who also has expectations.

- Understand your supervisor's strengths, weaknesses, and blind spots as well as your own. Identify ways your strengths can complement each other.

- Understand similarities and differences between you and your supervisor's communication style. Adhere to your supervisor's communication style (e.g., he or she may prefer one-page executive summaries on projects or issues rather than a lengthier document).

- Develop a trusting relationship with your supervisor by being dependable and honest and delivering on your commitments.

- Be the eyes and ears for your supervisor. Be sure issues or concerns you are aware of come from you and not the grapevine.

- Use your supervisor's time wisely. Be selective with how you spend your supervisor's time. Take care of trivial issues on your own.

Managing Down

The position of a clinical coordinator may or may not have formal direct reports, but it will always involve leading individuals.[20] Managing down involves all of the same concepts as managing up, but now the focus is on your team with you as the supervisor. Your role is to assist with problem solving, removing obstacles, and processing ideas. Building good relationships with direct reports, formally and informally, is essential to meeting your patient care goals and those of the organization.

- ***Managing by wandering around.***[21] This concept, used by those in formal management positions, is a hands-on approach to management. To be clinically effective, you must understand departmental operations. Establish mutually beneficial relationships with the people working in the central pharmacy. Regular visits to the area to check for issues that need to be resolved, such as problem orders or relaying information to the team regarding a complex patient, are essential in maintaining good relationships.

- **Knowing everyone's name.** Although this is challenging in large departments, calling individuals by their name is important to ensure you see people as more than numbers. By addressing individuals by name, we demonstrate that we appreciate, empathize with, and respect them.

- **Ask their opinion.** Ensure that team members feel their contributions are valued. Asking their opinion regarding a decision, or how they would have handled a situation or a clinical judgment, will ensure your team feels valued and builds trust. Fostering this type of atmosphere encourages the free flow of ideas and creates a safe environment for staff to communicate with you.

- **Teach them what you know.** Just as you are a lifelong learner, so are the pharmacists and technicians on your team. Take every opportunity to teach those around you. Think about succession planning. Who can fill your position if you are promoted? Training your successor will not only effectively fill a vacancy, but will also create a supporter for you in your new role.

Managing Across

Clinical coordinators are in a position to build trust and influence others including individuals in other departments and key stakeholders. To be successful, you must have a partnership of others within the organization to support your initiatives. Keep in mind the skills used in managing across are identical to those used with the team. Every member needs to feel valued, be a part of the decision process, and have common goals.

- **Act in the best interest of the patient/organization.** When working across the organization, avoid working with self-interest in mind. Shared goals are integral to obtaining broad support. The organization's goals or the patient's interest should be the common ground to work on.

- **Focus on them.** Remember, it is a two-way street. You will find yourself in the position of supporting others with their initiatives. You must be willing to assist others to foster and grow long-term relationships. Although your plate may be full, assisting someone today could build their support tomorrow.

- **Do not burn bridges.** Be careful on severing relationships. This could happen for a variety of reasons including being dishonest, being misleading with information, supplying bad information, or being overly aggressive. You may not always gain support for an initiative or recommendation. Look for a compromise, if possible, or find another supporter. Treat others as you would like to be treated. Burning bridges can lead to future obstacles, and you may acquire a reputation of being uncooperative.

Clinical coordinators must have the ability to shift between managing up, down, and across, as the situation dictates. Team members in each of these areas clearly have a different set of needs. Knowing the individuals and the situation you are dealing with is instrumental to deciding the way to communicate. Leading from the middle is not an easy task. However, effectively managing communication in these three directions will ensure developing strong relationships and will gain you influence and importance in the organization, and thereby garner support for your initiatives.

Professional Organizations and Your Network

Relationships Outside of Your Organization

Engagement in professional organizations, such as ASHP, the American College of Clinical Pharmacy, or the American Pharmacists Association, can be extremely rewarding. By establishing relationships outside of your organization, you expand your professional network. Casting a wider net keeps you abreast of developing trends.

Mike Sanborn, who is now the CEO at a Dallas hospital in the Baylor system, gave some relationship-building advice with broad applicability during ASHP Council Week. At a social gathering, Mike said, "Talk. Don't talk too much. And get to know the chair, the vice chair, and the ASHP staff member on your committee. They are the ones who decide who will stay on the committee and who becomes the vice chair the following year." This simple rule transcends the initial situation for which it was originally intended. It relates to almost any group setting where you are getting to know people, building credibility, and establishing relationships.

Here is a little more on each part of this concept.

- *Talk.* You are put on a committee or task force for a reason. Most often, it is because you represent a particular demographic. It could be your profession, your unit, or your state. The expectation is that you will represent your demographic through thoughtful input. You have an obligation to wisely add to the discussion, and this is your opportunity to establish credibility as an intelligent, thoughtful participant. You only have one chance to make a first impression.

- *Do not talk too much.* Thoughtful input is expected; however, monopolizing the conversation and tediously droning on is not acceptable. Everyone has been in a group where a person monopolizes the conversation. As a simple rule: do not be that person. If you are, your input may be dismissed. The group exists to bring together different perspectives, but it is not a forum for verbose individual monologues.

- *Get to know the chair, the vice chair, and the committee staff.* They decide who will be on the committee and in leadership roles the following year. This is a broadly transferrable statement. Whenever you are part of a group, there is a hierarchy. There is also an assessment of the group function, whether it is formal or informal. What you say and how you say it will be remembered. Were you insightful? Were you overly aggressive? Did you listen as well as you spoke? Did you demonstrate an appreciation for the issues? Performance drives perception, and perception drives value, which

is essential to becoming a valued member of the group.

Keep these simple principles of group dynamics in mind whenever you are part of a committee within or outside of an organization. Nurture the group's relationships, complete work offline, volunteer to lead a group project, and, most of all, deliver on your commitments.

Sharing Your Network

Relationships build networks; networks enable professional linkages. These connections expand your sphere of influence and your ability to tap into colleagues who are subject experts for advice. Sharing your professional network with the team helps enhance the depth of professional collaborations. When entering a formal mentoring relationship, begin the conversation with the statement, "My network is your network." Opening your network to others demonstrates trust and makes people feel valued. It exhibits an altruistic desire to invest in them.

Sharing your network does not end with employees. Students and residents also will benefit from being introduced to an established network. Perhaps they are seeking residencies. Or perhaps they were not until encountering your practice and your enthusiasm, which inspired them. Share your network with them, and introduce them to residency directors. If they do a good job, write letters of recommendation. When they accept residency positions, keep in touch because they will become your peers and some may even become your supervisors.

Investing time in these relationships is both benevolent and self-serving (in a positive way for society). These young learners will inevitably go to other institutions. When they do, you will have someone you can collaborate with on protocols or best practices.

Colleges of Pharmacy

Education should be a key part of a clinical coordinator's job. How do you keep yourself in the loop of a teaching and learning environment? Establishing meaningful relationships with colleges of pharmacy is central to ensuring that your team matures academically. How do you nurture these relationships? To begin with, you do not develop relationships with colleges but with the people who work there. Start small. Take students. Working as a clinical coordinator allows for giving back to the profession through training students and residents. It is a professional responsibility to serve as a positive role model to others in lifelong learning.

As a professional role model, you have the opportunity to deepen your involvement with the colleges of pharmacy by sharing your personal expertise. Volunteer to give lectures and attend student career events. Like every other relationship in life, start small and then work yourself into more advanced roles.

Closing Thoughts

Every Day Is a Job Interview

Treat every day and every interaction as an interview for a future job. Do not be so overly protective that you precisely sell every word in every conversation, but be aware that everyone is constantly evaluated. Your medical team is judging you. The doctor on rounds may become a department head, or the P&T Chair, or even the hospital CEO. The pharmacy student for whom you wrote a letter of recommendation may someday become the director of pharmacy at a major health system. The staff member you encouraged to get an MBA may become your colleague at another hospital or even your supervisor. People remember how you treated them, if you advocated for them, or if you stifled them.

Do Not Forget Where Your Paycheck Comes From

Professional involvement is the key to having a career and not just a job. The fact that we are part of something bigger than ourselves is motivating. Sharing our successes through presentations, posters, and publications is extremely gratifying. However, a key tenant of success as a clinical coordinator is balancing your job's interesting and exciting things with the fiduciary responsibilities of being a good steward of the organization's resources. Be sure you do not make so many commitments outside of work that it negatively impacts your ability to implement positive change in your organization.

This is where you need to manage your bias for saying yes, and be a strategic opportunist.

When success breeds success, and the opportunities start to come in, you need to effectively manage this newfound success. You must prioritize these opportunities within the context of your job responsibilities. As a leader, one of the best things is to share your successes. If your plate is too full, but a good opportunity presents itself, pass it on to a peer or a protégé. Pay it forward, and suggest someone from your team who has shown leadership in the residency interview process. It is like giving a referral. The recipient will appreciate this and may reciprocate when the opportunity presents itself.

Summary

Building and leveraging key relationships within and outside of your organization is critical to the success of any clinical coordinator. Remember, life is about relationships, and the best thing about life is that there are people in it.

PRACTICE TIPS

1. Establish credibility and trust when building relationships. Respond to requests appropriately, follow through, and meet and hopefully exceed expectations.

2. Spend time learning about yourself. Relationships are a two-way street, which requires a complete understanding of oneself.

3. Always do the right thing for the patient.

4. Focus on sharpening your communication skills. Review past emails and communications. Are they conveying the message as intended? Communication is essential in relationship building.

5. Challenge yourself to handle uncomfortable situations in a timely and respectful manner. Crucial conversations assist in building strong relationships.

6. Listen to the suggestions of others. Invaluable contributions are made to patient care by both direct and nondirect caregivers.

7. Take time to identify key individuals including peers, leaders, and subordinates,

to assist in meeting your goals. Managing up, down, and across the organization is required to function successfully.

8. Pay attention to the needs of your team. True leaders selflessly develop their teams and share their networks.

References

1. Brainyquote.com. http://www.brainyquote.com/quotes/quotes/a/alberteins133991.html?. Accessed December 15, 2014.

2. The Myers & Briggs Foundation. MBTI basics. 2014. http://www.myersbriggs.org/my-mbti-personality-type/mbti-basics/. Accessed December 15, 2014.

3. The Insights Group Limited. Insights discovery. https://www.insights.com/564/insights-discovery.html. Accessed December 15, 2014.

4. Inside Inspiration. What colour energy describes you best? http://www.inside-inspiration.com.au/insights-discovery/insights-colour-energies.html. Accessed December 15, 2014.

5. Covey SMR. *The Speed of Trust: The One Thing That Changes Everything.* New York, NY: Free Press; 2008.

6. Integrity. Merriam-Webster.com. http://www.merriam-webster.com/dictionary/integrity. Accessed December 15, 2014.

7. Brelund BD. Believing what we know: pharmacy provides value. *Am J Health-Syst Pharm.* 2007; 64(12):e18-e29.

8. Evans L. Less is more: why you're saying too much and getting ignored. http://www.fastcompany.com/3030659/less-is-more-why-youre-saying-too-much-and-getting-ignored. Accessed December 15, 2014.

9. Oswald Y. *Every Word Has Power: Switch on Your Language and Turn on Your Life.* New York, NY: Atria; 2008.

10. Haig KM, Suttton S, Whittington J. SBAR: a shared mental model for improving communication between clinicians. *Jt Comm J Qual Patient Saf.* 2006;32(3):167-175.

11. Mehrabian A. *Silent Messages.* Belmont, CA: Wadsworth; 1971.

12. Tone. Dictionary.com. http://dictionary.reference.com/browse/tone. Accessed December 15, 2014.

13. Orcajada E, Rao LT. The art of active listening. *Nursing Spectrum (New York/New Jersey Metro Edition).* 2005;17A(21):17, 30.

14. Robeznieks A. Hospitals hire more doctors as CEOs as focus on quality grows. http://www.modernhealthcare.com/article/20140510/MAGAZINE/305109988/. Accessed December 15, 2014.

15. Willson M. The growth of the physician CEO. http://www.healthleadersmedia.com/page-1/MAG-258908/The-Growth-of-the-Physician-CEO. Accessed December 15, 2014.

16. Merritt Hawkins. Review of physician and advanced practitioner recruiting incentives. 2015. http://www.merritthawkins.com/physician-compensation-and-recruiting.aspx. Accessed December 15, 2014.

17. NEJM Career Center. Understanding the physician employment movement. http://www.nejmcareercenter.org/article/understanding-the-physician-employment-movement-/. Accessed January 4, 2015.

18. Etkin JJ, Holm CE. Physician employment is here to stay. PEJ Career Center. http://www3.acpe.org:8082/docs/default-source/pej-archives-2011/physician-employment-is-here-to-stay.pdf?sfvrsn=4. Accessed January 4, 2015.

19. Gabarro JJ, Kotter JP. Managing your boss: a compatible relationship with your superior is essential to being effective in your job. *Harv Bus Rev.* 1980;58(1):92-100.

20. White SJ. Leading from a staff or clinical position. *Am J Health-Syst Pharm.* 2009;66(23):2092-2096.

21. Peters T, Austin N. *A Passion for Excellence: The Leadership Difference.* New York, NY: Warner Books; 1985.

Suggested Reading

Covey SMR. *The Speed of Trust: The One Thing That Changes Everything.* New York, NY: Free Press; 2008.

Kotter JP. *Leading Change.* Cambridge, MA: Harvard Business Review Press; 1996.

Patterson K, Grenny J, McMillan R, et al. *Crucial Conversations: Tools for Talking When Stakes Are High.* 2nd ed. New York, NY: McGraw-Hill; 2012.

CHAPTER 3

P&T Committee, Formulary Management Basics, and Medication-Use Evaluations

Bob Lobo and Mark Sullivan

KEY TERMS

FMEA—Stands for **f**ailure **m**ode and **e**ffects **a**nalysis. A process used to mitigate risk. FMEA involves choosing a process for investigation; forming a multidisciplinary team charged with the review; mapping out the processes; calculating risk priority for each step in the process; selecting an area for improvement based on the calculated risk priority; and implementing actions and outcomes measures.

Formulary—A continually updated list of medications and related information, representing the clinical judgment of physicians, pharmacists, and other experts in the diagnosis, prophylaxis, or treatment of disease and promotion of health.

Formulary System—The ongoing process through which a healthcare organization establishes policies regarding the use of drugs, therapies, and drug-related products and identifies those that are medically appropriate and cost-effective to best serve the health interests of a given patient population.

Medication-Use Policy—Refers to the decisions made by the P&T committee that impact how medications are used throughout the medication-use system. Often refers to how the P&T committee has decided to restrict medications.

MUE—Stands for **m**edication-**u**se **e**valuation. A performance improvement method that is used to assess and improve medication-use processes. MUEs are criteria-based assessments that incorporate institution-specific guidelines to retrospectively review how a medication was used in a population.

SBAR—Stands for **s**ituation, **b**ackground, **a**ssessment, and **r**ecommendations. A simple and efficient format that should be used to present a proposal with a solution.

Introduction

The clinical pharmacy coordinator is frequently called on to serve on the organization's pharmacy and therapeutics (P&T) committee and, in many instances, may serve as secretary of the committee. The P&T committee is always a very high-profile committee with tremendous influence throughout the organization. Membership on the P&T committee provides the clinical coordinator with a tremendous opportunity to advance and direct the **medication-use policy** of the organization. It is important that the clinical pharmacy coordinator understands and appreciates the importance of the P&T committee and uses membership on the committee to advance medication safety and quality initiatives.

The Pharmacy and Therapeutics Committee

The clinical coordinator often serves as the secretary of the P&T committee, which provides an opportunity to set the agenda for the meeting. Even if not serving as the secretary, the clinical coordinator still has a major influence on the agenda and provides input into important agenda items. The P&T committee is responsible for much more than simply managing the **formulary system**. It is charged with overseeing the entire medication-use process, including all of the policies and procedures, practices, and costs. It has the potential to shape how medicine, pharmacy, and nursing are all practiced at the institution.

ASHP has published several official documents that define the key terms and parameters around P&T committee functions.[1,2] The *ASHP Guidelines on the Pharmacy and Therapeutics Committee and the Formulary System* is a good overview of the functions of the P&T committee (see http://www.ashp.org/doclibrary/bestpractices/formgdlptcommformsyst.pdf).

ASHP defines **formulary** as "a continually updated list of medications and related information, representing the clinical judgment of physicians, pharmacists, and other experts in the diagnosis, prophylaxis, or treatment of disease and promotion of health."[1] ASHP suggests that health systems view the formulary more broadly than as a simple list of medications. They state that a formulary system is "the ongoing process through which a healthcare organization establishes policies regarding the use of drugs, therapies, and drug-related products and identifies those that are most medically appropriate and cost-effective to best serve the health interests of a given patient population."[1] In practice, the clinical coordinators will help to establish the formulary system, and if done well their efforts will have a significant and positive impact on the health system and the patients they serve. The term *medication-use policy* refers to the decisions made by P&T committees with respect to the formulary.

It is essential that you understand the place of the P&T committee in the hierarchy of the health system. The P&T committee's scope, organization, and authority are typically described in the medical staff bylaws and/or medical staff rules and regulations. It is a prestigious committee to serve on, and therefore members of the medical staff usually enjoy their role on the committee because they have an opportunity to influence practice at the institution. A key issue is that the P&T committee is first and foremost a committee of the medical staff. For this reason, the committee should be comprised of medical staff members that represent the major medical service areas for the health system. Decisions made at the P&T committee are decisions made by medical staff to promote the optimal use of medications throughout the health system. The P&T committee chairperson is most often an influential medical staff leader in the organization. Effective and respected leadership helps to ensure that P&T decisions are followed and less likely to be subject to second guessing.

The P&T committee generally reports directly (or indirectly through another medical staff committee) to the medical executive board of the health system. The medical executive board may not review each P&T agenda item and may only review P&T minutes from a high-level perspective. For this reason, decisions made at the P&T committee are usually the final word and are not further vetted by medical staff. In some cases, more controversial medication policies may be selected for review at the medical executive board level. If a particular P&T decision is likely to provoke controversy among the medical staff, the clinical coordinator may discuss the issue with the chair in advance and recommend that the chair discuss with colleagues at the medical executive level. This additional vetting and support at the medical executive level will help to avoid conflict and controversy after the policy goes into effect.

P&T Meetings

P&T committee meetings should be held on a regular, predictable schedule to facilitate the best possible medical staff attendance. For example, a recurring date such as the third Friday of the month is ideal. Frequent changes to the meeting schedule may result in poor attendance. The optimal meeting time may depend on the availability of key medical staff committee members. This can sometimes mean that the meeting is held early in the morning before surgeries are scheduled if surgeons comprise an important component, or in the evening after the medical staff members have finished rounding. Most health systems will find it advantageous to provide a meal during the meeting. This is a small expense that is well worth the cost to ensure optimal medical staff attendance, which is essential for a P&T committee to function effectively. Another important consideration is the meeting venue. The room should comfortably accommodate all members including guests and have a projector and screen because some agenda items will need to be presented in PowerPoint format. If the P&T committee serves a hospital system, then facilities for teleconferencing and video-conferencing should be available. An online webinar format would also allow participants to be engaged from their offices or homes, which encourages participation.

Most health systems find that monthly meetings are needed to meet the needs of the institution. When meetings are held less often than monthly, important decisions regarding medication-use policy may be delayed. The P&T meeting itself should be well structured, with the agenda and packet of meeting materials distributed well in advance of the meeting to provide members adequate time for review and to do their own research. Distribution of the agenda and packet of materials approximately 1 week in advance of the meeting is ideal. The meeting agenda should have a standard format, and there should be adequate time allotted to follow up on previous business (see

Figure 3-1). Some of the agenda items should recur monthly, such as approval of subcommittee meeting minutes, new drug reviews, medication shortage issues, new medication-use policy issues, Food and Drug Administration (FDA) alerts, and therapeutic interchanges. Special reports, such as medication-use evaluations (**MUEs**), pharmacist intervention reports, adverse drug event (ADE) reports, drug class reviews, and an annual review of the formulary may be presented quarterly or annually as appropriate. To accomplish the goal of distributing the packet in advance of each meeting, the committee secretary may need to obtain meeting materials several weeks ahead of the scheduled meeting. If the secretary waits until the last minute to assemble the agenda and meeting materials, it will not provide P&T committee members with enough time to review and consider key issues, making the meeting less efficient.

Agenda items should come from a variety of sources. The clinical coordinator should have an understanding of the various problems that are occurring within the medication-use system, and these issues should be identified and brought forward to the committee with recommended solutions. For example, if problems are occurring during the ordering or prescribing process, new ordering protocols or policies may be needed. When there are problems with medication ordering, it is ideal if the clinical coordinator works with a physician champion, especially if pushback from medical staff is expected. If the medication-use problem is occurring during the dispensing process, the clinical coordinator may need to collaborate with members of the pharmacy operations team to bring solutions forward. This is essential because operational pharmacists are most likely to understand the reasons underlying dispensing-related problems within the health system. Likewise, if the problems are occurring during drug administration, then nursing input will be necessary. Note that if the P&T committee serves a multihospital system, then the clinical coordinator should reach out to the other hospitals for agenda items regularly.

Presenting Medication-Use Problems and Solutions to the P&T Committee

A simple, efficient, and effective way for the clinical coordinator to summarize and present

FIGURE 3-1. Sample P&T Committee Meeting Agenda

Pharmacy Conference Room
December 1, 2014; Noon–1:30 p.m.

Lunch will be served during the meeting.

I.   Call to order

II. Review of corporate P&T committee minutes

III. Medical executive committee decisions

IV. Review of subcommittee meeting minutes
    a.   Medication safety committee
    b.   Medication policy committee
    c.   Children's hospital P&T committee
    d.   Antibiotic subcommittee

V.   Routine business
    a.   Follow-up from previous meeting
    b.   Medication shortages
    c.   Review of nonformulary medication use
    d.   FDA medication safety communications
    e.   Review of new FDA drug approvals
    f.   Policy and procedure reviews
    g.   New medication protocol reviews

VI. Quarterly reports
    h.   MUEs
    i.   Pharmacist intervention report
    j.   ADE stats
    k.   Formulary removals
    l.   Drug expense report

VII. Annual reports
    a.   Formulary review
        ii.   Drugs added
        iii. Drugs deleted
    b.   Medication-use system improvements

VIII. Meeting adjournment

ADE = Adverse drug event; FDA = Food and Drug Administration; MUEs = medication-use evaluations; P&T = Pharmacy & Therapeutics.

medication-use problems and solutions to the P&T committee is to use the situation, background, assessment, and recommendations (**SBAR**) format (see **Figure 3-2**). Nursing departments commonly use SBAR to identify potential patient care problems that must be presented to medical staff. The *situation* section states the problem; *background* presents evidence that supports the problem statement; *assessment* synthesizes and summarizes the information presented in the situation and background sections; and *recommendations* present specific and actionable items that the appropriate medical staff leadership will support. Recommendations should be evidence-based, so references are essential.

P&T Subcommittees

Today's health systems have a large amount of business related to medication use, and a single P&T committee may not have the time or resources to address all of the issues. Therefore, it is helpful to have various P&T subcommittees address the high volume of medication-related issues. P&T subcommittees also help to leverage more of the medical staff expertise in making policy decisions, and they should include experts who can assist with formulary and policy issues in a specialty practice area. The clinical coordinator should serve on these subcommittees to provide input or, at a minimum, review the meeting minutes to be aware of the subcommittee discussions and decisions. P&T subcommittees typically include antimicrobials, medication safety, oncology, and/or pediatrics. The most common P&T subcommittee is the antibiotic subcommittee, which is typically chaired by a leading infectious disease physician. The secretary may be an infectious disease clinical pharmacy specialist or clinical coordinator. Other subcommittee members may include representatives from the microbiology laboratory, epidemiology, infection control, pharmacy administration, and nursing. The antibiotic subcommittee generally provides oversight of the antimicrobial formulary and antimicrobial stewardship efforts of the hospital. This subcommittee has become increasingly important as both the Centers for Disease Control and Prevention and The Joint Commission (TJC) have national standards for antimicrobial stewardship. Antimicrobials are prone to misuse and usually comprise a significant percentage of the drug budget at most institutions, so it is very important that resources are dedicated to tracking and trending antimicrobial use. An example of an antibiotic subcommittee charter can be found in **Figure 3-3**.

Another key P&T subcommittee is the medication safety subcommittee. This subcommittee may report to another committee, such as a quality/safety committee at some hospitals. If the medication safety subcommittee reports to the P&T committee, it will provide synergy and an opportunity for the P&T committee to have a greater role with medication safety.

Hospitals with a large cancer center may have an oncology subcommittee, which can provide expertise in the rapidly evolving field of cancer pharmacotherapeutics. Chemotherapy has become a major driver of health-system drug expense, and having a subcommittee dedicated to this therapeutic area can provide the needed infrastructure to manage this expense.

Hospitals that have a large pediatric population will benefit from having a dedicated pediatrics subcommittee. This will ensure that the unique needs of this population are served by the appropriate experts. Other P&T subcommittees include the needs of special populations, cardiology, pain management, anesthesia/surgery, sedation, and critical care. If the clinical coordinator practices within a multihospital system, it is essential to have representation from as many hospitals as possible at each of the P&T subcommittees to have adequate buy-in throughout the system.

The Drug Review Process

An efficient mechanism is important for ensuring formulary requests for new drugs are processed in a timely manner to meet patient and institutional needs. It is a best practice to require physicians to complete a structured, standardized formulary request form (see **Figure 3-4**). The request form provides a permanent track record of who requested a drug and the rationale for the request and should be included in the packet of meeting materials to provide transparency to the request process. Without a formal and transparent request process, it is possible that an unscrupulous pharmaceutical vendor will initiate the formulary review.

FIGURE 3-2. Sample SBAR

Glyburide and First-Generation Sulfonylureas

Situation

First-generation sulfonylureas are rarely used anymore, and chlorpropamide use is strongly discouraged by diabetes experts due to the risk of severe and prolonged hypoglycemia. The efficacy of glyburide, glipizide, and glimepiride are equivalent, although glyburide poses a significantly higher risk of minor and major hypoglycemic events.

Background

Most clinicians have already abandoned the use of chlorpropamide and other first-generation sulfonylureas due to the widely recognized risk for prolonged, severe hypoglycemic episodes, especially in patients who are elderly or who have renal impairment. Like chlorpropamide, glyburide (Micronase, Diabeta) also has a long terminal half-life with active metabolites that accumulate in patients with renal insufficiency. The potential for severe hypoglycemia necessitating prolonged hospitalization is also a major concern with glyburide, although this problem is not as widely recognized as it is with chlorpropamide.

Assessment

Use of first-generation sulfonylureas has largely been abandoned. Glyburide is associated with severe, prolonged hypoglycemia; therefore, glipizide and glimepiride are preferred.

Recommendation

Recommend removal of glyburide and all of the first-generation sulfonylureas (chlorpropamide, tolbutamide, tolazamide, and acetohexamide) from formulary. Glipizide and glimepiride will remain on formulary as the only recommended sulfonylureas. This recommendation has been reviewed and endorsed by chief, division of diabetes, endocrinology, and metabolism.

References

1. Harrower AD. Comparative tolerability of sulphonylureas in diabetes mellitus. *Drug Safety.* 2000;22(4):313-320.
2. Asplund K, Wiholm BE, Lithner F. Glibenclamide-associated hypoglycaemia: a report on 57 cases. *Diabetologia.* 1983;24(6):412-417.
3. Seltzer HS. Drug-induced hypoglycemia. A review of 1418 cases. *Endocrinol Metab Clin North Am.* 1989;18(1):163-183.
4. Shorr RI, Ray WA, Daugherty JR, et al. Individual sulfonylureas and serious hypoglycemia in older people. *J Am Geriatr Soc.* 1996;44(7):751-755.

FIGURE 3-3. Sample Charter

Antibiotic Subcommittee of the Pharmacy and Therapeutics Committee

Purpose and Scope

Serves in an evaluative, educational, and advisory capacity to the P&T committee in all matters pertaining to the use of anti-infective medications. Provides oversight of the performance improvement activities of the medication-use system as it pertains to anti-infective medications. Provides mechanisms for communicating any changes to the formulary or medication policies and recommends educational programs on matters of medication-use for providers, staff, and others involved with the use of anti-infective medications.

Functions

Formulary management, medication safety, policy development, communication, and education for anti-infective therapies. Promotes the appropriate use of anti-infective medications in a safe, cost-effective manner through quality improvement processes including performance of MUEs, cost-benefit analysis and other systematic reviews. Institutes temporary anti-infective medication management protocols in response to drug shortages.

Reporting

Reports to the P&T committee whose recommendations are subject to approval by the organized medical staff and administrative approval process.

Membership and Process

Decisions are based on group consensus. Three voting physicians must be present to establish a quorum for voting to proceed. If consensus is not achieved, the subcommittee chair may forward to the P&T committee. Voting membership of this subcommittee is appointed by the chair and consists of physician representation from the division of infectious diseases (chair), infection control, critical care, pediatrics, surgery, medicine, pharmacy, pharmacy administration, clinical microbiology laboratory, and informatics. Nonvoting members may participate in an ad hoc basis, based on the needs of the committee. Voting members with potential conflicts of interest may be asked to abstain from voting.

Roles/Responsibilities

The chairperson is responsible for conducting meetings, communication of the subcommittee work to the P&T committee no less than quarterly, support of the subcommittee's work, and recruitment of appropriate members of the subcommittee. The secretary of the subcommittee is responsible for assembling and drafting the agenda, recording minutes of the meeting, and dissemination of the minutes. All subcommittee members are responsible for active participation, decision making, offering of needs, appropriate communication of subcommittee decisions, and commitment and support of the subcommittee's work. Subcommittee members sign a conflict of interest statement annually, which is kept on file with committee documents.

Consultants to the subcommittee are responsible for participation in review of medications and devices, attendance at selected meetings, and communication of actions for the subcommittee as needed.

Meeting Schedule

Meetings occur no less than six times per year.

MUEs = medication-use evaluations; P&T = Pharmacy & Therapeutics.

FIGURE 3-4. Sample Nonformulary Request Form

This form should be used when requesting a P&T committee review of a medication for inclusion on the formulary. A physician must complete the form and submit to the P&T committee secretary.

Physician name _____

Physician email _____

Generic name of requested medication _____

Brand name of requested medication _____

Reason for request (which indication) _____

Will the medication be used off-label? Yes or No? _____

Should the medication be restricted to a specific patient population? Yes or No? _____

Specify patient population for use _____

Estimated number of patients to be treated per month _____

Is there a similar medication already on formulary? Yes or No? _____

If yes, please specify _____

Are there any special medication safety concerns? Yes or No? _____

If yes, please specify _____

Please state why this medication should be added to the formulary _____
_____
_____

Check one of the following disclosure statements and sign below:

_____ Yes, I have received research support or will receive support from the manufacturer.

_____ Yes, I have a consulting agreement or currently plan to seek a consulting agreement from the manufacturer.

_____ Yes, I, my significant other, or dependent has a financial interest with the manufacturer of the medication I am requesting.

_____ Yes, I currently have no potential conflicts of interest with the manufacturer of the medication I am requesting.

Physician signature _____ Date _____

_____

P&T = Pharmacy & Therapeutics.

The clinical coordinator should watch out for potential conflicts of interest, such as when the requesting physician has a consulting agreement or other financial interest with the manufacturer. The drug should only move to the review stage after the formulary request form with disclosure statements has been submitted. The ideal way to manage potential conflicts of interest is to require a written disclosure on the formulary request form and to state the potential conflict of interest before the discussion of the agenda item at the P&T meeting.

The clinical coordinator should ensure that the new drug review is conducted in a timely manner. In many cases, it is the role of the P&T committee secretary or clinical coordinator to write up the P&T committee drug review monograph. Sometimes this responsibility is delegated to various clinical pharmacists who practice in the area where the drug will be used. Students and residents may also be assigned this responsibility. In any case, the clinical coordinator should review the monograph prior to distribution to the committee to ensure that the recommendations are appropriate.

Once a request has been made to add a drug to the formulary, the review should occur at the next P&T committee meeting if possible and generally no more than 2 months after the request. In some instances, a new drug therapy will offer a significant treatment advance, and the drug review may need to be expedited. The issue of urgent review of breakthrough treatments is becoming increasingly common, especially with newer chemotherapeutic agents. A potential solution to the problem of breakthrough treatments requiring urgent reviews is to allow limited nonformulary use of the breakthrough therapy on a case-by-case basis until the formal P&T committee review can be completed. The clinical coordinator may need to scan the horizon for potential new breakthrough drugs to be prepared for an expedited review. In practice, it is not easy to predict when breakthrough drugs will be marketed, and the amount of lead time to prepare for a breakthrough drug review may only be a matter of days. Nevertheless, when possible, the clinical coordinator may actually want to begin developing the formulary monograph for breakthrough therapies before the drug is formally requested.

Facts & Comparisons provides structured formulary monographs for many new drugs as a subscription service. These reviews are typically well written and unbiased. However, some of these preprepared reviews may be out of date by the time the medication is on the market. The busy clinical coordinator may benefit from using this service on occasion, as preparing new drug monographs is a time-consuming task. At least several hours of work are typically required for each new drug review even if there is a preprepared monograph to work from. This is because the clinical coordinator should thoroughly review any new data on the medication and should work to identify potential safety issues with the new medication. Estimating the budgetary impact on the hospital is a critical function as well. New drug reviews should be handled with a standard P&T review process. Review and approval of new drugs by email should be strongly discouraged because P&T committee members are unlikely to take the required time to review and consider all of the data and potential clinical, safety, and cost issues with an email vote. In addition, there is less of an opportunity to gain a group consensus on important decisions through email.

The new drug review will contain a number of standard elements that are defined in policy. In fact, TJC requires written criteria to be used for determining which drugs are selected for inclusion on the formulary.[3] TJC states that at a minimum the criteria for selecting new medications should include the indications for use, effectiveness, drug interactions, potential for errors and abuse, ADEs and other risks, sentinel event advisories, patient population served, and costs. The clinical coordinator should ensure these criteria are specified in a formal policy and procedure (see a sample policy in **Appendix 3-A**). In addition to the standard written formulary monograph, the clinical coordinator may want to summarize key monograph points in a PowerPoint presentation. This is especially important when the new drug review has the potential to make a large impact on patient care or the finances of the institution. The presentation itself should last no more than approximately 10 minutes and should conclude with specific formulary recommendations. The presentation should be included along with the formulary monograph in the P&T packet and distributed in advance of the meeting so that members can follow along during the presentation. An outline containing all of the elements of a P&T committee formulary monograph for a new drug review can be found in **Figure 3-5**. The clinical coordinator should ensure that anyone who presents a new drug review to the P&T committee understands the policy and follows the standard formulary monograph.

Formulary Restrictions

Formulary recommendations should be carefully considered, and the decision is often not a simple "add to formulary" or "deny addition to formulary." In some instances a new drug should be conditionally accepted and/or restricted to serve a particular population. Some drugs may require specialized knowledge to prescribe appropriately. For example, a new antibiotic may offer a very broad spectrum of activity, leading to overuse by general practitioners who do not take the time to carefully consider a narrow-spectrum drug. This type of drug may need to be restricted to specific providers, such as infectious disease specialists. Another approach may be to restrict the drug to a specific patient population, such as those who have failed a 72-hour course of appropriate antimicrobial therapy. Restriction to a specialist group for use in a specific disease or patient population may also be appropriate. Once a precedent is set for using a particular type of restriction, the clinical coordinator will find it easier to use the same strategy for restricting the use of other drugs at the hospital.

Other types of restrictions that may be implemented include limiting use to particular geographic areas of the hospital. For instance, a new sedative drug may be restricted to only intensive care units or procedural areas. An expensive new chemotherapeutic drug may be restricted to clinic areas only. Restricting expensive new therapies to clinic areas increases the likelihood of obtaining appropriate reimbursement and minimizing the impact on the inpatient drug budget. A potential political pitfall is to restrict a drug to a specific physician when it may be more appropriate to restrict use to a particular patient population or specialty practice. If the medical staff believes that a particular physician is receiving special consideration from the committee, they may lose confidence in the committee's decision-making ability. Restricting use to an order set or protocol is commonly used for complex or high-risk medications such as chemotherapy. The order set or protocol will ensure important baseline assessments are completed, and monitoring protocols are followed. Order sets and protocols will ensure the most optimal and safe care is "hard wired" into the drug ordering, dispensing, administration, and monitoring process.

The clinical coordinator may need to make sure representatives from all hospitals within a multihospital system are onboard with how a drug will be restricted, as managing formulary restrictions is often a challenge for pharmacies. The clinical coordinator must carefully consider how any restrictions will affect pharmacy workflow. Some restrictions place a heavy burden on pharmacy resources, especially if the pharmacist must screen each order to ensure compliance with the restrictions. In a multihospital system, there may be one or more hospitals that struggle with enforcing compliance if resources are inadequate or if work flow differs significantly from the other hospitals. The clinical coordinator will ensure the proposed restrictions are thoroughly vetted by representatives at all hospitals prior to the P&T meeting to increase the likelihood that the medication will be used safely and optimally once it is available for ordering.

Managing the Formulary

Having an easily retrievable formulary is essential to ensure providers, pharmacists, and nurses will adhere to the hospital formulary. When clinicians do not know whether a medication is formulary or not, it will result in unnecessary phone calls between pharmacists and prescribers. Computerized physician order entry (CPOE) systems offer the benefit of having the formulary hard wired into the system, effectively eliminating formulary misunderstandings. Use of CPOE is a vital piece of health-system technology when it comes to managing the formulary. The Leapfrog Group (www.leapfroggroup.org) tracks CPOE adoption, and in 2014 there were 1,339 hospitals using CPOE in at least one inpatient unit versus 384 in 2010. There is a growing expectation for hospitals to implement clinical decision support that will reduce risk for ADEs, and the clinical coordi-

FIGURE 3-5. Sample Format—P&T Committee Formulary Monograph

I. Presenter

II. Drug names: generic, brand

III. Manufacturer

IV. FDA approval rating

V. ISMP high-risk category

VI. Drug class

VII. Therapeutic indication

VIII. REMS requirements

IX. Basic pharmacology

    a. Pharmacokinetics

    b. Pharmacodynamics

X. Comparative efficacy and safety literature review

XI. Safety analysis

    a. Adverse effects

    b. Drug interactions

    c. Warnings/precautions

    d. Contraindications

    e. Other safety concerns

        i. Clinical decision support for CPOE system

        ii. Look-alike/sound-alike concerns

        iii. Complexity of use and potential for errors

XII. Dosage forms and dosing

XIII. Cost comparison and budgetary impact

XIV. Target patient population/proposed restrictions

XV. MUE criteria if applicable

XVI. Informatics requirements

XVII. Educational requirements

XVIII. Conclusions and recommendations

XIX. References

CPOE = computerized physician order entry; FDA = Food and Drug Administration; ISMP = Institute for Safe Medication Practices; MUE = medication-use evaluation; P&T = Pharmacy & Therapeutics; REMS = risk evaluation and mitigation strategy.

nator should be engaged in this process. To properly leverage this technology, the clinical coordinator should collaborate closely with the staff members who maintain the CPOE system to ensure the most efficient practice.

In areas that do not use CPOE, having an electronic formulary reference is essential. Like CPOE systems, an electronic formulary will require ongoing maintenance to ensure it is continuously updated with the latest formulary information. An electronic formulary must be comprehensive and able to provide policy decisions regarding restrictions and protocols that are unique to the institution. An electronic formulary system, Lexicomp FORMULINK, is commercially available by subscription from Wolters Kluwer. It allows hospitals to integrate the hospital formulary, policies and procedures, and therapeutic guidelines. It may be useful to use this tool as a P&T website for communicating P&T decisions and policies.

The clinical coordinator may be faced with a number of challenges involving the management of the formulary, and one of the most common is the handling of nonformulary drug requests (see **Figure 3-6** for an example of a process for handling nonformulary drug requests). A nonformulary request is usually a request for a one-time use of a nonformulary medication and does not necessarily mean the medication should be reviewed for formulary status by the P&T committee. Inherent in the formulary system, hospitals should not stock and provide all medications. The clinical coordinator should have an effective system to handle nonformulary drug requests that the P&T committee supports. This system should be recognized and well-understood by medical staff providers as well as pharmacy staff. It should have adequate flexibility to deal with legitimate nonformulary needs when they arise. Some latitude is required to meet the needs of specific patients. At the same time, pharmacists must be empowered to challenge nonformulary drug requests and to offer alternative formulary solutions when appropriate. If there is no reasonable formulary alternative and the medication is medically necessary while hospitalized, the pharmacy should have a mechanism for obtaining the drug as required by TJC.[3] Instances of nonformulary drug requests should be documented so that the clinical coordinator can track and trend these requests. In some cases a nonformulary

medication may be frequently requested, which creates a burden on the pharmacy operations, and its formulary status should be re-evaluated. These instances should be referred to the P&T committee for review. An alternative to obtaining the nonformulary medication is to allow the patient to use home medications. Some patients and providers may feel more comfortable using their own medications than switching to a nonformulary alternative, even for a short period of time. If home medication use is allowed, then a process for verifying the integrity of the medication will be required. This can place a burden on pharmacy resources if home medication use is a frequent occurrence.

Safety Assessment

When a new medication is reviewed for formulary inclusion, a comprehensive evaluation of the medication safety profile to assess risk:benefit should be conducted. Premarketing studies of dosing, efficacy, and safety in populations with small sample sizes may not translate to the general population. New adverse reactions and drug interactions with combinations of drugs and disease states continue to be reported for many years after a medication is placed on the market. Once added to the formulary, an ongoing surveillance process is needed to monitor for known and potentially new adverse effects. A number of quality and safety assessments should be included in the formulary review process. General operational issues such as checking packaging, barcoding, and labeling of new formulary medications for look-alike/sound-alike/scan-alike errors is supportive of safe onboarding of new formulary additions. If additional precautions are required for storage or during the dispensing or administration step of the drug's medication use, these should be incorporated into existing training for staff. Evaluation of the drug's hazard classification can support inclusion of appropriate staff training and disposal procedures. Use of a drug safety checklist during the formulary approval process is a good tool for addressing issues with a formalized process. Including these steps in the education and implementation plan can help address additional resources that may be needed to use the new medication from a people, process, or technology perspective.

An example of a formulary checklist for safety, the SAFE Tool, developed at the Univer-

FIGURE 3-6. Process for Handling Nonformulary Drug Requests

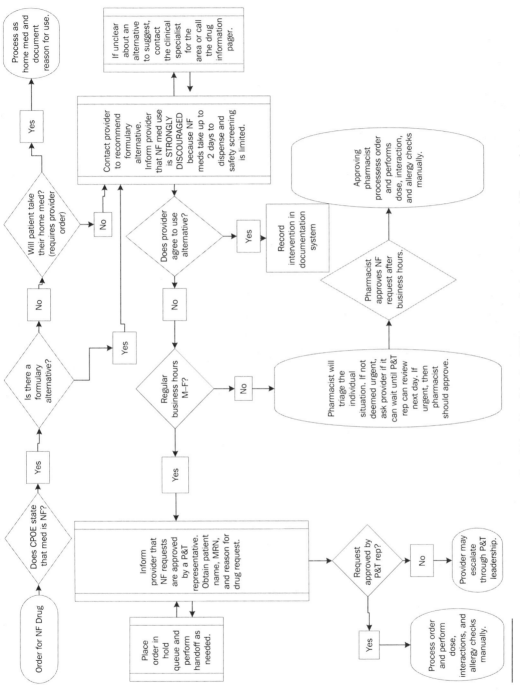

CPOE = computerized physician order entry; F = Friday; M = Monday; MRN = medical record number; NF = nonformulary; P&T = Pharmacy & Therapeutics.

sity of Nebraska, is a formal process for evaluating new drug safety profile (see **Figure 3-7**).[4] The SAFE Tool is a checklist that systematically reviews each step of the medication-use system for process errors. Pharmacists with expertise in the drug class are used to support a scoring process with high reliability. Once the assessment is completed, a scoring process can guide additional measures recommended for successful implementation of putting the drug in use (see **Figure 3-8**). A proactive risk assessment process will allow risk points to be identified and mitigated before they cause harm. Failure mode and effects analysis (**FMEA**) is a proven process used to mitigate risk.[5] It involves choosing a process for investigation; forming a multidisciplinary team charged with the review; mapping out the processes; calculating risk priority for each step in the process; selecting an area for improvement based on the calculated risk priority; and implementing actions and outcomes measures. This process can be applied in an iterative fashion to the medication-use process governed by the P&T committee to minimize risk. The Veterans Affairs National Center for Patient Safety website (www.patientsafety.va.gov) and the Joint Commission on Accreditation for Healthcare Organizations (http://www.jcrinc.com/assets/1/14/FMEA10_Sample_Pages.pdf) both have resources for learning about and applying FMEA principles in the P&T process.

Nonformulary medication ordering can create potential safety issues and add unnecessary costs if not managed. Nonformulary orders may be entered into some CPOE systems in a variety of methods depending on the file structure used in the system. Users may be able to enter nonformulary orders using "miscellaneous" or free text, thus bypassing decision support tools provided for formulary maintenance and safety. When free text entries are allowed, medication names can be entered incorrectly, look-alike/sound-alike errors and dosing errors can be made, and patients can be exposed to unrecognized drug–drug interactions. In their study on nonformulary medication use, Pummer et al. noted a majority of the nonformulary medication orders were for formulary medications and patients' own medications.[6] Most of the formulary medications were order-entry errors most likely due to the prescribers' lack of knowledge of the formulary

system. A required educational program for all prescribers was implemented to support use of formulary management tools. Educational programs should include direction on where formulary lists are maintained as well as how decision support may be used in CPOE systems for safe ordering. Provider education in the appropriate use of clinical systems has been noted to be a gap in many organizations with residency training programs. Informal survival-type education may be happening without the knowledge of the P&T coordinator. Pharmacy involvement in these training programs can assist new providers in understanding the formulary and the systems that support it. Another decision support tool created in the Pummer study was a new patient's home medication order screen. This was built as a strategy to require pharmacy verification and labeling and alert nurses and pharmacists that home medications are being used.

Because decision support tools are used to manage the medication-use process, clinical support decisions should be part of the P&T oversight process where systems allow the use of such tools. Safety and efficacy of these tools can be supported by an oversight/approval process managed via the P&T committee. This approval can be done in subcommittee with pharmacists, physicians, nurses, informatics, and other participants. Inappropriate medication use can result when a formal approval process is not in place. Many systems have struggled to rein in private order sets or manage use of medications for unapproved indications. Another facet of this oversight is clinical alerts. Systems may allow use of commercial or locally customized clinical alerts that may be maintained by informatics, pharmacy, or other staff.[7] The oversight process should include criteria for how clinical alerts should be deployed in the prescribing, pharmacy, and medication administration systems in use within the facility. Clear indications for how the medication is prescribed and standards for medication ordering—including standardized units for weight-based dosing if applicable—must be included in the implementation plan.

It is also recommended to include all of the medications reviewed by the P&T committee even if they were approved, approved with restrictions, or denied formulary status. When something is determined as nonformulary or

FIGURE 3-7. SAFE Tool

Process Errors				
Ordering and Transcribing	**Order Entry**	**Storage and Order Verification**	**Compounding and Dispensing**	**Administration and Monitoring**
☐ Name looks alike ☐ Name sounds alike ☐ Dosing difficult ☐ Decimal in dose ☐ Abbreviated name ☐ Calculated dose ☐ Renal concern ☐ Hepatic concern ☐ Lab required ☐ Monitoring needed ☐ Class duplicate ☐ Black-box warning ☐ >5% adverse effects[a] ☐ Drug–drug reactions ☐ On market <6 mo	☐ Name looks alike ☐ Name sounds alike ☐ Decimal in dose ☐ Abbreviated name ☐ Critical omission ☐ Nurse order entry ☐ Secretary order entry ☐ Pharmacy order entry[b]	☐ Drug–drug reactions ☐ Renal concern ☐ Hepatic concern ☐ Dosing difficult ☐ Decimal in dose ☐ Calculated dose ☐ Lab required ☐ Monitoring needed ☐ Black-box warning ☐ Hazardous drug ☐ On market <6 mo	☐ Drug looks alike ☐ Packaging issues ☐ Compounding ☐ No barcode ☐ Multiple strengths ☐ Pyxis loading ☐ Medication cart[c] ☐ Nurse servers ☐ Special storage ☐ Floor stock[c] ☐ Hazardous drug ☐ Blood product	☐ Food interactions ☐ Lab interactions ☐ Monitoring needed ☐ >5% adverse effects[a] ☐ Special storage ☐ Black-box warning ☐ Multiple routes ☐ IV pump dosing ☐ Epidural dosing ☐ Patient-controlled analgesia dosing ☐ Irrigation ☐ Inline filter ☐ On market <6 mo ☐ Hazardous drug ☐ Blood product
Process risk:	Process risk:	Process risk:	Process risk:	Process risk:
Cumulative SAFE score:				

IV = intravenous; mo = month; SAFE = safety assessment formulary evaluator.

[a]Other medications may be required to minimize these adverse effects at the original time of prescribing; they may need to be given at the time of administration or at onset of symptoms.

[b]A double-check system of all orders helps reduce risk of error. Our institution prefers secretary order entry and pharmacist verification of the entry.

[c]Our institution does not use medication cart exchange. Instead, the majority of medications are dispensed from Pyxis. Floor stock and medication carts bypass the security checkpoint of Pyxis medication profiles.

FIGURE 3-8. SAFE Tool Scoring System

SAFE Score System

SAFE Score	Potential Error	Recommendations
0–10	Low	Provide healthcare professional education before addition
11–25	Medium	Provide healthcare professional education before addition; have multidisciplinary evaluation plan to establish need for protocols, specialist prescriptive authority, and enhanced education before addition
≥26	High	Provide healthcare professional education before addition; have multidisciplinary evaluation plan to establish need for protocols, specialist prescriptive authority, and enhanced education before addition; implement medication safety process before use within the hospital before addition

SAFE = safety assessment formulary evaluator.

Source: Originally published in Pick AM, Massoomi F, Neff WJ, et al. A safety assessment tool for formulary candidates. *Am J Health-Syst Pharm.* 2006;63(13):1269-1272. © 2006, American Society of Health-System Pharmacists, Inc. All rights reserved. Reprinted with permission.

restricted, hard stops or other language should be added to the entry so that the prescribers and pharmacy know the prohibited status of the medications. If you do not add these to your informatics system, then a prescriber may order it but the pharmacist may not know and might try to order the medication from the wholesaler or borrow it from another institution (bypassing all the sound work from the P&T committee in developing guidelines or restrictions for the medication). If the medication is built into the informatics system, then the pharmacist will know not to process the medication.

Risk Evaluation and Mitigation Strategies

Risk evaluation and mitigation strategies (REMS) programs were authorized following the passage of the FDA Amendment Act of 2007. These programs are implemented if the FDA feels that safety measures beyond the professional labeling are needed to ensure a drug's benefits outweigh the risks. REMS programs can be required during the preapproval or postapproval process if new information becomes available, and the FDA deems a postapproval program necessary. These programs may require provision of a medication guide, a medication-specific communication plan, and/or specific steps to ensure safe use and an implementation system. Depending on how position responsibil-

ities are structured in a given facility, the clinical coordinator may be responsible for reviewing REMS programs associated with a new formulary addition, which may include such tasks as arranging training for providers, nursing, and pharmacy staff; monitoring needed documentation; and reporting to the pharmaceutical company. In some instances, compliance with these programs can be a resource-intensive process, requiring the clinical coordinator to seek additional resources for support. This can be through a subcommittee process, where REMS programs are managed centrally on behalf of the P&T committee, or a decentralized process, where the clinical coordinator delegates medication-specific REMS program responsibilities to the local clinical or operations staff. Either way, the coordinator retains oversight responsibilities that program compliance is maintained.

Managing Drug Shortages

Clinical coordinators may be tasked to work with the P&T committee to establish criteria for how drug shortages should be managed. The coordinator may have a significant role in monitoring communication from procurement staff and repackaging, including communication with therapeutic substitution information for prescribers, discussing system drug file changes with informatics and operations staff, and helping providers assess strategies for mitigating patient impacts based on limited therapy availability. The coordinator may have a role in working with medical staff for special patient populations such as oncology or pediatrics, where facilitation of ethical discussions may be required to determine which patients receive limited therapies. The consensus statement on managing drug shortages from a pediatrics chemotherapy perspective offers several guidelines for the P&T coordinator to consider.[8] The first, optimize and efficiently use supplies to mitigate the effects of future shortages, can be operationalized via the P&T committee at the local level by enacting restrictions that limit use to only approved indications and scheduling doses on the same day or time of day to mitigate wastage. The guidelines also foster equal use of scarce medication resources for evidence-based use whether that use is internal or external to a clinical trial. Finally, establishing central clearinghouses for information on drug shortages that connect to local communication tools is critical for appropriate notification of prescribers when drug shortages occur.

Supply chain communication continues to be variable, with no supply of a key medication noted in the supplier's system when an order is placed but an adequate supply noted minutes later when checking back on alternatives. Coordinators can mitigate adverse impacts of false alarms when communicating drug shortages by maintaining open lines of communication with procurement staff to validate product status and with operations staff to monitor inventory when multiple storage sites may be consolidated to maintain system-wide supplies. Good faith communication of what is known as soon as it is verified is a valid strategy in addressing these instances.

A coordinated drug shortage situation, where patient care impact is mitigated, requires collaboration between the clinical coordinator, pharmacy procurement, informatics, and operations staff. They should communicate key shortages and timeline projections (based on recent utilization for when therapeutic substitutions should be implemented); update inactivate/reactivate drug files; coordinate inventory in pharmacy and unit-based, automated dispensing cabinet storage; and educate staff and providers about the drug shortage. Coordinators may also need to help develop

and educate the prescribers on how to dose and use the alternative agents as well as how to write a memo for distribution and/or meet face-to-face with the prescribers. Due to the complexity required to integrate people, processes, and systems, many facilities use checklists to ensure appropriate coordination is in place. One such checklist can be accessed at http://patientsafetyauthority.org/educationaltools/patientsafetytools/shortages/documents/checklist.pdf.

Protocols, Policies, and Procedures— P&T Role

Protocol use is a type of decision support that enables efficient patient care. Unfortunately, the development of physician-based private protocols or written protocols that have not gone through P&T review can result in inappropriate medication use, potentially unsafe medication use, and expose the facility to regulatory issues due to unapproved abbreviations, unclear dosing directions, and therapeutic duplications.

The clinical coordinator's role is to develop criteria for development and institution of protocols under the oversight of the P&T committee. Open communication is needed for appropriate oversight, such as with pharmacy staff who review protocol-based orders; nurses who enact protocol orders under verbal or written provider orders; and informatics staff who may be asked to build unapproved protocol orders. Regulatory requirements related to protocol use in hospitals require documented provider initiation, policy to direct the implementation, and oversight to verify appropriate use. Pharmacy law in some states may preclude the use of protocols, and a check of local regulations is necessary as these policies begin to be used. Written versus unwritten protocols must be considered because the unwritten unit-based protocol that is embedded in culture on a particular unit will only be uncovered by local knowledge and reporting.

The clinical coordinator that handles medication-use management may be responsible for oversight of policy development related to medication use, which may also require facilitation of policy approval by the P&T committee. The coordinator will need to provide oversight of the policy development by working with content experts to craft the policy based on templates in use within the facility. A clear policy approval process, with buy-in from affected parties, may require the coordinator to use previously mentioned SBAR tools to summarize the clinical issue being addressed by the policy and the resolution that the policy provides. These summary documents support an efficient review-and-approval process during presentation to the P&T committee, which may also be used to solicit approvals via email processes without taking time from other formulary considerations during the P&T meeting.

Managing Conflicts

Making choices in a resource-constrained healthcare system can generate conflict between impacted parties. The traditional P&T processes facilitated by the clinical coordinator are based on best practice guidelines using an evidence-based approach, with a pharmacist generally providing a monograph along with comments from a physician and a recommendation for addition or deferment based on efficacy, safety, and cost. Navigating conflicts of interest in the P&T process, aggressive medication positioning by influential physicians, or influential pharmaceutical firms remain challenges for the clinical coordinator. Committee charters, stated goals, and criteria for medication-review processes are helpful, but managing competing interests in the P&T process requires excellent communication skills, maintenance of strong working relationships with key physician and administrative staff, ability to help competing interests find common ground, and the ability to address bias should it enter into considerations.

The recent advent of specialty pharmacy drugs in the formulary process has thrown the traditional P&T process askew. These expensive, limited distribution agents that are life extending, not disease treating, require different processes in today's healthcare economic environment. The clinical coordinator will need to bring together input from not only medical staff to facilitate assessment of these agents, but also finance, patient accounting, patient assistance, and other parties to define the value these agents will have for the organization and how best to introduce, prescribe, obtain payment, and monitor outcomes. In addition to efficacy, risk, and cost assessments, societal benefit is a way to assess medication value if added to the formulary process. Some facilities choose to enlist members outside the healthcare area for this assessment. Pastors, university professors of theology or ethics, community activists, and teachers are some of the team members used for this assessment. The teams developed criteria for their assessment and regularly discuss rankings with the P&T healthcare team. This approach serves to balance the focus on the individual patient versus the population at large in an environment with limited resources. Moving to a formulary approval process that considers the population impacts of such decisions may be an effective way to manage this new wave of specialty medications, which focus on providing high-cost, limited distribution products with some measurable individual value but minimal population value. This value philosophy can drive interactions with decision-making related to pharmacy practice, advance medication safety, and address protocols for dealing with industry.

Medication-Use Evaluations

When the P&T committee is tasked with outcome assessments of medication therapies, the clinical coordinator may be responsible for facilitation of routine, ongoing medication class review. MUE is an effective tool for facilitating this process, which is a performance improvement method used to assess and improve medication-use processes. MUEs are criteria-based assessments that are essentially retrospective reviews of how a medication was used in a population. Pharmacy departments have used MUEs as a quality improvement technique with great success over many decades. An MUE can be a very simple and effective tool when used correctly. MUEs should generally be conducted on medications that are high volume, high cost, or high risk. Other reasons for conducting MUEs include highly complex ordering or monitoring requirements, legal requirements, or regulatory/compliance issues. In some cases, an MUE may need to be conducted to ensure compliance with an FDA or manufacturer's prescribing recommendations, such as REMS. Or, an MUE may be conducted to ensure an institutional protocol is being followed correctly. For example, compliance with a pharmacy-to-dose protocol or a medication protocol conducted by nurses should be assessed to ensure the protocol is followed correctly. Another benefit to assessing protocol use is to determine if the protocol is produoing the intended outcomes. If pharmacy or nursing staff are not following the protocol, it may suggest that the protocol needs to be revised or the process needs to be improved.

The clinical coordinator should strive to include a variety of P&T committee members in the identification and prioritization of MUE ideas. The clinical coordinator should enlist the help of students and residents in the MUE process. MUE data collection can be time-consuming, and students will benefit from instruction and mentoring in this process. Input should be sought from across the health system to identify high-priority drug therapy issues that should be evaluated. This can be done by speaking with front-line pharmacy, nursing, and medical staff who are using the drugs. Ideas may also come from medication variance reports. Obtaining input from an array of medical staff leaders ensures the overall medication-use system is being evaluated in an ongoing basis. After identifying several of the key issues that should be addressed through the MUE process, the clinical coordinator should bring the proposed list of MUE ideas to the P&T committee for endorsement (see **Figure 3-9**).

A koy to using MUEs successfully is to have a clear proposal including the specific criteria for appropriate or inappropriate medication use (see **Appendix 3-B**). Once the proposal is written, the clinical coordinator should consult with a physician champion or thought leaders in the area to obtain their buy-in and make any suggested changes to the criteria. The full proposal with criteria may then be taken to a subsequent P&T committee meeting, giving the clinical coordinator a "green light" to begin data collection. If this is not done before conducting the MUE, the clinical coordinator risks wasting a great deal of time collecting data that may not be useful to the P&T committee. The MUE criteria should state what is considered appropriate and inappropriate for drug prescribing, dispensing, monitoring, and administering. In many cases, it is appropriate to conduct an MUE that is focused on a particular area, such as appropriate prescribing.

Another important step to consider before beginning the data collection is the need for exemption from the institutional review board (IRB) review or an expedited review. MUEs

FIGURE 3-9. Example of MUE Ideas Submitted to P&T Committee

MUE Priorities for 2014

First Quarter

QT prolonging antiarrhythmic drugs and electrolyte abnormalities

New oral anticoagulant dosing

Second Quarter

Warfarin protocol

Third Quarter

Proton pump inhibitors—transitions from ICU to home

Linezolid—compliance with formulary restrictions

Fourth Quarter

Inhaled epoprostenol

ICU = intensive care unit; MUE = medication-use evaluation; P&T = Pharmacy & Therapeutics; QT = measure of delayed ventricular repolarization.

usually do not require a full or even expedited review, but a formal exemption from review is usually appropriate as the purpose of the MUE is quality improvement. Most IRBs have a simple form that can be used for this purpose. A benefit of obtaining IRB clearance before conducting the MUE is that the clinical coordinator may find that the results are compelling enough to share with other institutions in the form of a published abstract, poster presentation, or manuscript. In this way, many other institutions may benefit from the process. However, if the MUE is to be shared only internally for quality improvement, most institutions do not require IRB approval.

The MUE presentation format will vary depending on the size and scope of the MUE. A small MUE can be presented in a simple SBAR format as seen in **Appendix 3-C**. A more complex MUE may be presented to the committee in a PowerPoint format. The basic elements of the presentation should have a consistent format (**Figure 3-10**). The clinical coordinator should ensure there is appropriate follow-up to close the loop. In general, the clinical coordinator should approach the MUE as a PDSA (**p**lan, **d**o, **s**tudy, **a**ct) cycle. It is not enough to identify problems with the way a medication is being used within the health system; the clinical coordinator must also identify potential solutions to the problems that were identified with the MUE. It is also not enough to identify problems and leave them for the P&T committee; the clinical coordinator should

FIGURE 3-10. MUE Presentation Template

1. Rationale/background
2. MUE objectives
3. MUE criteria—appropriate and inappropriate
4. Methods
5. Results
6. Limitations
7. Recommendations
8. Plan for follow-up

MUE = medication-use evaluation.

always have a plan to reassess the problem identified by the MUE and provide follow-up to ensure the issues were minimized or resolved.

Summary

The clinical coordinator is uniquely positioned to have a significant impact on the safety and quality of the medication-use system by working closely with the P&T committee membership. Every clinical coordinator should have at least some role with P&T committee functions, although it is ideal for the clinical coordinator to have a leadership role on the committee, either formal or informal. The clinical coordinator should seek to increase the involvement of other department members with the P&T committee to distribute the large workload and to increase buy-in from others within the department. The savvy clinical coordinator will be sure to collaborate with key medical staff members on controversial issues. The value an effective P&T committee brings to the health system, in terms of improved medication safety, quality, and cost-effectiveness, cannot be overestimated.

PRACTICE TIPS

1. As the P&T committee is a major driver of medication safety, quality, and cost-effectiveness, clinical coordinators should be integrally involved in all P&T activities.

2. SBAR is a simple and efficient way for clinical coordinators to present a problem and solution to the P&T committee.

3. Clinical coordinators should distribute the P&T workload among a variety of pharmacy staff to increase participation and to improve staff recognition of the committee's functions.

4. Clinical coordinators should seek input and involvement of key medical staff members to ensure that P&T initiatives are accepted and therefore successfully implemented.

5. MUEs are effective tools for assessing the quality and safety of medication use in the health system. Clinical coordinators should seek input from key medical staff members on the most appropriate criteria for use and report findings to the P&T committee.

References

1. Tyler LS, Cole SW, May JR, et al. ASHP guidelines on the pharmacy and therapeutics committee and the formulary system. *Am J Health-Syst Pharm.* 2008;65(13):1272-1283.

2. ASHP statement on the pharmacy and therapeutics committee and the formulary system. *Am J Health-Syst Pharm.* 2008;65:2384-2386.

3. The Joint Commission Medication Management Standard MM.02.01.01 The hospital selects and procures medications. https://e-dition.jcrinc.com/ASearch.aspx. Accessed October 20, 2015.

4. Pick AM, Massoomi F, Neff WJ, et al. A safety assessment tool for formulary candidates. *Am J Health-Syst Pharm.* 2006;63(13):1269-1272.

5. Adachi W, Locolce AE. Use of failure mode and effects analysis in improving the safety of iv drug administration. *Am J Health-Syst Pharm.* 2005;62(9):917-920.

6. Pummer T, Shalaby KM, Erush SC. Ordering off the menu: assessing compliance with a nonformulary medication policy. *Ann Pharmacother.* 2009;43(7):1251-1257.

7. Phansalkar S, Desai A, Choksi A, et al. High priority drug-drug interactions for use in electronic health records. *J Am Med Inform Assoc.* 2012;19(5):735-743.

8. Decamp M, Joffe S, Fernandez CV, et al. Chemotherapy drug shortages in pediatric oncology: a consensus statement *Pediatrics.* 2014;133(3):e 716-e724.

Appendix 3-A

Sample P&T Committee Policy

I. *Purpose*:

To provide safe and cost-effective medication therapy through the development and enforcement of medication-use policies and restrictions, which are rational, evidence-based, and clinically appropriate.

II. *Policy*:

A. The formulary is approved by the P&T committee and published electronically for faculty/staff access.

B. Medications available for dispensing or administration are selected and listed in the formulary based on established criteria.

C. Medications on formulary are reviewed at least annually by the designated pharmacy representative based on emerging safety and efficacy information.

D. Approved indications for medications on formulary include those approved by the Food and Drug Administration (FDA) as well as those listed in designated dosing references including *AHFS*, *Lexi-Comp*, *Micromedex*, *NeoFax*, *the Harriet Lane Handbook*, and the National Comprehensive Cancer Network (NCCN) *Drugs and Biologics Compendium* unless otherwise specified. Restrictions identified by the P&T committee take precedence over these references.

III. *Definition*:

Formulary is the official approved listing of medications available for use throughout inpatient and outpatient services.

IV. *Procedures*:

A. P&T committee review and approval process:

1. Information on new pharmaceuticals approved by FDA is brought to the P&T committee for review. This information includes approved indications, expected position in the market, cost relative to conventional therapy when available, and any unique therapeutic effects.

2. Information utilized for review of medications includes clinical data collected from randomized, placebo-controlled, double-blinded trials or other sound and scientific information. Anecdotal evidence is not accepted when reviewing formulary considerations.

3. Pharmaceuticals having unique therapeutic qualities, particularly those costing less than conventional therapy, are reviewed thoroughly by the P&T committee. Criteria covered in this review:

a. Generic name

b. Proprietary name

c. Look-alike/sound-alike names

d. Similar drugs

e. Indications for use

f. Drug interactions

g. Potential for errors or abuse

h. Clinical pharmacology

i. Pharmacokinetics

j. Comparative

k. Contraindications

l. Warnings and precautions

m. Adverse drug events (ADEs)

n. Recommended monitoring

o. Dosing

p. Product availability, storage, and costs

q. Sentinel event advisories

r. Population(s) served (e.g., pediatrics, geriatrics)

s. Other risks

t. Costs

u. References

v. Electronic decision support (if needed)

4. Individual requests for review are made by contacting the designated pharmacy P&T committee representative. Requests are assessed for consideration before inclusion on a committee agenda. The requestor is asked to disclose any conflict of interest and to defend the request if the medication is placed on the agenda for review.

5. Pharmaceuticals that do not possess any unique therapeutic effect and/or are not less expensive than equivalent drugs are rejected until new information is presented to the committee that shows reason for a thorough review and/or approval.

6. Any appeal of a P&T decision is presented to the P&T committee chairman and/or the designated pharmacy P&T committee representative.

7. Medications reviewed and approved for inclusion on the formulary are classified by the following criteria:

a. Formulary (F): The medication can be prescribed without restriction in any location.

b. Formulary/restricted (R): The medication can be prescribed as limited by specific criteria including but not limited to facility, patient type (outpatient/inpatient), medical or surgical service, and clinical presentation.

8. Any medication that is reviewed and not approved by a P&T committee is considered nonformulary (NF). These items may be listed in the computerized provider order entry (CPOE)

system and pharmacy computer system to provide practitioners guidance on their exclusion from the formulary.

B. Formulary management:

1. Approved formulary medications are incorporated into the drug master files in the billing system, pharmacy computer system, and the CPOE system.

2. Formulary items are routinely stocked throughout the appropriate pharmacy locations.

3. P&T committee approved generic or therapeutic substitutions are made through informational pages in the CPOE system describing the substitution to the practitioner at time of order entry.

4. Nonformulary requests from practitioners are considered and processed by the pharmacist involved in processing the order. An escalation plan is instituted for unresolved requests that may include clinical pharmacy staff, the designated pharmacy P&T committee representative, or the P&T committee chair as deemed necessary.

5. If the decision is made by the practitioner and pharmacist to provide the nonformulary request, pharmacy provides the medication through coordination with the pharmacy buyers or available staff when a buyer is not available.

6. The designated pharmacy P&T committee representative is notified of and reviews nonformulary requests.

C. Medication-use evaluation (MUE):

1. Specific medications or medication classes may be further evaluated by a pharmacist by analyzing patient-specific data to provide optimal medication therapy to patients. Rationale may include, but not limited to, medications posing safety risk to a patient

or staff member, high-utilization medications, or high-cost medications.

2. When a medication or medication class is reviewed, a recommendation is presented to the P&T committee when requested.

3. Evaluations are performed in accordance with ASHP guidelines.

4. Evaluations obtain IRB approval when appropriate.

5. Evaluations are retained in the pharmacy for reference and are re-evaluated as applicable.

Appendix 3-B

Example of MUE Proposal

Proton Pump Inhibitor Use at Discharge from the ICU

Background:

Proton pump inhibitors (PPI) are medications commonly seen in both the inpatient and outpatient setting today. Although many patients are appropriately initiated on therapy by their primary care physician or in the hospital, there is a significant problem with patients continued on PPI therapy after hospital discharge without an appropriate indication. The purpose of this project is to evaluate the appropriateness of PPI therapy at discharge from the intensive care unit (ICU).

The indications for PPIs in the hospital include peptic ulcer disease including bleeding peptic ulcers, chronic nonsteroidal anti-inflammatory drug use, *Helicobacter pylori*, erosive esophagitis, gastroesophageal reflux disease, and Barrett esophagus. The use of PPIs in these disease states have shown benefit and are appropriate indications for these medications.

Although PPIs are generally considered safe, they do have adverse effects, both with short-term and long-term use. Short-term, class adverse effects include headache, diarrhea, constipation, nausea, and rash. Chronic PPI use is associated with significant adverse effects, including increased risk of bone fractures and osteoporosis due to altered mineral absorption and metabolism.[3] Chronic use may also lead to an increased risk of infection, including community and hospital-acquired pneumonia and *Clostridium difficile*, due to lack of sterilization by stomach acid. One major concern with PPIs is the well-defined drug interactions, especially with clopidogrel. Finally, chronic use may cause hypomagnesemia, which should be monitored prior to and during therapy.

Purpose:

The purpose of this study is to evaluate the appropriateness of PPI therapy at discharge from the intensive care unit, in patients initiated on PPI therapy in the ICU.

MUE Criteria:

Presence of appropriate indication for PPI at ICU discharge: stress ulcer prophylaxis, bleeding ulcer, peptic ulcer disease, gastroesophageal reflux, mechanical ventilation, and coagulopathy, considered INR >1.5 or platelets <50.

Specific Measures to Be Reported:

Percentage of patients discharged inappropriately on PPI after being started on PPI in ICU:

- Includes patients started appropriately, but inappropriate indication for PPI at discharge
- Only includes patients started on PPI in ICU, not those who were admitted on PPI

Methods:

Retrospective medical record review from March 2013–September 2013. Randomly select patients admitted during this time were initiated and discharged on PPI therapy from ICU.

Target Sample Size:

50 patients

Patient Population:

Patients admitted to ICU from March 2013–September 2013

Patients both initiated on, and discharged from, the ICU on PPI therapy.

Exclusion Criteria:

Patients <18 years old

Prisoners

Pregnant women

Committee for Presentation:

P&T

References

1. Ahrens A, Behrens G, Himmel W, et al. Appropriateness of proton pump inhibitor recommendations at hospital discharge and continuation in primary care. *Int J Clin Pract.* 2012;66(8):767-773.

2. Chubineh S, Birk J. Proton pump inhibitors: the good, the bad, and the unwanted. *South Med J.* 2012;105(11):613-618.

3. Yachimski PS, Farrell EA, Hunt DP, et al. Proton pump inhibitors for prophylaxis of nosocomial upper gastrointestinal bleeding: the impact of standardized guidelines on prescribing practice. *Arch Intern Med.* 2010;170(9):779-783.

Appendix 3-C

Medication-Use Evaluation SBAR

Immediate-Release Nifedipine

Situation:

Immediate-release (IR) nifedipine is commonly ordered for treatment of acute and chronic hypertension, but the practice should be regarded as inappropriate for either condition. There are numerous alternative antihypertensive agents available with better efficacy and safety data to support their use.

Background:

The medical literature contains numerous reports of serious adverse effects associated with the use of IR nifedipine. Most of these adverse events are correlated with a rapid decrease in blood pressure (within 15 minutes of administration) produced by the IR formulation. Specifically, IR nifedipine (oral or sublingual) has been associated with severe hypotension resulting in changes in neurological status, transient ischemic attack, stroke, conduction disturbances, myocardial ischemia, angina pectoris, and acute myocardial infarction, fetal disturbances, and death.

The manufacturer of IR nifedipine (Procardia) states "Several well-documented reports describe cases of profound hypotension, myocardial infarction, and death when immediate-release nifedipine was used in this way. PROCARDIA capsules should not be used for the acute reduction of blood pressure." Furthermore, in 1985, the FDA warned that IR nifedipine was neither safe nor effective to treat hypertensive emergencies and therefore should not be used. The manufacturer also states "PROCARDIA and other immediate-release nifedipine capsules have also been used for the long-term control of essential hypertension, although no properly controlled studies have been conducted to define an appropriate dose or dose interval for such treatment. PROCARDIA capsules should not be used for the control of essential hypertension." In addition to the warnings provided by the FDA and manufacturer, numerous experts and the Joint National Committee (JNC) guidelines strongly advise against the use of immediate-release nifedipine for treatment of any stage of hypertension. Specifically, JNC-7 states "Short-acting nifedipine is no longer considered acceptable in the initial treatment of hypertensive emergencies or urgencies." Furthermore, JNC-7 states "short-acting calcium channel blockers are not appropriate for treatment of essential hypertension."

Assessment:

This MUE shows that over the past 3 months, 47 adult inpatients received IR nifedipine. Of these, 43 patients received the medication for blood pressure control and four for preterm labor. Two of the 43 patients receiving IR nifedipine for blood pressure experienced serious adverse effects that resulted in rapid response team consults and/or transfer to a higher level of care for hypotension-related problems. Chart review did not identify any other indications for IR nifedipine use.

Recommendations:

Use of IR nifedipine for blood pressure reduction should be prohibited. Immediate-release nifedipine use should be restricted only to obstetrics-attending physician management of preterm labor.

References

1. Burton TJ, Wilkinson IB. The dangers of immediate-release nifedipine in the emergency treatment of hypertension. *J Hum Hypertens.* 2008;22(4):301.

2. Grossman E, Messerli FH, Grodzicki T, et al. Should a moratorium be placed on sublingual nifedipine capsules given for hypertensive emergencies and pseudoemergencies? *JAMA.* 1996;276(16):1328-1331.

3. Stason WB, Schmid CH, Niedzwiecki D, et al. Safety of nifedipine in angina pectoris: a meta-analysis. *Hypertension.* 1999;33(1):24-31.

4. Varon J. Treatment of acute severe hypertension: current and newer agents. *Drugs.* 2008;68(3):283-297.

5. Mansoor AF, von Hagel Keefer LA. The dangers of immediate-release nifedipine for hypertensive crises. *Pharm Ther.* 2002;27(7):362-365.

CHAPTER 4

Finance: Focusing on the Bottom Line

Robert P. Granko

KEY TERMS

Benchmarking—A process for comparing practices across peer or like organizations to ultimately implement best practices with a focus on efficiency and quality.

Budget—A plan for future expenses and revenue, typically over a 12-month period to measure the financial and operational performance over a defined period of time.

Budget Timeline—A timeline for budget-related activities due at a specific time.

Capital Budget—Capital budget is defined as an asset that costs more than a fixed dollar amount (e.g., $5,000) per item (or a composite of individual items that comprise a $5,000 asset) and has a minimum useful life of 3 years.

Cost Center—A defined business unit (e.g., inpatient pharmacy) within the department of pharmacy financial summary, which may have direct expenses and revenue specific to that business unit.

Facility Improvement Project (FIP)—Large, complex project with an estimated construction cost greater than a fixed dollar amount (e.g., $200,000).

Group Purchasing Organization (GPO)—An organization whose role is to develop purchasing contracts for products and nonlabor services that member hospitals can access. By pooling the purchases, the members of the GPO can negotiate more competitive prices from suppliers and manufacturers.

Hospital Consumer Assessment of Healthcare Providers and Systems—A standardized survey for measuring patients' perspectives on hospital care.

Operating Budget—A forecast of daily expenses required for a department to operate, including—but not limited to—labor, drugs, and supplies. An operating budget includes the revenue budget and expense budget.

Note: Parts of this chapter appeared previously in Granko PR, Lamm MH. Promoting pharmacy business through the implementation of a departmental operating review series. *Am J Health-Syst Pharm.* 2015;72(8):610, 612-613.

Operating Review Series (ORS)—The framework for pharmacy area-specific presentations that include pharmacy area or service line finances, employee engagement efforts where applicable, clinical practice metrics, and ongoing clinical and operational projects and educational and research initiatives, which affect the overall health of the area or service line.

Revenue—Monies received for products or services provided to customers and patients.

Service Line—A service line organizes the approach to clinical management of patient care around like patients (e.g., cardiovascular services).

Introduction

Hospital and health-system leaders face increasing pressures today, and these broad pressures extend to the **service lines** where pharmacy coordinators practice. Specifically, many hospitals and health systems are continuously looking to generate sufficient operating margin for clinical, educational, and research programs for indigent patients. Information system implementations are costly ventures that allow integrated care for our patients and ensure strong clinical sharing, but these ventures must be financed appropriately.

Many executive and service line leaders struggle with the ever-evolving standardization of operating models, clinical integration, and care delivery transformation to stabilize current and new affiliate operations. As experts in medication management across the continuum of care, coordinators must plan for sustained pressure to contain costs, ensure clinical and operational efficiencies, search for new **revenue** sources, and provide marketable value-based care.

Leading the Business of Pharmacy, Its Areas, and Service Lines Using an Operating Review Series

Business-specific and service line knowledge is essential to the development of competent coordinators. Traditionally, back-end business aspects of pharmacy routinely involve billing and reimbursement. Although those aspects are critical to running a successful area or service line, progressive pharmacy healthcare stressors—

such as increasing medication and practice model cost control—continue to mount. More than ever, coordinators must ensure that the totality of pharmacy business is reviewed and discussed in an all-encompassing manner.

Coordinators should position themselves to effectively market pharmacy services and, more importantly, know how areas or service lines support and contribute to departmental and organizational goals. Because departments of pharmacy and their corresponding areas and service lines manage large revenues and expenses, coordinators must demonstrate a broad and in-depth understanding of—and be able to effectively communicate—the core business value of their areas and service lines. By using departmental data to drive meaningful pharmacy business insight, skilled coordinators can ensure a strong, vibrant, and sustainable platform for the organization.

Tenets of the Pharmacy Operating Review Series

Given the dynamic, integral, and critical part the department of pharmacy plays in patient care—coupled with the growing complexity and scope of existing business nuances—coordinators are encouraged to institute a framework for the successful deployment of an area or service line **operating review series** (ORS). Functionally, an ORS is an in-depth and objective review of an area within a larger department. The series allows leadership, both internal and external to the host department, to be a useful forum for defining and discussing key areas within that unit.[1] The purpose of creating the ORS was to establish a framework for pharmacy area-specific presentations while ensuring continual area readiness and preparedness for what occurs at most organizations (e.g., a larger, more comprehensive quarterly organizational ORS held with hospital or health-system executive leadership).

Applied to the level of area or service with the pharmacy department, topical ORS agendas should be developed to include pharmacy area or service line finances, employee engagement efforts, clinical practice metrics, ongoing clinical and operational projects, and educational and research initiatives that affect the overall health of the area or service line.

To culturally embed an ORS, a department of pharmacy should create central governing and anchoring series tenets. For example:

- Define area-specific goals as a means to improve operational standards under the organization (e.g., pillars of excellence such as finance, growth, innovation, people, quality, and service).

- Provide pharmacy departmental leadership and external customers with routine performance reports for defined operational groups while promoting and demonstrating connectivity across all areas (e.g., cost centers) housed within the department.

- Promote the creation of dashboards illustrating best practices and current standards with the area or service line.

- Serve as a venue to plan and discuss future avenues for revenue growth and expansion of the pharmacy practice model.

- Encourage staff involvement in operational objectives and initiatives by having them take part in the ORS presentation—both in assembly and conveyance of the final presentation deliverables—thus supporting and upholding the employee engagement and partnership values of the department.

Planning for the Pharmacy Area-Specific or Service Line Operating Review Series

ORS should be introduced and refined before deployment with staff in the area. In some cases, the structure and identification of required and essential data streams will take time to mature. To ensure go-live readiness with the ORS, this planning phase should be spread over 3 to 6 months with one or more 2-month preparatory phases.

Each of the coordinator's areas of management and leadership should have its own detailed ORS so that each area can create and maintain, among other deliverables, functional area-specific dashboards. These dashboards target features of area or service line–specific performance within the pillars of excellence and provide a visual business reference for review

during larger, external audience presentations. Illustratively, performance metrics for an area or service line–specific ORS presentation may include the following:

- **Finance** (budget updates and variance explanations). Departmental monthly financial summary: operating revenue, net inpatient/outpatient revenue, income from operations, operating expenses, income trends, and variance explanations.

- **Growth** (expansion of clinical services or cost savings associated with value-based initiatives). Growth of clinical pharmacist(s) in the ambulatory care setting to support specialty pharmacy practice; revenue generation from prescriptions filled from the strategic placement of a clinical pharmacist; intravenous to oral conversion cost-saving tracking; cost savings due to contract renegotiation; expense optimization through bulk buy purchases of pharmaceuticals; establishment of mail-order services; establishment of reinsourced sterile compounding preparation savings, etc.

- **Innovation** (deployment of a new inventory management system). Improvement in the number of inventory turns, which reduces expense of tracked and expired medications. Identify cost savings and value-based initiatives from information via the hospital's wholesaler and **group purchasing organizations** (GPOs). Examples may include switching to less costly but therapeutically equivalent medication, examining uses and purchases to ensure medications are used in accordance with establishment guidelines, and following procedures that are rooted in the latest evidenced-based practice.

- **People** (employee engagement updates). Other examples may include trending of employee satisfaction scores by area and/or department, employee action planning results, etc.

- **Quality** (medication turnaround time performance). Other examples may include number of orders verified, number of doses dispensed by category or product, clinical pharmacist interventions, percentage of doses dispensed from automated dispensing cabinetry, etc.

- **Service** (Hospital Consumer Assessment of Healthcare Providers and Systems score updates).

As departments of pharmacy grow in size, number, and complexity, it becomes increasingly difficult for members of the leadership team to stay up-to-date on the performance metrics of areas outside of their respective **cost centers**. Past practice was such that each pharmacy leader singularly focused on his or her cost center and area of influence; thus, specific expectations were only known by the coordinator who oversaw them.

The ORS has afforded each member of the pharmacy leadership team, as well as the pharmacy's customers, to broadly and inclusively discuss key areas of focus within the area or service line, including finance, employee engagement, clinical practice, and ongoing operational projects and initiatives, which affect the overall health of the area. Moreover, the ORS allows for the creation of transparency within the area or service line and helps the coordinator market all of the pharmacy services.

Series Schedule for the Pharmacy Departmental Operating Review

A *departmental operating review* (DOR) is scheduled as a recurring monthly meeting with defined area-specific pharmacy presentation groups who present to the pharmacy leadership team and pharmacy staff on a rotating basis. This allows pharmacy leadership to evaluate the performance of these areas or service lines over the previous period and gives other coordinators the opportunity to learn about ongoing and potential future projects and initiatives throughout the department.

Presenting teams for the area-specific pharmacy DOR series represent four main groupings: (1) administrative services and acute care services core operations; (2) ambulatory care services; (3) acute care services and medication-use advancement; and (4) pharmacy hospital and clinic affiliates not directly housed on the main campus who have

a reporting relationship to leaders within the hospital's department of pharmacy. The areas or service lines under the management of the coordinator will determine the scheduling of his or her area-specific ORS.

Where applicable, hospital or health-system executive leadership may hold a larger organizational quarterly DOR session. Using the cumulative pharmacy area-specific business data and trends presented over the past months by each of the coordinators, senior pharmacy leadership will assemble the pharmacy departmental presentation, including many of the thematic trends and area-specific data to highlight the department and drive-trending insight. The monthly pharmacy DOR series allows senior pharmacy leadership, their teams, and their staff to be in an ever-present and recurrently readied state to review and discuss the department's business.

Ideally, each member of the pharmacy leadership team should know, understand, and be able to articulate the functional metrics of each area within the department. At the same time, the pharmacy DOR series serves as an effective tool for allowing coordinators to market the accomplishments of their teams, creating an open and inviting environment for other pharmacy leaders to ask questions, give suggestions, and understand the complexities of different operational areas within the department and across the continuum of each cost center. Additionally, it promotes a culture of data awareness and reporting—something that is often missing in progressive departments of pharmacy.

Budgeting Procedures

Building from the ORS, coordinators should have an in-depth appreciation of the budgeting preparation process, procedures, and overall responsibilities for the department of pharmacy's **budget**. They should also know how that process aligns with the overall organizational budget process. As we continue to educate our coordinators and other departmental leaders, we must ensure they are working at the top of their licenses and certifications. The transference of these skills rests with the organization's finance department, the pharmacy department's finance leaders, and with those leaders that have full or partial responsibility for specific areas and service lines.

The following information has been adapted from an amalgamation of different institutional practices. Although the details of each institutional budget practice may differ, the essential themes of the budget process should be broadly applicable regardless of the institution's setting or size. The intent of the following information is to provide coordinators with a framework from which to work and ultimately develop their area-specific or service line guidelines. Additionally, coordinators should partner with the organization's department of finance to clarify the budget process. This integral relationship, once established, is key to the sustainable success of each department and the organization as a whole.

Budget Timeline

Budget planning and preparation is typically led by the organization's pharmacy finance team each fiscal year (beginning in November in the following example). The starting month will vary and is correlated with the beginning of the actual month prior to the start of the organization's fiscal year (July in the following example).

The budget calendar is typically published by the fiscal or finance department and distributed at a meeting of executives and departmental directors. Once the budget calendar is made available, the pharmacy finance team or other designated member will distribute the important dates to pharmacy department leadership.

Key dates in a typical schedule may vary slightly between fiscal years (see **Figure 4-1**). Internal dates for the department of pharmacy are also included in this schedule.

Capital Budget Requests

Capital is defined as an asset that costs greater than a fixed dollar amount (e.g., $5,000) per item (or a composite of individual items that comprise a $5,000 asset) *and* has a minimum useful life of 3 years. Understanding what is included in the **capital budget** is essential to understand what is or is not included. In this case, the capital budget does not include personal computers, printers, or telecommunication items.

Facility improvement projects (FIPs) are large, complex projects with an estimated construction cost greater than a fixed dollar amount (e.g., $200,000). Design and construction are generally completed by outside services with oversight by a hospital project manager. FIPs may typically require approval from the board of directors as part of the annual budget request, and they may also be referred to as *capital projects*.

Following a similar schedule as above, FIP request reminders may be sent out in November/December to system vice presidents. Official FIP request forms must be submitted by a specified deadline. The scope of the project and cost estimates are further developed in January/February. FIP refinements, cuts, and additions are generally made by an oversight body (such as an operations council) in the March/April timeframe, and then they are submitted to the board of directors for final approval in May.

Although not common for the department of pharmacy, some leases for equipment may be capitalized. The expense associated with the lease will be set up on a depreciation schedule by fiscal or financial services. It is necessary to review each newly requested equipment lease to determine if it qualifies for a capitalized lease. If the equipment lease is capitalized, it should be submitted with the capital equipment budget. For example—and this may not represent your institution—if at its inception a lease meets one or more of the following four criteria, the lease can be classified and accounted for as a capital lease:

1. The lease transfers ownership to the lessee (hospital) by the end of the lease term.

2. The lease contains a bargain purchase option (as opposed to a fair market value option).

3. The lease term is equal to 75% or more of the estimated economic life of the leased property. However, if the beginning of the lease term falls within the last 25% of the total estimated economic life of the leased property (i.e., leasing well-used equipment), including earlier years of use, this criterion shall not be used for purposes of classifying the lease.

4. At the inception of the lease, the present value of the minimum lease payments,

FIGURE 4-1. Sample Typical Budget Schedule

Nov 10	Pharmacy capital requests email and sends memo to pharmacy leadership
Dec 2	Pharmacy capital requests are due
Dec 3	Capital equipment files are sent to departments
Dec 3	Computer and communication email and memo are sent to pharmacy leadership
Dec 3	Pharmacy business manager begins creating operating expense cost center templates
Dec 5	Pharmacy business office prioritizes department capital requests
Dec 5	Pharmacy business office completes department capital spreadsheet
Dec 12	Department of pharmacy holds mock capital budget hearing
Dec 19	Executive pharmacy leadership finalizes capital budget request priority levels
Dec 27	Capital files are due to budget department
Jan 3	Pharmacy computer and communication requests are due
Jan 3	Pharmacy finance team requests 6-month budget trends from business office
Jan 5–20	Pharmacy business manager or designee prepares operating revenue budget
Jan 5	Hospital managers and directors receive operating expense cost center templates
Jan 9	Executive pharmacy leadership reviews communication requests
Jan 9	Pharmacy information services department reviews computer requests
Jan 15	Pharmacy business office completes computer, ergonomics, and communication files
Jan 21	Cost center operating expense templates are due
Jan 20–30	Pharmacy business office reviews revenue projections
Jan 25	Computer, ergonomics, and communication requests are due
Feb 1	Operating budget files (budget software such as Kaufman Hall) are sent to departments
Feb 1–13	Pharmacy finance team reviews operating expenses and prepares workbooks
Feb 13	Operating budget files are due
Feb 13	Submitted files are distributed to team
Mar 21	Initial-draft budget is returned for review by executive pharmacy leadership (budget hearing)
Mar 31	Second-draft budget returned for review by executive pharmacy leadership
April 7	Third-draft budget returned for review by executive pharmacy leadership
April–May	President/COO/CFO and board review and finalize budget

CFO = chief financial officer; COO = chief operating officer.

excluding executory costs, to be paid by the lessor, including any profit, equals or exceeds 90% of the excess of the fair value of the leased property to the lessor at the inception of the lease over any related investment tax credit retained by the lessor and expected to be realized by the lessor. However, if the beginning of the lease falls within the last 25% of the total estimated economic life of the leased property, including earlier years of use, this criterion shall not be used for purposes of classifying the lease. Again, the department of fiscal services can help define how these should be handled. Certainly, consulting the department of fiscal services is the prudent action to take if there are questions or necessary clarifications regarding a capitalized lease.

In this example timeline, capital budget requests are due by the fourth week of December each year. Each coordinator will be asked to submit capital requests for his or her cost center to be reviewed and prioritized by the department. In many cases, a mock pharmacy capital request and review meeting will be conducted to aid in prioritization and capital budget requests. Capital requests must be complete with vendor quotes and clear justifications. The final capital budget request should be succinct to clearly communicate its necessity (e.g., **s**ituation, **b**ackground, **a**ssessment, and **r**ecommendations [SBAR] document), and coordinators should make sure that all details of the submission are ready for discussion/presentation.

Requests for Renovations

Requests for renovations may be made through the plant engineering or facilities department, and they include all in-house projects less than a certain dollar amount (e.g., $200,000). Funding should be available (1) in the appropriate fiscal year's **operating budget** to support requests for renovations, and (2) in the month that the project will begin.

Computer Requests

The computer budget includes requests for additional equipment, such as personal computers, monitors, printers, docking stations, and site-licensed software for new personnel or other expansions. Examples of applicable site-licensed software include Visio, Project, and Adobe products. Items that are not customarily included in the computer budget include batteries and styluses for laptops/tablets. Typically, replacement of existing equipment may not be included in this budget as the information services division (ISD) of the hospital or health-system budgets separately for these replacements. The ISD may budget computer software access on all computers. Coordinators should work with ISD to ensure all necessary items are included in this budget.

Computer equipment purchase requests must include the planned month of purchase. Additional documentation may be provided for justification. Following budget allocation of the computer equipment purchases, areas will need to specifically request equipment delivery and installation via ISD.

Final computer request submissions are due to ISD around the fourth week of January. In advance of the ISD deadline, coordinators may be asked to submit computer requests for their cost center to be reviewed and approved by a pharmacy information services department manager.

Ergonomic Equipment Requests

The institutional ergonomic budget is intended for unplanned ergonomic needs during the fiscal year. Ergonomic equipment typically includes office or workstation chairs, keyboard trays, document holders, task lights, foot rests, and worksite assessments. This ergonomic equipment request is not intended to replace departmental budgets for replacement of existing equipment, staff relocations within a department, new programs, new personnel, or departmental moves or renovations.

Ergonomic requests, like computer requests, are due around the fourth week of January. In advance of the ergonomic equipment request deadline, coordinators may be asked to submit ergonomic requests for their cost centers to be reviewed and approved by the pharmacy information services department manager or designee. The pharmacy finance team will likely submit the ergonomics request each year, if needed, on behalf of the department.

Telecommunications Equipment Requests

Telecommunications equipment often includes phones and headsets, new telecommunication lines, single-line telephone sets, wireless phones, wired headsets, wireless headsets, and miscellaneous telecommunications equipment. Wiring expense typically does not need to be addressed by individual departments.

Recurring costs for phone lines, pagers, and cell phones are not included in this budget but are often included in the departmental operating budget. Telecommunication requests are due around the fourth week of January. Coordinators will be asked to submit a telecommunications equipment request for their cost center to be reviewed and approved by executive pharmacy leadership.

Operating Budget

The department of pharmacy operating budget includes the revenue budget and expense budget. The revenue budget typically is comprised of primarily drug revenue, which is often predicted and forecasted by the pharmacy finance team but may involve other outside parties (e.g., finance).

Coordinators should, after proper tutorial from the pharmacy finance team or their designee, be responsible for drafting, reviewing, and submitting their respective expense budget. A pharmacy operating budget typically includes pharmaceutical expenses (approximately 23.6%), labor (approximately 5.3%), equipment rental and maintenance (approximately 0.01%), and other expenses (approximately 0.1%).

Revenue Budget

The pharmacy finance team, in conjunction with content experts including the coordinator, will be responsible for compiling the revenue budget for each fiscal year.

The revenue budget should be developed first and serve as a crosscheck against the drug expense budget because the two must correlate.

Any increase in expense must be supported by a corresponding and identifiable increase in revenue. Thus, it is critical to maintain a detailed list of revenue increases, which specifically identifies the drivers of the increases.

Revenue Cost Centers

The following areas (e.g., cost centers) may have associated drug revenue. Directors and coordinators in each area should help predict drug revenue for each of these cost centers for the upcoming fiscal year.

Examples of cost centers may include central inpatient pharmacy, sterile products and manufacturing, and retail pharmacy locations, etc.

In many cases, but not all, both drug cost and associated revenue may be allocated to the cost center bearing the expense of the medication. Coordinators should understand their cost center's flow of expense and revenue. This information can be readily retrieved on the monthly financial reports that are often distributed by finance.

Cost Center Establishment

Revenue and expense should match within a cost center. If a cost center exists that contributes revenue to a different cost center, revenue should be aligned accordingly. Customarily, the department of fiscal services creates cost centers on request. The need for new cost centers should be identified early in the budget process so that templates can be created within the budgeting software. The pharmacy finance team should be contacted if changes are needed to a cost center or a new cost center needs to be established.

Revenue Calculations

To accurately forecast revenue, the previous year's calculations and subsequent revenue should be considered. At least 6 months of current fiscal year data should be reviewed, when available. In January, the pharmacy finance team should obtain a spreadsheet of the current revenue including the institution's charging methodologies. These methodologies can assist in the modelling of gross revenue for the upcoming fiscal year.

Revenue projections are often calculated by the pharmacy finance team with the help of the revenue charge model. The model serves as a tool to determine which drug charging categories (e.g., blood product), drug pricing markups, and/or other applied fees should be adjusted to meet projected revenue targets for the upcoming fiscal year.

After revenue projections are made, the pharmacy finance team will review the projections for quality assurance and data integrity. The following should be considered when finalizing revenue projections:

- **Seasonality.** In some institutions, both gross revenue and expenses may be up to 5% to 10% higher in the second half of the fiscal year (for an example fiscal year running July 1–June 30) than in the first half, due to price inflation, the impact of new drugs, first-half holidays, and certain patient volume increases.

- **Introduction of drug budget drivers.** Accelerated specialty pharmacy growth, inflation, and drug shortages can have a major impact on the overall expenditures of a drug budget. Coordinators should be aware of drug launch and expenditure trends that affect their areas and should consider service line budget drivers when assembling their budgets.

Revenue Assumptions

The budget department will often provide volume assumptions for the department to utilize for projections. The department must also make its own assumptions and consider the following:

- The coordinator should determine volume increases (inpatient and outpatient), why, where, and when they may occur. Each increase translates to a percentage increase in revenue for that particular area, and this can be estimated and totaled into a data-supported form. For example, a volume increase in a chemotherapy clinic will provide more revenue than a volume increase in labor and delivery because chemotherapy drug revenue and expense is higher.

- The following should also be considered in projecting revenue growth and can be included in an annual service line compendium that should provide qualitative and quantitative information to best understand drivers and other service line influences:

- Service line growth (e.g., transplant, cardiac, etc.)
- Clinic growth, new clinics, and clinic conversion from or to hospital-owned classification
- Ambulatory/retail pharmacy growth
- Specialty pharmacy growth (Revenue is estimated based on prescription volume growth. Realize that new drugs may drastically affect revenue.)
- Projected increases in charge markups and other associated fees
- Drug cost inflation (The annual AJHP inflation article may not conform to your hospital's experience but can serve as useful general reference.[2])

Expense Budget

The expense budget will be completed by the coordinator for each cost center and finalized in conjunction with the pharmacy business manager. Where applicable, the business manager will review each expense budget with each cost center coordinator. Customarily, any growth in expenses must be supported by revenue. The department must produce sufficient new net revenue to cover any increased expense in the budget.

Calculating Expense Budget

For each expense, coordinators and directors should take year-to-date expense through the most recent month and extrapolate to 12 months. This should be used as the base from which to adjust the expense for the upcoming fiscal year.

If the extrapolation differs widely from the prior year's budget, calendar-year expense, or present-year extrapolation, reasons why should be researched.

Specific Expense Budget Considerations

Minor equipment. The coordinator should carefully review and consider all minor equipment requests (e.g., equipment costing less than $5,000).

Personnel. Coordinators may be planning to add additional personnel for the coming fiscal year. The personnel budget can only include current personnel approved. Often misapplied, a reasonable vacancy rate should be used for the area. Reviewing the historically applied vacancy rate in addition to current scheduling and vacancy rate changes should be considered. A "normal" rate would not exceed 7% to 10%.

Drug budget. Although the drug budget may often be viewed from departmental perspective, it is prudent for coordinators to accurately work to forecast area-specific expenditures for their respective departments. The drug budget should include an extrapolation from the prior 6 or 7 months, an allowance for seasonality, a volume increase, additions to the formulary, and possibly a number for expanded use of existing drugs.

ASHP provides guidance on drug cost inflation that could be reviewed, and several GPOs also develop predictions as well.

Often, drug purchases and drug usage information obtained from the pharmacy or enterprise-wide information system is obtained. This information serves as the starting point for drug budget forecasting and can be viewed in several ways including by service, by prescriber, by AHFS drug category and, importantly, by charge description.

Coordinators play an integral role working with physicians and other clinicians for medications to be added or deleted from the formulary. Key to successful area-specific and drug budget forecasting is a trusting relationship with physicians and other prescribers that is often built though embedded pharmacists on clinical teams.

Often, due to wide fluctuations in blood factor utilization, the blood factor budget may be constructed differently than the drug budget. An average of the prior year's actual expense may be used to approximate expense. Additionally, because blood factors may comprise a large expense, chief financial officers may require this expense portion of the budget to maintain its own budgetary line for trending and tracking purposes.

Some departments of pharmacy employ the internal practice of conducting class-wide and new-to-market therapeutic reviews by their clinical and administrative staff. Although beneficial to understanding the drug market over the coming year, shortages and sweeping price fluctuations have made some of these reviews outdated the minute they are completed. Some leaders turn to their GPOs to help provide some of the information or use a combination of both methodologies to help frame the drug expenditures for the year.

Coordinators should review the utilization of medications to determine if there are more cost-effective alternatives or opportunities to use evidence-based medicine while still ensuring optimal patient outcomes to develop restrictions or guidelines for use. The coordinator can then work the pharmacy and therapeutics (P&T) committee on therapeutic interchanges or restricted medication policies. Examples: With the rising price of nitroprusside, are there clinical alternatives and/or restrictions to using this medication? With all of the antibiotics on the market, are there restrictions or alternatives that should be used in different patient scenarios?

Equipment rental and maintenance. Equipment not included in the capital budget (leased equipment) may be included in this budget. The coordinator should work with his or her team to understand the specific agreements and terms of such leases and how the institution prefers to apply their costs to the overall budget. Permission is granted for coordinators to review and understand contract terms and conditions.

Labor contracts. It is not uncommon for certain pharmacist staff members to be funded from external sources, such as a school of pharmacy or school of medicine. It is important that these labor contracts are funded in the correct cost center and are applied to the correct general ledger code. Although these contracts may not be directly funded from their area or service line, coordinators should understand in detail the funds flow and general terms of such contracts and budget for them accordingly. It is prudent to work with the department of finance representative to ensure the funds flow remains accurate and timely.

Productivity and Benchmarking—Labor and Efficiency

Many organizations support and closely follow the productivity of overall efficiency of the pharmacy department. Within the department, each corresponding cost center or area is subject to its own productivity measure. Although institutions vary in what productivity tools they use, coordinators must have an in-depth understanding of this tool to ensure success for their areas in the long term. Internal pharmacy reference documents should be made available for understanding how productivity is calculated and what drivers can impact the productivity of a specific area or service line.

As an example, there is an assigned workload statistic for each cost center or area throughout a department of pharmacy. Commonly used statistics: daily average adjusted patient days (APD) or calendar days (CD). APD is a variable metric, while CD is a fixed metric. APD is an endorsed organizational metric that, in this example, considers gross revenue, inpatient revenue, and volume of inpatient days. This figure is selected for a large number of organizational departments across the hospital. APD or CD may not be an exact match to determine actual pharmacy volume. Often, there is not one metric that captures the work completed by all of those in a pharmacy department or area; nevertheless, a metric must be selected from a standardized **benchmarking** perspective.

Reading and understanding productivity reports is essential. Typically, productivity reports are distributed on a biweekly basis and reflect the productivity index, which is the overall productivity for the identified reporting period. Typically, there are target ranges at, below, or above designated ranges. Additionally, the reporting results are usually available for the current pay period (e.g., every 2 weeks) and feature the reporting period, historical periods, and the fiscal year-to-date views.

Often, other graphical, metrics, or both are displayed. These graphs can include staffing-to-volume, overtime usage, skill mix, paid time off, and education. Ultimately, these reports and trending information can be used to justify variances or aberrations within the reporting period. Guiding productivity materials should highlight the criteria for writing a variance report, when a variance report is required, and to whom the variance report should be submitted.

Finally, in most organizations, there is an internal committee that provides productivity

and operational benchmarking oversight. Benchmarking is commonly used to ensure best practices among peer organizations. Bench marking statistics are used to efficiently and effectively run and improve the utilization of all resources across an area or department.[3] Benchmarking might also occur using external comparators such as Truven or Action OI data. Coordinators should familiarize themselves extensively with how the organization defines, collects, and aggregates pharmacy and other data that will ultimately feed into the vendor-generated benchmarks. Critically, coordinators must become experts with a thorough understanding of these vital details and an exceptional understanding of vendor formulas and calculations, which are used to derive the final reported numbers and percentiles.[4,5] Also, assuming an owner mentality, rather than a renter mentality, of the business of your pharmacy or area is paramount. See **Table 4-1** for common internal benchmarking productivity monitoring ratios.[3]

It is prudent for coordinators to schedule dedicated time with the leadership responsible for administering the productivity (e.g., decision support) monitoring tool. Coordinators should understand the peer hospitals against which their hospital is benchmarked. Importantly, the administration of external benchmarking and internal productivity monitoring will ultimately drive the brand image of pharmacy services.

Summary

The impact of healthcare industry reform is giving pause to many leaders across health systems and their departments. The department of pharmacy is often one of the largest departments within a hospital, typically comprising millions of dollars in drug and personnel expense along with strong revenue

Table 4-1. Common Internal Benchmarking Productivity Monitoring Ratios

Total cost/ admission	Drug cost/ admission	Labor expense/1,000 doses billed
Doses/ admission	Inventory turns/year	Clinical interventions/ pharmacist shift(s) worked

and profit margin generation. The astute coordinator must have the education, training, and experiences to lead the business of pharmacy, as well as a solid understanding of financial management, including budgeting, forecasting, productivity/benchmarking, and marketing.

PRACTICE TIPS

1. Review resources that include financial and business terminology along with general principles and practices of financial management for pharmacists.[3] See how those principles and practice are generally applicable to the areas you lead.

2. Begin having the conversation with your departmental pharmacy leaders about an ORS, and put together a team to develop the framework and a deployment schedule for your area ORS. Be the first area in your department to showcase how it contributes to the department and more broadly to the organization's goals.

3. Invest time in understanding the overall organizational budget process, starting with the department of pharmacy's policies and procedures. Spend time with the department of pharmacy's finance and business leaders, review the materials they find valuable, and educate yourself on the overall process and accompanying timelines. Meet with your front-line clinical leaders and see how the process can be further broken down to reveal new insights from your area that can go on to be used to support the larger pharmacy budget process.

4. Educate yourself to understand the external operational benchmarking and internal productivity monitoring for your area or department. Start by networking with those leaders who administer the program(s) and work to apply the benchmarking and productivity lessons learned to better direct, apply new, and reapply existing resources throughout your area(s).

References

1. Granko RP, Lamm MH. Promoting pharmacy business success through the implementation of a departmental operating review series. *Am J Health-Syst Pharm.* 2015;72(8):610, 612-613.

2. Hoffman JM, Li E, Doloresco F, et al. Projecting future drug expenditures in US nonfederal hospitals and clinics—2013. *Am J Health-Syst Pharm.* 2013;70(6):525-539.

3. Wilson AL. *Financial Management for Health-System Pharmacists.* Bethesda, MD: ASHP; 2009.

4. Rough SS, McDaniel M, Rinehart JR. Effective use of workload and productivity monitoring tools in health-system pharmacy, part 1. *Am J Health-Syst Pharm.* 2010;67(5):300-311.

5. Rough SS, McDaniel M, Rinehart JR. Effective use of workload and productivity monitoring tools in health-system pharmacy, part 2. *Am J Health-Syst Pharm.* 2010;67(5)380-388.

Suggested Reading

National trends in prescription drug expenditures and projections. Annually in *Am J Health-Syst Pharm.*

Rough SS, McDaniel M, Rinehart J. Effective use of workload and productivity monitoring tools in health-system pharmacy, part 1. *Am J Health-Syst Pharm.* 2010;67(5):300-311.

Rough SS, McDaniel M, Rinehart JR. Effective use of workload and productivity monitoring tools in health-system pharmacy, part 2. *Am J Health-Syst Pharm.* 2010;67(5);380-388.

Wilson AL. *Financial Management for Health-System Pharmacists.* Bethesda, MD: ASHP; 2009.

CHAPTER 5

Medication Safety Essentials for the Clinical Coordinator

Lynn Eschenbacher

KEY TERMS

Employee Assistance Program (EAP)—A service offered by most employers to assist employees in times of need with counseling or other support.

Failure Mode and Effects Analysis (FMEA)—A problem-solving tool used to analyze a process or system to identify possible modes of failure and potential consequences before the failures occur.

Just Culture—A culture that recognizes the contribution of systems in error, focuses on behavioral choices and accountability, and distinguishes between acceptable and unacceptable behavior as well as between unsafe acts and the blatant disregard of safety procedures with which most peers would comply. Just culture is one component of an overarching safety culture.

Mistake-Proofing or Poka-Yoke—A device or method that prevents people from making mistakes or implementation of fail-safe mechanisms to prevent errors from occurring with a process (e.g., an ATM that gives the debit card back before the cash so that the card is not forgotten).

Near Miss—An error process that is stopped or interrupted either by chance or through a check-and-balance in the medication-use process, such as recognition of the problem and intervention by an experienced practitioner before it reaches the patient. Other similar terms include close call and good catch.

PDSA (plan, do, study, act)—A quality improvement methodology involving plan-do-study-act steps for planning, implementing, evaluating, and changing a process or system.

Root Cause Analysis—A systematic process utilized to determine the primary cause of system failures that has already occurred. The goal is to define the root causes and develop an action plan to prevent recurrence or mitigate a future event.

Second Victim—A healthcare provider involved in an unanticipated adverse patient event, medical error, and/or a patient-related injury who becomes victimized in the sense that the provider is traumatized by the event. Frequently, second victims feel personally responsible for the unexpected patient outcomes and doubt their clinical skills and knowledge base.

Introduction

As a clinical coordinator, it is important to have a solid understanding of the pharmacy department's role in medication safety. If the department has a medication safety officer (MSO), it is also important to know how to interact with the MSO; if there is no MSO, you will need to be the medication safety leader and know how to lead these efforts. This chapter will outline the critical information about being an effective leader in medication safety whether you are complementing someone else's efforts or leading the efforts.

Medication safety is important to incorporate into everything that you do as a clinical coordinator. If you make decisions and lead with the patient at the center, this will help you make sound decisions and remove emotion from discussions. This chapter provides a high-level overview of medication safety for the clinical coordinator. For more detailed information about medication safety, I recommend Larson and Saine's *Medication Safety Officer's Handbook*.[1]

Medication safety-related errors will happen in the organization, and you need to know how to address these from a clinical coordinator's perspective. Sometimes you will be asked to be the expert to explain the medication's clinical aspects; sometimes you will have a staff member involved and need to learn what happened from them; and sometimes you will be the expert for the pharmacy medication management processes. You may be asked for this information via email, sidebar in the hallway, or in a more formal setting such as a **failure mode and effects analysis** (FMEA), **root cause analysis** (RCA), or during the medication safety committee meeting. Whatever the situation, it is important to make sure you have all the facts and always look for the story behind the story. It can be tempting to just ask a few questions and make a conclusion, but you need to keep digging and ask probing questions. One good technique is to continue to ask "why" several times until the root cause or the underlying reason is discovered. It is

important to ask objectively and tactfully. Try not to lead the employee to the answer you want them to give, but instead let them talk and share what they know.

Talking with Staff and a Culture of Safety

Addressing medication errors with the staff can be challenging and should be approached thoughtfully. You will need to ask staff members for their recollection of what happened. Remember, they may be worried about getting in trouble or need help remembering what happened. Have discussions in a private area rather than in the middle of the patient care unit or where others are around. You can go to their work area rather than calling staff members to your office, which might place them on the defensive because they may be scared or concerned about the discussion's outcome. Having a good culture of safety at your organization will help to facilitate this conversation. In a strong culture of safety, employees know that medication errors may happen as a result of a system failure or due to something more pervasive than an individual's mistake. If your organization does not have a strong culture of safety, I recommend investigating **just culture**.[2] A just culture supports a learning organization focused on improving processes and systems to develop a safer environment for employees and patients.

To promote a culture in which we learn from our mistakes, organizations must re-evaluate how their disciplinary system fits into the equation. Disciplining employees in response to honest mistakes does little to improve overall system safety. In a just culture, it is important to determine if the error was human error, negligent conduct, reckless conduct, or an intentional violation of the rules.[3] Once this determination is made, it is possible to hold the employee accountable for his or her actions, to help coach and console, and, most importantly, to review the system that led to the error so as to prevent future occurrences. By understanding the reason behind the error, you can build trust with your staff members. They will see that they will not be penalized for something beyond their control, but if they knowingly violate rules, they will be held accountable. Tell your staff members you support them when support is needed, and hold them accountable when required; this will go a long way to build trust and demonstrate transparency in ensuring a safe environment for staff and patients.

When you approach staff members, they may be upset by hearing about the error. They may be concerned that the patient was harmed or wonder how they could have made an error without realizing it. If they need to be consoled, make sure you provide support and listen to them. Other options include contacting your **employee assistance program** (EAP). You can make a referral, or if the situation is severe enough and an employee needs immediate help, the EAP representative could come to the hospital. The patient is the *first victim*; the healthcare provider who was involved in the error is the **second victim** (in the sense the provider is also traumatized by the event). Frequently, second victims feel personally responsible for the unexpected patient outcomes and may doubt their clinical skills and knowledge base.[4]

If staff members are extremely upset, you may consider letting them go home for the day or longer depending on the severity and outcomes of the error. If they are distracted by the error, they may be more prone to making another error. Another option might be to have them take a break. You can provide or arrange the coverage during the break. Another aspect you may consider is whether employees will have to go to the board of pharmacy as the result of the error. Some questions you may need to ask: Does your organization provide a lawyer? Does an employee require a lawyer? What is your role with the board of pharmacy investigation? What does this mean for the employee while the board of pharmacy investigation is going on? This situation would be extremely rare, but it is good to be prepared.

Also, consider that information may spread quickly, so you need to act quickly to get accurate information to staff as soon as possible. Work with your human resource department and risk manager to determine what you can share regarding a serious event. If it is minor, you may not need to share the details, but help the staff understand what is needed to prevent future errors. Determining the root cause is essential in developing a solution to ensure other patients are not harmed by future errors.

Determining Root Cause of the Error and Fixing the System

After the details have been obtained and staff members are supported, you need to determine if the error was human error, a violation of the rules, or reckless behavior. Your human resources department can help with the assessment as well. If it was human error that was a result of a system error, you should work with your staff and other departments or hospital leadership on a solution to the problem. If the system is not fixed, then the error could recur. If it did not reach the patient the first time, it would be a **near miss** or close call, but if the system is not fixed, then the error could reach the patient and cause harm. As a coordinator, it is important to look for those near misses (even those that reach the patient) and develop a solution that will truly fix the root cause. Methods to reach the root cause include an RCA, risk assessment, **PDSA** (**p**lan, **d**o, **s**tudy, **a**ct), Six Sigma, etc.[1] It is important to involve a multidisciplinary team for identifying the root causes and ensure that all the aspects of the error and the solution are considered rather than just a one-sided view. If you do not get to the root cause, you will have spent time, energy, and money on a solution that has no impact on patient safety. You will have to start over again, and patients could be harmed in the interim.

The sessions to reach the root cause are usually limited to those directly involved in the event. If staff members are involved, you should ensure attendance by providing coverage for their patient care assignments. In addition, you should ask other staff members for their ideas and solutions. Be careful not to disclose every detail and exactly who was involved, but give enough information so that others understand the issue and can be involved in the solution. Discuss the event at a staff meeting, and then take the ideas to the RCA sessions. Involving staff members helps them to feel included and part of the solution, and it also helps to determine more robust drill downs to the root cause with stronger solutions developed.

Developing a Solution

Once the root cause is identified, it is important to work with a multidisciplinary team to develop the solution. **Mistake-proofing** techniques can be employed to make long-lasting significant changes. Mistake-proofing, or **Poka-Yoke**, is a way that prevents people from making mistakes.[1] The following are suggested methods, in order of strongest potential, to prevent future errors:

1. *Eliminate part of the process or the step that is causing the error.* For example, if the error is selection of the wrong patient-controlled, analgesia narcotic concentrations and several concentrations are available, the strongest mistake-proofing technique would be eliminating one or more of the concentrations and having only one concentration. This would dramatically reduce the opportunity for selecting the wrong concentration if only one concentration is available.

2. *Replace the error-prone step with a less error-prone step.* For example, using premixed heparin bags rather than mixing your own, which could lead to the wrong amount of heparin put in the bag or wrong base fluid.

3. *Use facilitation.* For example, use a checklist or other tool to help make the right decision and take the correct actions each time.

The next two steps would occur after the error has happened but would help to identify the error quickly so as to reduce patient harm.

1. *Detection* is putting in a step that would create an alert if something has gone wrong. An example of detection is to get a blood glucose level at a predefined time after administration of insulin. If the blood glucose is too low, then the patient caregiver can quickly intervene and avoid a possible seizure.

2. *Mitigation* is how quickly after the error is detected you alleviate or lessen its effects. In the insulin and blood glucose error, having a hypoglycemia protocol is a good example of a mitigation process. As soon as the adverse outcome is detected, the patient caregiver can proceed with the protocol, and patient harm may be minimized.

As a clinical coordinator, you know your department's workflow. You should be a leader in brainstorming ideas based on these different human factors and mistake-proofing techniques. Also, provide feedback to the committees to help them refine the recommendations. You would not want to say *no* to all of the recommendations without valid reasons. Because you do not want to do it or it might be additional work for your department should not be reasons to rule out the solutions. It is important that other disciplines see you as a collaborative partner. If there are serious concerns, then bring those forward in a professional manner. Ask your director or chief pharmacy officer for their opinions as well. Pharmacy often takes on additional responsibilities and work without additional resources. There may be situations where it is okay not to add additional resources, and other times it may be essential to request additional resources. Knowing your audience and your organization is key to deciding how to approach the resource conversation. Above all, make sure you are a leader in helping to design the solutions and provide authentic feedback to staff and administrators in a timely manner.

Getting the Staff Involved

Staff involvement is also essential in the development of proposed solutions. Make sure to include your staff members in the brainstorming for a solution or ask them for feedback. Hold sensing sessions where you review the root cause and ask for ideas. What might sound good in a conference room of the RCA or FMEA meetings might not work in the real world. The front-line staff knows the workarounds and direct application of the ideas. Getting their thoughts will help with their buy-in for successful implementation. Another way to address this with your staff is to have a mini-proactive risk-assessment session, sometimes called an *initiative review session* (IRS). The IRS is a concentrated systematic review of the proposed solution or for the development of solutions (see **Figure 5-1**). You can schedule these sessions, lasting from 30 minutes to 1 hour, at lunch time or during shift changes. At the start of a session, explain the error that occurred and circumstances surrounding it.

FIGURE 5-1. IRS Document Template

Initiative Review Session (IRS)

Initiative _____

Date _____ Facilitator _____

Attendees: _____

Opportunities for Improvement Identified by the Attendees:

1. _____

_____

2. _____

_____

3. _____

_____

4. _____

_____

Proposed Solutions for Each Opportunity for Improvement:

1. _____

_____

2. _____

_____

3. _____

_____

4. _____

_____

Additional Ideas and Suggestions from the Staff:

1. _____

_____

2. _____

_____

3. _____

_____

Does the staff in attendance support the proposed solutions?

1. _____ YES _____ NO

2. _____ YES _____ NO

3. _____ YES _____ NO

4. _____ YES _____ NO

This should make staff members more comfortable with the idea of change. If they are initially resistant and unsure why something needs to change, further explain why and share the proposed solution. Then, ask them for their initial reactions:

- Is this solution feasible?
- Will this solution solve the problem?
- What issues do you see with the proposed solution?
- Are there any other solutions?

Allow staff members to brainstorm ideas. If they are quiet, try to stimulate the conversation by passing out note cards and asking them to write their ideas down. You may want to have two or more sessions at different times of the day to make sure all staff members have the opportunity to participate. After the sessions, you can send out the suggested solutions via email to those who could not attend. After all of the feedback is received and incorporated, send out another email and ask for final comments.

Implementation and Measuring Outcomes

Once the root cause and solution are identified, it is important to implement the change and check if the solution has made a difference. As clinical coordinator, you may be responsible for the implementation; thus, you should ensure that the pharmacy staff is educated, the nursing department is prepared, and all necessary supplies or new processes are obtained and in place. You may need to set a go-live date and work with the public relations team or develop your own communications. Explain to your pharmacy staff why you are implementing the change so they understand and can adhere to the new process.

To ensure that the solution is in place and is making a difference, you need to create the metrics to measure or monitor the solution's effectiveness. A defined timeframe for collecting data is necessary to determine if the solution resolved the problem. Medication safety events are usually rare and infrequent, so it might be hard to use future events as a metric (e.g., outcome measure). Finding a *process measure* (a measure that is part of the steps prior to the final outcome) can show

if there is a breakdown in the process that will lead to an adverse medication event. Tracking and trending process measures can allow you to be more proactive and address issues in the process prior to reaching the patient and causing harm. If the measure you select is too difficult to collect, then it might not be collected. Also, make sure that it is meaningful. Often measures are selected that are easy to collect but do not give us substantial information. Make a dashboard that can be shared with the staff members so they know how they are doing with the new process. If they know they are doing well, this helps to maintain morale; and if they know there are opportunities for improvement, it provides a process for accountability. Post the dashboard electronically or physically in the department and review it at staff meetings. The more transparent you are with your staff members, the more they will trust you, and the more successful you will be.

If the error was a result of a violation or disregarding the rules, then disciplinary action must be considered and human resources consulted. Consider if the employee is a right fit for your organization. In a just culture, reckless people must be held accountable for their actions. Look for patterns. Is this something that you have already coached and consoled the employee on in the past? Has this same situation occurred several times, and the employee is not applying lessons learned? This may be a difficult discussion to deliver to the employee, but if you remember to put the patient at the center of the discussion, it will help diffuse the conversation and keep your message on target.

Communication for Success

Communication is essential to ensure your staff learns from previous medication safety issues. Share these events at staff meetings, and start the meeting with *great catches and errors*. Great catches is a proactive method to help you to identify possible errors before they reach patients and cause harm. Ask staff members to share any great catches they have witnessed, and then later post a great-catch board in your department. Having a theme for great catches—such as a baseball diamond, a dog catching a Frisbee, or a star that is being caught—is a fun way to attract attention and encourage staff participation.

Also, ask staff members to share their medication safety stories from the past month, and describe what is listed in the official report from your organization's reporting system. Remember to deidentify medication safety events so that no one feels singled out or embarrassed, and maintain a positive, not demeaning, tone. Share the steps that are being taken to fix problems and improve patient safety outcomes. By sharing and communicating with your staff members, you will build their confidence in your organization's ability to improve patient care.

Being Proactive Rather Than Reactive

Several other resources and tools can be used to identify opportunities and prevent adverse medication events reaching patients and causing harm. One resource is the Institute for Safe Medication Practices' (ISMP) newsletter.[6] The ISMP newsletter reviews errors that have occurred and provides suggestions to ensure safety at your organization. Although not all of the events in the newsletter might apply to your organization, it a good source of information for you in reviewing and making sure you have a strong system in place to support medication safety. Also, on a quarterly basis, the ISMP newsletter contains the Quarterly Action Agenda, which you can use to formally review these recommendations. It is set up as a grid and allows you to document your findings and access the issues (see **Figure 5-2** for a sample ISMP Quarterly Action Agenda). You can share this information with your medication safety committee, within your department of pharmacy, and with your pharmacy and therapeutics (P&T) committee.

In addition, ISMP has several self-assessment tools available. If your organization has not completed these or has not done them in a long time, they are excellent tools to systematically and objectively review your organization's processes and identify areas for improvement. The self-assessments cover topics such as automated dispensing cabinets, smart pumps, and anticoagulation. Complete the assessments with a multidisciplinary team to ensure a robust and accurate assessment; if they are completed with only pharmacists, then you will

get only one perspective and may miss key information that could prevent a patient safety error (see **Figure 5-3** for an example of the ISMP self-assessment tool).

Performing a gap analysis based on The Joint Commission (TJC) Sentinel Events is another proactive tool.[6] TJC does not publish these alerts on a predefined schedule but rather as issues arise, which are considered dangerous enough to raise concern. You can create a grid from the alert and address each of the recommendations using the techniques previously described: having a multidisciplinary team, developing mistake-proofing solutions, involving staff in the brainstorming, and ensuring successful implementation. Also, share these alerts with your medication safety committee, the pharmacy department, and the P&T committee (see **Figure 5-4** for an example of how to take the alert and create a gap analysis).

You can also create a dashboard or balanced scorecard with metrics where you select a variety of medication safety measures to monitor, track, and trend. Medication-related events are voluntarily reported through an online, telephone, or paper system, and they can be a great measure of the culture of safety. However, there are some disadvantages such as relying on end users to remember to report and the time it takes to receive such reports. Because this does not guarantee a systematic process with a consistent denominator, it is hard to trend the data and make conclusions about how to improve safety. Therefore, it is important to implement a systematic process that is reliable and consistent. The new National Action Plan for Adverse Drug Event Prevention, Centers for Medicare & Medicaid Services (CMS), and the Partnership for Patients can provide guidance on what to collect.[7] In addition, three metrics that several of the Hospital Engagement Networks, as part of the Partnership for Patients, have used include blood glucose <40 mg/dL, international normalized ratio >5, and naloxone for opiate reversal.

As a clinical coordinator, you might be responsible for determining who collects data, where the data are kept, and how data are shared. An MSO might do this, but you also might be asked to help staff collect data. Such information should be shared on an elec-

FIGURE 5-2. ISMP Quarterly Action Agenda

January–March 2015

ISMP Quarterly Action Agenda

ISMP One of the most important ways to prevent medication errors is to learn about problems that have occurred in other organizations and to use that information to prevent similar problems at your practice site. To promote such a process, the following selected items from the January—March 2015 issues of the *ISMP Medication Safety Alert!* have been prepared for an interdisciplinary committee to stimulate discussion and action to reduce the risk of medication errors. Each item includes a brief description of the medication safety problem, a few recommendations to reduce the risk of errors, and the issue number to locate additional information as desired. Look for our high-alert medication icon under the issue number if the agenda item involves one or more medications on the ISMP List of High-Alert Medications (www.ismp.org/sc?id=479). The Action Agenda is also available for download in a Microsoft Word format (https://ismp.org/newsletters/acutecare/articles/ActionAgenda1502.doc) that allows expansion of the columns in the table designated for organizational documentation of an assessment, actions required, and assignments for each agenda item. Continuing education credit is available for nurses at www.ismp.org/sc?id=480.

Key: ⚠ —ISMP high-alert medication

No.	Problem	Recommendation	Organization Assessment	Action Required/ Assignment	Date Completed
		Technology and error-prevention strategies needed to address the IV sterile compounding process			
(1,5) ⚠	Sterile compounding is a significant core pharmacy practice in dire need of improvement. However, it is routinely relegated to low priority until a significant error occurs. Variability in practices, a failure to identify and teach best practices, learned workplace tolerance of risk, routine practice deviations, and a host of cultural issues have led to harmful errors that should cause pharmacy to examine every task involved in sterile compounding. IV workflow technology with barcode scanning is available to help prevent many errors but only 6%—7% of hospital pharmacies employ this technology.	All staff involved in sterile compounding should be taught the safe, detailed steps associated with sterile compounding along with the reasons behind these steps to reinforce the need to follow these standards. Pharmacy staff should be knowledgeable of the best practice standards required by USP <797>. IV workflow technologies or barcode scanning that's integrated with the pharmacy and hospital information systems can also help prevent sterile compounding errors (www.pharmacyautomation.com). ISMP is up-dating its sterile compounding guidelines to better guide those involved in these processes.			

IV = intravenous.

FIGURE 5-3. ISMP Self-Assessment[a]

A	No activity to implement
B	Considered, but not implemented
C	Partially implemented in some or all areas
D	Fully implemented in some areas
E	Fully implemented throughout

I.   PATIENT INFORMATION

	A	B	C	D	E
Core Characteristic #1 Essential patient information is obtained, readily available in useful form, and considered when prescribing, dispensing, and administering medications, and when monitoring the effects of medications.					
1 *Prescribers* and *nurses* can easily and electronically access *inpatient* laboratory values while working in their respective clinical locations.					
2 *Pharmacists* can easily and electronically access *inpatient* laboratory values while working in their respective clinical locations.					
3 *Prescribers* and *nurses* can easily and electronically access *outpatient* laboratory values while working in their respective clinical locations.					
4 *Pharmacists* can easily and electronically access *outpatient* laboratory values while working in their respective clinical locations.					
5 Recent inpatient and outpatient laboratory values are automatically displayed on **COMPUTER ORDER ENTRY SYSTEM** screens for medications that typically require dose adjustments based on pending laboratory results (e.g., if warfarin is ordered, the most recent INR is displayed).					

[a]The full assessment is available at https://ismp.org/selfassessments/Hospital/2011/full.pdf.

INR = international normalized ratio; ISMP = Institute for Safe Medication Practices.

tronic dashboard, posted in the department, or discussed at a staff meeting. You need to determine how to keep these topics active for your staff members to consider and understand in their daily practice.

Collaboration with Other Departments

The final aspect of medication safety is collaboration with others, such as with risk management, your patient safety officer, or the quality department. You may be asked to collect data or describe the department's workflow. It is important to be proactive when you meet various individuals so that you can develop successful relationships. If you are new to the clinical coordinator position, you should set up meetings with representatives from these departments. In addition to them requesting information from you, there are times you will need their expertise. For example, if patients want to use their home total parenteral nutrition and your organization's policy does not allow this, you might need to discuss it with risk management. Or, if a medication error happens and you need to determine who is going to disclose it to the patient and family, you might want to talk with risk management or the patient safety officer.

Summary

Medication safety concerns all pharmacists and their organizations. Whether you have an MSO or medication safety pharmacist at your

FIGURE 5-4. Joint Commission Sentinel Event Gap Analysis[a]

Sentinel Event Risk Reduction Strategy	Current State	Opportunities for Improvement	Person Assigned	Updates and Follow Up	Date Completed
Establish and maintain a functional pediatric formulary system with policies for drug evaluation, selection, and therapeutic use.					
To prevent timing errors in medication administration, standardize how days are counted in all protocols by deciding on a protocol start date (e.g., Day 0 or Day 1).					
Limit the number of concentrations and dose strengths of high-alert medications to the minimum needed to provide safe care.					
For pediatric patients who are receiving compounded oral medications and total parenteral nutrition at home, ensure that the doses are equivalent to those prepared in the hospital (i.e., the volume of the home dose should be the same as the volume of the hospital prepared products).					
Use oral syringes to administer oral medications. The pharmacy should use oral syringes when preparing oral liquid medications. Make oral syringes available on patient care units when "as needed" medications are prepared. Educate staff about the benefits of oral syringes in preventing inadvertent intravenous administration of oral medications.					

[a]For more information, see http://www.jointcommission.org/assets/1/18/SEA_39.PDF.

organization, a clinical coordinator has many responsibilities related to medication safety. You are the workflow expert and can represent pharmacy at safety discussions, help determine root causes and develop solutions, coach and counsel staff, and share events and lessons learned to ensure patient safety. You are really the hub of all the information; thus, you need to be aware of what is happening as well as what could happen.

PRACTICE TIPS

1. Create an environment of trust and transparency with your staff members. Once you do, you will be able to have critical and sensitive conversations with them, and they will not question your motives.

2. If a medication safety error occurs, you need to completely understand why it

occurred, which involves talking with the staff involved as soon as possible and then getting to the root cause rather than guessing or assuming what happened.

3. Once you know why the error occurred, you need to take action to ensure it does not happen again or be proactive and review new processes before they are implemented to mitigate and mistake-proof any potential errors.

4. It is important to implement the new solution(s). Ideas cannot just be developed in a conference or as the result of overanalyzed data; they need to be implemented in the real world. Otherwise, patient safety and outcomes are not impacted.

5. Get to know your colleagues in different departments before you need to work with them so as to establish strong relationships. This allows for better communication and resolution in the event of an error or crisis.

References

1. Larson CM, Saine D. *Medication Safety Officer's Handbook*. Bethesda, MD: ASHP; 2013.

2. Marx D. *Patient Safety and the "Just Culture": A Primer for Health Care Executives*. New York, NY: Columbia University; 2001.

3. http://www.safer.healthcare.ucla.edu/safer/archive/ahrq/FinalPrimerDoc.pdf. Accessed July 9, 2015.

4. Scott SD, Hirschinger LE, Cox KR, et al. The natural history of recovery for the healthcare provider "second victim" after adverse patient events. *Qual Saf Health Care*. 2009;18(5):325-330.

5. Institute for Safe Medication Practices. www.ISMP.org.

6. http://www.jointcommission.org/sentinel_event.aspx. Accessed July 9, 2015.

7. http://www.health.gov/hai/pdfs/ADE-Action-Plan-508c.pdf. Accessed July 9, 2015.

Suggested Reading

Agency for Healthcare Research and Quality. www.ahrq.gov.

Institute for Healthcare Improvement. www.IHI.org.

Institute for Safe Medication Practices. www.ISMP.org.

Joint Commission Journal on Quality and Patient Safety. http://www.jointcommissioninternational.org/the-joint-commission-journal-on-quality-and-patient-safety-jci/.

Joint Commission Sentinel Events. www.jointcommission.org/sentinel_event.aspx.

Larson CM, Saine D. *Medication Safety Officer's Handbook*. Bethesda, MD: ASHP; 2013.

National Patient Safety Foundation. www.npsf.org.

Norman DA. *The Design of Everyday Things: Revised and Expanded*. New York, NY: Basic Books; 2013.

CHAPTER 6

Accreditation, Medication Management, and the Clinical Coordinator

Trista Pfeiffenberger

KEY TERMS

Accreditation—A voluntary process through which an organization is subject to external review and receives recognition for meeting established, high-quality standards.

Mock Survey—An internal, preparatory review that is meant to simulate the components of a full, external accreditation visit.

Standards—Rules or criteria that establish an acceptable level of quality, are objectively developed from existing subject matter knowledge, and are adopted by a consensus of experts and stakeholders.

Tracer Methodology—A means of conducting an accreditation survey that follows a patient throughout the episode of care and reviews compliance with accreditation standards.

Introduction

As a clinical coordinator, a solid understanding of the pharmacy department's role in hospital **accreditation** processes is critical. This is true both because you are a formal leader in the pharmacy department and because you manage staff members that have a high likelihood of being directly involved in accreditation surveys. Additionally, proper medication use and storage are highlighted throughout the accreditation **standards**, and the pharmacy department is often considered the owner of these standards regardless of the setting of care (e.g., inpatient, emergency department, procedure areas, outpatient clinics). This chapter outlines the critical accreditation information that is specific to the role of a clinical coordinator.

Hospital Accreditation 101

Why Do Hospitals Seek Accreditation?

The Centers for Medicare & Medicaid Services (CMS) established a set of requirements, **Conditions of Participation** (CoPs), that hospitals must meet if they wish to seek reimbursement for care provided to beneficiaries covered by Medicare or Medicaid. Accreditation bodies such as The Joint Commission (TJC) and DNV GL Healthcare were created to periodically verify that hospitals are indeed meeting these requirements. These accreditation agencies periodically survey hospital performance against their latest standards, which are based on the CMS CoPs.[1]

What Organizations Certify Accreditation?

Three organizations currently hold deeming status from CMS. TJC, as one of the original hospital accreditation bodies dating back to 1965, is used by the vast majority of U.S. hospitals.[2,3] For that reason, TJC will be the basis of most information and use cases presented in this chapter. DNV GL Healthcare, which was established in 2008, has approximately 500 hospitals accredited through its program but takes a unique approach to their standards by building the CMS CoPs into a larger quality management program.[4] Likewise, the Healthcare Facilities Accreditation Program (HFAP)

established by the American Osteopathic Association is an option for hospital accreditation, but it is also used by fewer hospitals than TJC.[3]

What Is Part of an Accreditation Survey?

Accreditation surveys are usually a combination of reviewing policies and procedures, directly observing care provision and patient care areas, interviewing staff and administrators, and following patients throughout their course of care (**tracer methodology**). For this reason, your preparedness efforts in the pharmacy department, which are discussed later in this chapter, should parallel the survey process. Your hospital may choose to engage a consulting firm to conduct a mock accreditation survey to assess your hospital's readiness for the official survey. **Mock surveys**, if done either internally or with an external agency, are a great preparedness tool because they simulate all or most components of the real survey process. The results are only for quality improvement purposes and have no official impact on your hospital's accreditation status. Your hospital's leadership and the accreditation department typically make the decisions about accreditation agencies, mock surveys, and other strategic decisions related to accreditation. Even though you are unlikely to be involved in the decision-making process, you should know the hospital's chosen accreditation agency and related standards, general plans for survey preparedness and mock surveys, and the expected involvement of you and your pharmacy staff.

Although DNV GL Healthcare has established an annual survey process, TJC and HFAP surveys occur every 3 years.[5] Triennial TJC surveys are unannounced, but there is a survey window within which the surveyors will usually arrive. Regardless, it is important that survey preparedness be a continuous process because patient safety events could occur and result in an unannounced survey at any point in time. Additionally, your state government has an agency linked to CMS at the federal level, and it may choose your hospital to survey so as to validate the results of your hospital's chosen accreditation agency (called a *validation survey*).

How Are the Standards Developed?

There are a few key points to understand about TJC standards development. First, new standards are created only when one or more of three scenarios exist: (1) there are emerging issues related to patient safety or quality of care; (2) new processes or procedures have been documented to have a positive impact on health outcomes; or (3) new laws or regulations have been approved. Importantly, standards are developed only around these scenarios if they are measurable. The process of developing standards is robust and includes input from healthcare professionals, providers, subject matter experts, consumers, government agencies (including CMS), and employers. The standards are informed by scientific evidence and consensus of subject matter experts.[6]

You may ask, "Why do I need to know how and why standards are developed by TJC?" The reason is that accreditation efforts have the potential to feel like an administrative exercise (and, therefore, a burden) to front-line staff focused on providing patient care. You, as the clinical coordinator, have the potential to frame all accreditation activities around the notion that they help the organization and all departments within it adhere to common standards of safety and quality, thereby creating an infrastructure for the best possible patient care. Also, incorporating aspects of accreditation preparedness into the regular job responsibilities of clinical pharmacists can also help avoid perceptions that it is an additional responsibility that occurs during the accreditation window.

Accreditation Standards Related to Medications

It is helpful to know there are not any standards labeled as the specific responsibility of the pharmacy department; however, hospitals commonly see the pharmacy department as having responsibility for oversight of all standards related to medication use in any setting (e.g., inpatient, operating room/procedure areas, emergency department) and by any care provider. Along those lines, a number of accreditation standards specifically relate to medication use. They address everything from medication storage and security to medication reconciliation, safe handling of high-alert

medications, and use of medications in special populations, such as pediatric patients.[7]

Although TJC has a set of National Patient Safety Goals, which usually contain a few new standards related to safe medication use, the majority of the standards related to pharmacy appear in the medication management chapter of TJC's accreditation manual. If you read the medication management standards cover-to-cover, you will likely discover the rationale behind some of your pharmacy department's policies. However, you will probably also be left with questions because the standards set the bar for performance but do not tell you how to get there.

As a clinical coordinator, you have several resources available for more information about the standards and how they will be surveyed. First, the accreditation standards themselves provide additional information with a fairly succinct and easy-to-understand description of what is required and a more detailed section with specific implementation requirements. TJC refers to the more detailed sections as *Elements of Performance*; the CMS CoPs call them *Interpretive Guidelines and Survey Procedures*.

Second, you should have a designated person in the pharmacy department who is responsible for accreditation. Depending on the size of your hospital and department, your pharmacy accreditation lead may be your director or assistant director of pharmacy, a manager, or a staff member. Because your pharmacy lead for accreditation should have an in-depth understanding of the standards and what is required to meet them, he or she should be your first point of contact if you have a question. In addition to having specific knowledge on the subject, your pharmacy accreditation lead can point you to publications by accreditation agencies that are not in the standards themselves, such as frequently asked questions and newsletters. Your hospital should also have a key person identified to lead the organization's accreditation efforts. Like your pharmacy department liaison, the hospital accreditation lead is a wealth of information and knows who to contact at your hospital's accreditation organization (TJC, DNV GL Healthcare, or HFAP) to get more information if a question or issue comes up that cannot be answered. It is important to note that as a clinical coordinator, you should not independently make the decision to contact the accreditation organization about a question without first speaking to the internal resources described.

Preparing for Accreditation Survey

Staff Education

Preparing staff to successfully assist with and participate in the accreditation survey process is arguably one of the more difficult activities of a clinical coordinator. Because staff members are probably not immersed in policies and accreditation standards as part of their daily work, they will need to learn a number of things to enable them to respond to a surveyor's questions. Although a number of different ideas will be presented in this chapter about how to increase your staff members' knowledge of your pharmacy department and hospital policies, it is essential for you to understand what your staff members need to know and do during a real accreditation survey visit. Clinical pharmacy staff members based in the patient care units should be able to perform the following:

- Assist with reviewing the patient care unit(s) that they cover for proper medication storage and related procedures
- Follow established policies and procedures that relate to accreditation standards
- Respond to a surveyor's questions

Consider the case examples below:

Case Example 1

An accreditation surveyor is using tracer methodology to follow a patient from the emergency department to the cath lab to the cardiology floor, where your clinical pharmacist is covering. It is now the patient's second day in the hospital, and the surveyor is on the cardiology unit reviewing the medication administration record, which shows that the patient is taking two of her own medications because they are nonformulary. The surveyor asks to see a copy of the hospital's policy related to patient's own medications and asks the pharmacist to describe

the proper procedure that must be followed. The pharmacist's verbal description of the process must align with the policy, and perhaps more importantly, the medication storage and documentation for this particular patient should align with the policy for the surveyor to believe the standard is successfully met.

Case Example 2

A different surveyor is following a patient who was directly admitted from clinic for scheduled chemotherapy. Because chemotherapy is considered a high-alert medication at your hospital and also has its own policy regarding safe use, the surveyor wants to observe that the proper procedures are being followed in the delivery of care for this particular patient. Although the pharmacist has already reviewed the chemotherapy orders that are now being prepared in the pharmacy, the surveyor asks the clinical pharmacist to describe the procedure for reviewing chemotherapy orders. The clinical pharmacist describes what is reviewed on the order and that it is a double validation process, with the intravenous (IV) room pharmacist serving as the second check. The surveyor asks to see documentation of the double check and then proceeds to the pharmacy to observe the preparation of the chemotherapy. The surveyor will expect to see that high-alert medication procedures as well as the chemotherapy-specific procedures are followed throughout the medication-use process and will likely ask questions of the IV room pharmacist and nurse(s) administering the medications as well. Finally, one of the medications in the patient's chemotherapy protocol is currently in short supply, and the surveyor wants to understand how the hospital handles shortages and communicates to staff.

These examples illustrate the importance of staff knowing your hospital and pharmacy departmental policies related to medication use and following those policies on a daily basis. As a clinical coordinator, this probably sounds simple enough, but often seasoned staff train new staff members by describing traditional handling of procedures without tying the orientation back to the most recent policies. Keeping all of your staff well educated on changes to medication-use policies and ensuring they know and follow these policies in their daily tasks will make survey preparedness efforts much easier.

In addition to medication-use policies and procedures, your pharmacy and/or hospital lead for accreditation can provide you with a complete list that is customized to your facility. Here are some examples:

- The hospital's mission and vision statements

- Examples of performance improvement projects (pharmacy-related or ones that they were personally involved with are best)

- The PASS (**p**ull, **a**im, **s**queeze, **s**weep) and RACE (**r**escue, **a**larm, **c**ontain, **e**xtinguish) acronyms for fire safety

Here are some ideas for educating your staff about policies and procedures (and hopefully incorporating a little bit of fun along the way).[8] These activities should be considered a regular part of your job as the clinical coordinator but can be intensified in the year leading up to your anticipated accreditation survey date. In the intense phase of accreditation preparation, it may be worthwhile for you to plan ahead with your educational efforts so that you cover all relevant topics and rotate the types of activities you use. These plans could be documented in a calendar format and shared with your department's accreditation coordinator and your manager so that they are aware of your efforts and can assist you with alignment of unit-specific preparations to anything the department or hospital may be doing more globally.[9] (See **Figure 6-1**.)

- **Daily Work Group Huddles.** You may already have work group huddles with your team each day or each shift to communicate critical and timely information. If so, consider adding one question to each huddle that is related to accreditation surveys.

- **Signs/Posters.** Put signs up on the walls with tips or reminders related to accreditation standards. Make them brightly colored so they stand out, and change both the sign content and color often so staff members notice the change.

- **Pocket Resource Guides.** Provide booklets with key information and consolidated versions of policies for staff members to keep in the pocket of their lab coats. This effort could be coordinated with other hospital departments.

- **Flashcards.** Create flashcards that can be used during clinical coordinator walking rounds or staff meetings.

- **Daily Clinical Coordinator Walking Rounds.** Walk to the patient care units where your staff members are based each day to check in on how they are doing and incorporate accreditation survey questions into your discussion.

- **Regular Email Tips or Newsletters.** Send emails with an accreditation survey tip of the day/week. Include accreditation-related items in existing department newsletters.

- **Bulletin Boards or Table Tent Cards.** Similar to the signs and posters above, use a bulletin board or table tent cards in the break room or other area where staff periodically congregate to post education about accreditation survey-related items. Regularly rotate posted items.

- **Computer Screen Savers.** If possible, coordinate with your hospital accreditation and IT departments to use computer screen savers as a place to put critical policy reminders that would be important for all or most staff.

- **Assessments.** Use a short quiz before and after an educational blitz to measure progress. Incentivize participation (and competition among work units) by providing prizes for the work units with the highest amount of participation and the highest rate of correct answers.

- **Use Social Media.** Post questions to Twitter, Instagram, etc., and award prizes to a staff member who is the first one to answer correctly. (Note: Hospital policies related to use of social media should be followed. This idea should not be implemented without approval from your pharmacy director.)

FIGURE 6-1. Education Calendar Example

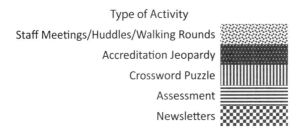

Topic	Medication Management Standard	Jan	Feb	Mar
High-alert medications	MM.01.01.03			
Nonformulary medication orders	MM.02.01.01			
Shortages	MM.02.01.01			
Medication security	MM.03.01.01			
Patient's own medications	MM.03.01.05			

Type of Activity

Staff Meetings/Huddles/Walking Rounds

Accreditation Jeopardy

Crossword Puzzle

Assessment

Newsletters

• **Games.** Make learning the standards and related policies and procedures fun! Use a portion of a staff meeting to play accreditation Jeopardy or create an accreditation-themed crossword puzzle. Award prizes to staff members with the highest score.

Additionally, you may want to consider assigning clinical pharmacists to staff-level oversight of various policies and procedures to accomplish the following:

• It creates ownership among the front-line staff for correct policy knowledge and procedural accuracy.

• It gives other staff members a peer to go to for assistance or to give feedback about the ease of policy implementation.

• It gives you and other managers in the department someone to assist with policy updates, monitoring, and education.

Review of Patient Care Areas

Reviewing patient care areas for survey readiness basically occurs in two forms: (1) routine unit inspections; and (2) coordinated tracers

or mock surveys. Ideally, all of the elements of regular unit inspections are covered during mock surveys/tracers, but there are some components of mock surveys/tracers that are unique to that activity.

Routine Patient Care Area Inspections

Your hospital and pharmacy departments probably have a patient care area inspection form for staff to regularly (typically monthly at a minimum) review compliance with medication-storage policies on each nursing unit. The form should contain questions about expired medications, unsecured medications, unlabeled medications, unlocked crash carts, refrigerator temperature logs, etc. An example can be found in **Appendix 6-A**. What you may not have realized is that many of the questions on that form are directly related to accreditation standards. As a clinical coordinator, you should understand the process of these monthly patient care area inspections—who completes them, where to find the most updated form, where the results are stored, and with whom the results are shared. If you and your clinical pharmacy staff are knowledgeable about or involved in the unit inspection process, the participation in survey readiness efforts will be more straightforward; otherwise, it will be much more difficult.

In addition to using the patient care area/nursing unit inspection form on a monthly basis for each patient care area in the facility, the form is useful to guide pharmacy staff participation on mock surveys/tracers and as a checklist for the day surveyors arrive.

Mock Surveys/Tracers

Most hospitals have mock surveys and/or tracers scheduled for each patient care area by their accreditation lead (see **Appendix 6-B** for an example). These internal surveys are meant to be somewhat impromptu from a staff perspective (just like an unannounced survey would be), so they are scheduled only a couple of days in advance. The internal surveys include the hospital's accreditation lead and the nurse manager of the patient care unit being surveyed, plus one representative from infection control, engineering, pharmacy, and potentially other departments such as respiratory therapy. If you are given the option to attend these internal surveys, you in turn may wish to delegate attendance to one of your clinical pharmacists (ideally, not the same staff member that works in the patient care area because that person may need to participate in the staff aspects of the mock survey). You should attend the first survey with the clinical pharmacist and demonstrate how to participate.

When you report to the internal survey, you may find that the rest of the team is there and ready to get started as a group, which would indicate you will probably do the tracer portion first. Alternatively, you may report at the correct time and place and find that you are the only team member there; in this case, others may be doing their own department or area-specific reviews of the unit before coming together for the team tracer, or they may not be conducting a team review at all. If the latter is the case, you can feel free to get started with the medication-related assessments that you alone will be evaluating, then transition to the team-based tracer if you see the group forming.

Before attending any type of internal survey, you should familiarize yourself with all of the medication-related standards and understand what findings constitute a successful survey. This can be accomplished by reading the standards and, if needed, solidifying your knowledge by communicating with your desig-nated pharmacy department accreditation lead. You should bring a blank patient care area inspection form with you to fill out during your assessment as well as a copy of the last routine inspection of that same patient care area so you can assess if previously documented issues are resolved. For example, if the last routine inspection found that the crash cart contained expired medications and was unlocked, you would want to check that same crash cart to make sure that the expired meds were updated and the cart is now locked. Although the questions on the patient care area inspection form will guide you in what to look for (e.g., unlabeled syringes, unsecured medications), you should also consider the following locations:

- Medication room or preparation area, both on counter tops and in drawers commonly accessed by nursing
- Patient's bedside
- Tube station and medication delivery bin
- Supply rooms
- Medication storage refrigerators (and associated monitoring logs)
- Automated dispensing cabinet
- Crash cart (and associated monitoring logs)

For the patient-specific tracer review, the internal survey coordinator may let you know which patient(s) will be a part of the mock tracer in advance, or they may inform the group at the time of the survey. Either way, you can conduct the tracer part of the review with the group or on your own. Because the tracer is looking at one specific patient, it gives you the opportunity to survey items that are difficult to do at the level of a nursing unit, such as the following:

- Hospital-designated timelines for medication administration are followed.
- Instructions are listed for each taken as needed (prn) medication.
- Each medication has an indication listed in the chart.
- Verbal medication orders are minimized as much as possible and have timely co-signatures.

- Medications are appropriately reconciled at care transitions.

Because of the nature of this part of the review, it is often easiest to start with a review of the patient's medication administration record and physician orders. These sources also indicate whether the patient is using his or her own medications or self-administering medications, both of which are important procedures to be able to evaluate during some of the internal surveys.

The results of each internal survey need to be documented and communicated. Most hospitals have a standard form to document the mock survey or tracer findings similar to that found in Appendix 6-B. Once you have completed your assessment and made handwritten notes of all of your findings, you should communicate them to your pharmacy accreditation lead, your pharmacy director, and your hospital's accreditation lead within 2 to 3 business days. Although all of your findings must be included in the template for the sake of completeness, it would be helpful to your pharmacy director to also include a shortened version of the most significant findings in the body of your email message.

Activities in the Survey Window

Once your hospital reaches the timeframe when you are considered due for your next accreditation survey, the previously described readiness efforts should be implemented in high gear. To ensure everything is in the best order possible, staff should begin to take extra steps every day, including a regular profile review for the purposes of clean up (i.e., removing duplicate therapies, making sure the prescribed medication profile matches the one for dispensing and administration, and double checking for instructions on all prn medications). Also, staff can do regular sweeps of the patient care units to quickly look for red flags based on the patient care area inspection form (see Appendix 6-A).

Once it is announced that surveyors are on the premises, a final sweep of the patient care units is recommended and should be done at least daily while the surveyors are on site. Keep in mind that although this sweep sounds time-consuming, if staff have been involved during either the routine patient care area inspections or the mock surveys, they will be highly familiar

with what is required of them, and the sweep should take no longer than 5 to 15 minutes per unit.

While on site, the surveyors will be escorted by hospital administrator(s). This could possibly include the pharmacy director or, more rarely, the clinical coordinator. However, the surveyors will commonly separate and survey different areas during the day, coming together only for morning announcements, the end-of-day reports, and other important sessions. Thus, there is the potential for clinical pharmacy staff or clinical coordinators to be aware of survey activity when your director is not. It is critical that staff members immediately email their direct supervisor and the department director whenever they interact with the surveyor, describing what the surveyor was reviewing at the time of the encounter, what questions were asked, what answers were provided, and any necessary follow-up. Alerting the pharmacy director to an encounter may allow for some follow-up before or at that day's report-out meeting, and it has the potential to affect how the finding is perceived by the surveyor.

Finally, even if staff members have not interacted with the surveyors, they are likely interested in how the survey is going and want to understand any identified areas of concern. Although the accreditation survey is a very busy week for all staff—including the clinical coordinator—it is worth taking a few minutes at the end of each day to summarize the events in an email to your staff members. This will help them feel informed and prepared to participate in the next day's survey, should they be called to do so.

Summary

Staying abreast of medication-related accreditation standards and helping your staff do the same is a key part of the clinical coordinator's role. Ultimately, understanding and following accreditation-related policies and procedures are simply a part of providing quality patient care.

PRACTICE TIPS

1. Create a schedule or calendar of activities that you can do with staff to reinforce policies and procedures related to accredita-

tion standards. Ramp up the frequency of the activities when your hospital is approaching the accreditation window.

2. Involve staff members in unit inspection surveys so that they are knowledgeable about medication security standards and regulations.

3. Participate in mock surveys, and encourage your staff to do the same, so that everyone is familiar with the survey process prior to the official accreditation survey.

4. Frame accreditation-related education around the concept of safe and optimal patient care (i.e., compliance with standards is needed to provide high-quality patient care).

5. As much as possible, make staff education fun!

References

1. Centers for Medicare & Medicaid Services. CMS deeming authority requirements. https://www.cms.gov/Medicare/Provider-Enrollment-and-Certification/SurveyCertificationGenInfo/downloads/application requirements.pdf. Accessed June 7, 2015.

2. The Joint Commission. Facts about hospital accreditation. http://www.jointcommission.org/accreditation/accreditation_main.aspx. Accessed June 7, 2015.

3. American Society for Healthcare Engineering. Hospital accrediting organizations offer different approaches to the survey process. http://www.ashe.org/ashenews/2013/hosp_ao_article_131011.shtml. Accessed December 1, 2014.

4. DNV GL Healthcare. http://dnvglhealthcare.com. Accessed July 27, 2015.

5. Centers for Medicare & Medicaid Services. Comparison of accreditation organizations. http://cms.ipressroom.com.s3.amazonaws.com/107/files/20125/comparison-dnvhc_to_tjc_tcm4-358498.pdf. Accessed December 1, 2014.

6. The Joint Commission. Facts about Joint Commission standards. http://www.jointcommission.org/facts_about_joint_commission_accreditation_standards/. Accessed June 7, 2015.

7. The Joint Commission. *2013 Hospital Accreditation Standards*. Oakbrook Terrace, IL: Joint Commission; 2013.

8. Thompson EM, Pool S, Brown D, et al. JCAHO preparation: an educational plan. *J Contin Educ Nurs.* 2008;39(5):225-227.

9. Thurber R, Read LE. A comprehensive education plan: the key to a successful joint commission on accreditation of healthcare organizations survey. *J Nurs Staff Dev.* 2008;24(3):129-132.

Suggested Reading

Centers for Medicare & Medicaid Services. Conditions for coverage (CfCs) & conditions of participations (CoPs): hospitals. http://www.cms.gov/Regulations-and-Guidance/Legislation/CFCsAndCoPs/Hospitals.html.

Centers for Medicare & Medicaid Services. State operations manual: survey protocol, regulations and interpretive guidelines for hospitals. http://www.cms.gov/Regulations-and-Guidance/Guidance/Manuals/Downloads/som107ap_a_hospitals.pdf.

Joint Commission Hospital Accreditation Standards. *2013 Hospital Accreditation Standards.* Oakbrook Terrace, IL: Joint Commission Resources; 2013.

The Joint Commission. http://www.jointcommission.org/.

The Joint Commission National Patient Safety Goals. http://www.jointcommission.org/standards_information/npsgs.aspx.

Uselton JP, Kienle PC, Murdaugh LB. *Assuring Continuous Compliance with Joint Commission Standards: A Pharmacy Guide.* 8th ed. Bethesda, MD: American Society of Health-System Pharmacists; 2010.

Appendix 6-A

MEDICATION AREA INSPECTION

Location _____ Month/Year _____

	YES	NO	N/A	REMARKS
MEDICATION PREPARATION AREA				
Medication preparation area is clean, neat, and well organized.				
IV preparation area is clean, uncluttered, and functionally separate.				
PATIENT AND STOCK MEDICATIONS				
Only authorized medications are present. (There is no excess stock, unauthorized storage areas, or unidentified patient medications.)				
All medications are locked.				
Tops of automated dispensing cabinets and medication carts are free of medications.				
Medications to be returned to pharmacy are in the authorized location.				
All medications are within their expiration or beyond-use date. (Check bulk supplies, refrigerator, etc.)				
Check of two patient records and medications (automated dispensing cabinets, medication drawer, MAR, Kardex, chart) matched.				
Check of two MARs show nursing reconciliation documentation.				
Check of automated dispensing cabinets for two items reveal correct count and within expiration date.				
Internal and external bulk stock is separated.				
CONTROLLED SUBSTANCES				
Automated dispensing cabinets and manual systems are free of discrepancies.				
REFRIGERATOR				
Refrigerator temperature is between 36°F and 46°F. Note temperature:				
Freezer temperature is between –13°F and 14°F. Note temperature: Note freezer drugs:				
Refrigerators/freezers containing vaccines are monitored constantly or checked twice a day.				
Refrigerator is clean.				
Freezer is free from frost.				
Refrigerator and freezer logs are complete for every day this month.				

	YES	NO	N/A	REMARKS
Only drugs are stored in the refrigerator and freezer. (No food, lab reagents, or specimens are allowed.)				
Floor-stock insulins are in the appropriate bin.				
MISCELLANEOUS				
Single-dose vials are destroyed after one entry.				
Multiple-dose vials are dated with the beyond-use date of within 28 days (or shorted date if appropriate).				
The current formulary is present and can be located by a nurse.				
Only current (with 2 years) reference books are present.				
Saline syringes are appropriately stored.				
The necessary changes have been made since the last inspection. Note:				

IV = intravenous; MAR = medication administration record.

CORRECTIVE ACTIONS FOR ANY "NO"

_____

_____

_____

_____   _____

Pharmacy signature/date   Care unit signature/date

Appendix 6-A, continued

MEDICATION AREA INSPECTION—CLINICS

Location _____ Month/Year _____

	YES	NO	N/A	REMARKS
STOCK MEDICATIONS				
Only authorized medications are present. (There is no excess stock, unauthorized storage areas, or unidentified patient medications.)				
All medications are locked.				
Medications in treatment rooms are locked.				
Medications to be returned to pharmacy are in the authorized location.				
All medications are within their expiration or beyond-use date. (Check bulk supplies, refrigerator, etc.)				
Internal and external bulk stock is separated.				
MEDICATION PREPARATION AREA				
Medication preparation area is clean, neat, and well organized.				
IV preparation area is clean, uncluttered, and functionally separate.				
SAMPLE MEDICATIONS				
Sample cabinet/room is locked and accessible only to licensed individuals in the practice.				
Log is complete (check two items).				
Samples present reflect appropriate medications for type of practice.				
No controlled substances are present.				
All medications are within their expiration date.				
CONTROLLED SUBSTANCES				
Controlled substance records are complete. (Check count for two items.)				
Wastage is appropriately documented.				
REFRIGERATOR				
Refrigerator temperature is between 36°F and 46°F. Note temperature:				
Freezer temperature is between –13°F and 14°F. Note temperature: Note freezer drugs:				
Refrigerators/freezers containing vaccines are monitored constantly or checked twice a day.				
Refrigerator is clean.				

	YES	NO	N/A	REMARKS
Freezer is free from frost.				
High/low thermometer is properly reset.				
Refrigerator and freezer logs are complete for every day this month.				
Only drugs are stored in the refrigerator and freezer. (No food, lab reagents or specimens are allowed.)				
MISCELLANEOUS				
Single-dose vials are destroyed after one entry.				
Multiple-dose vials are dated with beyond-use date within 28 days (or shorted date if appropriate).				
Saline syringes are appropriately stored.				
The necessary changes have been made since the last inspection. Note:				

CORRECTIVE ACTIONS FOR ANY "NO"

_____

_____

_____

_____

_____   _____

Pharmacy signature/date   Clinic signature/date

Source: Adapted with permission from Uselton JP, Kienle PC, Murdaugh LB. _Assuring Continuous Compliance with Joint Commission Standards: A Pharmacy Guide._ 8th ed. Bethesda, MD: American Society of Health-System Pharmacists; © 2010:385-386.

Appendix 6-B

Medication Management Mock Survey Tracer

Follow Administered Medication Through Medication-Use Process

Element/Question	Resource	Yes	No	If No, Explanation	Action Plan
Prescribing					
Authorized prescriber?	P/P				
Ordering criteria followed?	P/P				
Complete order, no abbreviations					
If order set, approved and in-date					
If verbal order, meets criteria for use					
High-alert requirements followed if applies	P/P				
Patient information accessed used for medication (e.g., INR for warfarin)	P/P, medical record				
Diagnosis, condition, or indication for use documented	Medical record				
Procurement/Storage					
Medication on formulary	Formulary				
If not on formulary, NF policy followed	P/P				
If medication shortage: Evidence of communication Policy followed	Documents, P/P				
Medication stored at proper temperature/light	mfr, P/P				
Medication storage is secure	P/P				

Element/Question	Resource	Yes	No	If No, Explanation	Action Plan
Most ready-to-administer dosage form?	mfr, formulary				
If patient's own medication, stored per P/P	P/P				
If high-alert medication, requirements followed	P/P				
Pharmacist Review					
Review completed prior to dispensing or removal from ADC If not, exception criteria met?	PIS, P/P				
Any concerns regarding allergy, interactions, dose/route/frequency, duplications, contraindications, lab values	Reviewer, PIS				
If order was clarified, documentation exists Clarified directly with prescriber if appropriate	PIS, medical record, P/P				
If manual entry, transcription accurate	PIS, medical record				
If manual entry, two patient identifiers used	Observation				
Scheduled appropriately	P/P, eMAR				
Dispensing/Medication Preparation					
If ADC, fill process per P/P	P/P				
If sterile product, follows all standards	USP <797>, NIOSH, P/P, CDC Safe Injection Practice				
If high-alert medication, P/P followed	P/P				
If on hazardous substance list, P/P followed	P/P				
Product labeled appropriately	P/P, TJC				

Appendix 6-B, continued

Element/Question	Resource	Yes	No	If No, Explanation	Action Plan
Unit dose?	Product				
Ready-to-use form?	Product				
Administration					
Administered by authorized person?	P/P				
MAR accurate?	MAR				
Administered according to schedule or prn indication	MAR				
Observed administration process follows established process, including: ■ Two-patient identifiers ■ Barcode drug, patient wrist band ■ Correct medication verified prior to administration ■ Correct medication preparation, if required (for example, dilution) ■ Hold parameters followed if applicable	Observation, P/P, MAR				
Patient education completed	Observation, medical record, P/P				
Monitoring					
Documentation of patient response	Medical record				
If error occurred during process, was it reported?	P/P risk report system				

Element/Question	Resource	Yes	No	If No, Explanation	Action Plan
If ADR occurred, was it reported?	P/P, risk report system				

ADC = automated dispensing cabinets; CDC = Centers for Disease Control and Prevention; eMAR = electronic medication administration record; INR = international normalized ratio; MAR = medication administration record; mfr = manufacturer; NIOSH = National Institute for Occupational Safety and Health; NF = nonformulary; PIS = pharmacy information system; P/P = policy and procedure; prn = as needed; TJC = The Joint Commission; USP = United States Pharmacopeia.

Source: Adapted with permission from Larson CM, Saine D. *Medication Safety Officer's Handbook.* Bethesda, MD: American Society of Health-System Pharmacists; © 2013 117-120.

CHAPTER 7

Human Resources and People Management

Jennifer Burnette

KEY TERMS

Crucial Conversation—A discussion between two or more people where (1) stakes are high, (2) opinions vary, and (3) emotions run strong.

Emotional Intelligence—Skill in perceiving, understanding, and managing emotions and feelings whether your own or others.

Employee Assistance Program (EAP)—Voluntary, work-based program that offers free and confidential assessments, short-term counseling, referrals, and follow-up services to employees who have personal and/or work-related problems.

Employee Engagement—The extent to which employees feel passionate about their jobs, are committed to the organization, and put discretionary effort into their work.

Fair Labor Standards Act (FLSA)—Act that prescribes standards for wages and overtime pay, which affect most private and public employment. This act requires employers to pay covered employees, who are not otherwise exempt, at least the federal minimum wage and overtime pay of 1½-times the regular rate of pay. Exempt or nonexempt status depends on salary level, salary basis, and job duties.[1]

Family and Medical Leave Act (FMLA)—Act requires employers of 50 or more employees to provide up to 12 weeks of unpaid, job-protected leave to eligible employees for the birth or adoption of a child or for the serious illness of the employee or a spouse, child, or parent.

Introduction

Be Intentional

These words were continuously spoken by my coach when training for a triathlon with the Leukemia & Lymphoma Society team. Completing an Olympic-distance triathlon required both physical and mental strength. As I physically participated in each training session, my coach pointed out that she could see a decline in my performance when my mind was wandering compared to when I was solely focused on the task at hand. When these instances were noticed, she would tell me to "Be Intentional" in both my thoughts and actions in that moment. This served as a reminder to refocus my thoughts on the task at hand to produce the best result possible. Repeating this process many times helped me consistently align my thoughts and actions. Just like my coach, a clinical coordinator likely has a team to engage, motivate, and lead. I urge you to "Be Intentional" in all your actions and words to create a positive learning culture and engage your team in aligning and achieving the goals that support high-quality patient care. This chapter provides scenarios to learn from and tools to help you lead your team.

Getting Started

As a pharmacist, you are already well versed in medication-related laws. However, as a new coordinator who likely has supervisory responsibilities, it is imperative to have a baseline understanding of labor laws and how they apply to your direct reports. Acronyms such as **FLSA (Fair Labor Standards Act)**, **EAP (Employee Assistance Program)**, and **FMLA (Family and Medical Leave Act)** are part of the U.S. Department of Labor regulations to familiarize yourself with in the first 90 days of your new role. Schedule time with your supervisor or human resources (HR) representative to better understand how these laws and specific policies and procedures at your institution affect your direct reports. Here is a list of questions to ask:

- Are my direct reports exempt (hourly) or nonexempt (salaried)?
- What is our policy on overtime?
- What is the process to compensate employees for overtime work?
- What is our policy on working from home?
- How do my direct reports support other areas of our department? Or other departments?
- Do any of my direct reports currently have FMLA?
- When should I recommend EAP and/ or FMLA?

FMLA allows employees to balance their work and family life by taking reasonable unpaid leave for certain family and medical reasons. FMLA seeks to accomplish these purposes in a manner that accommodates the legitimate interests of employers and minimizes the potential for employment discrimination on the basis of gender, while promoting equal employment opportunity for men and women.[2] Below is a list of questions to ask your HR representative or FMLA administrator:

- How many hours or months must an employee work to be eligible for FMLA?
- How many weeks of unpaid leave can be granted to an eligible employee?
- What are the reasons or qualifying conditions for which FMLA may be approved?
- What is the institution's policy on substituting paid leave for an employee to continue receiving pay during unpaid FMLA leave?
- What is the institution's policy regarding maintenance of health benefits for unpaid FMLA leave when an employee receives benefits through the employer's group health insurance coverage?

The most challenging aspect of FMLA's impact to day-to-day functions is intermittent leave where an employee provides notice of absence the same day he or she is scheduled to work. A survey report by the Society for Human Resource Management revealed challenges including chronic abuse of intermittent leave by employees, morale problems with employees asked to cover for absent employees, and costs associated with lost productivity.[3] One option for fulfilling service needs during an intermittent FMLA absence may be to transition the employee to an area where work can be absorbed by existing or pool employees. There may be unforeseen barriers that your HR representative or FMLA administrator can help you address when determining the best coverage plan to maintain pharmacy services while employees are on leave. Although it is helpful to understand the general aspects of FMLA, it is important to identify the appropriate contact persons, such as the benefits office or FMLA administrator, to direct employees for more specific guidance regarding their individual situations. There are several qualifying conditions, such as the birth of a child, where there is a relatively new portion of the 2010 Patient Protection and Affordable Care Act (Affordable Care Act). Employers are required to provide a reasonable break time and place, other than a bathroom, for an employee to express breast milk for her nursing child for 1 year after the child's birth each time such employee has need to express milk. Similar to learning pharmacy law, learning the basics about the laws and regulations governing employees is important to your success as a coordinator. Remember to use your resources and seek guidance from your HR representative or FMLA administrator.

Recruit the Right Behaviors and Actions

Another important support person to meet is your recruiter. Schedule an introduction with your recruiter and ask for the specific criteria as to how candidates are identified. In collaboration with your recruiter, fellow leaders, and employees, develop a set of characteristics or qualities that a competitive candidate should exhibit. This exercise is quickly becoming a standard and often includes a section where the candidate completes a personality test or predictive index test prior to interviewing. Predictive index is a science-based assessment that provides managers with accurate, actionable data, which quantify the unique motivating needs and behavioral drives of each employee and potential employee.[4] The test serves as a comparison of the applicant to the ideal candidate, thus giving the employer a more objective method to determining whether the organization and the role is a good fit for the applicant. This is an opportunity to discuss and agree to criteria that will allow the recruiter to support you by screening for ideal candidates.

Discuss with your recruiter where to post advertisements about employment opportunities based on the type of position and whether the position should be posted internally or both internally and externally. It is important to recruit internally to promote career advancement opportunities among employees at your institution. Even if you are not aware of anyone in your institution that is interested or even a good fit for the position, you may be surprised. For example, Jill is an evening shift pharmacist, who reports to a different coordinator in your institution, and she applies for a day shift critical care clinical pharmacist position. Upon interviewing Jill, you learn that she completed five critical care rotations as a pharmacy practice resident and a quality improvement project to reduce delirium in critically ill patients, but she was not able to pursue a specialty residency in critical care. She explains that she would like to continue her career growth specifically in critical care and is currently participating in one of the department's initiatives related to this area of practice. Although Jill lacks the critical care specialty residency, her attitude, past experiences, and current involvement in critical care initiatives that she may be a good fit for your new role.

When discussing where to post positions externally, consider the type of role you are recruiting for and where the best candidate pool can be found. For example, if recruiting for a midnight pharmacist position, consider contacting local state societies. If recruiting for a pharmacist specializing in antimicrobial stewardship, consider contacting infectious diseases residency training programs and national professional societies such as ASHP and ACCP. Also, establish a personal network of pharmacists whom you trust and value as they may be a good resource for finding quality candidates. This often facilitates timely identification of talented candidates. Consider recruiting former residents that may be a good fit for the role and your institution.

Lastly, employers commonly ask for reference persons to complete a behavioral-based survey about the applicant. After you identify the recruitment strategies at your institution, work with your recruiter to develop a template for the applicant's interview day and an evaluation tool. Determine who will provide the applicant with directions and lodging information, greet the applicant, transfer the applicant between interviews, take the applicant to lunch, and close the day with the applicant. As an applicant, you may have experienced the unfortunate situation of not being provided adequate information for an interview, being left alone for lunch, or having multiple persons not show up for the interview. How did that make you feel? Unimportant? Not worth the person's time? This is typically the applicant's first experience at your institution, and you want the applicant to complete the interview process with a positive first impression. If you have time constraints, let your recruiter know who the applicant must interview with for both the applicant and the employer to gain enough insight to make an informed decision. It is imperative that applicants meet employees that they will work closely with on a daily basis. Depending on the culture and norms at your institution, this may be a formal interview session or an informal discussion among peers. Also, identify key information you need to know about an applicant to make an informed decision.

Sample of Focused, Behavioral-Based Interview Questions

Assess Prioritization

1. I am going to give you three situations, and I want you to list them in order of highest priority to lowest priority.

   a. A medical resident contacts you and states that his patient received 1 g intravenous (IV) cefepime instead of 1 g IV ceftriaxone yesterday in the emergency department; the patient is doing fine today.

   b. A nurse contacts you regarding a stat order for a dopamine infusion for a patient in the intensive care unit.

   c. A nurse contacts you for a missing metronidazole dose.

Assess Customer Service and Service Recovery

1. Judy, a nurse at your institution, calls you for the third time regarding a missing vancomycin dose due 2 hours ago. What is your response to Judy and your follow-up action(s)?

2. Describe a time where a prescriber disagreed with your recommendation. How did you respond and what was the outcome?

3. Tell us about a time when a prescriber requested a medication that was not on the formulary and how you handled the situation.

Assess Interpersonal Skills

1. What is the single greatest contribution you have made in your present (or most recent) position?[5]

2. What is something you have recommended or tried in your present (or most recent) position that did not work? What was the follow-up and final outcome?

3. Describe a time where you provided incorrect information to someone and how did you correct the situation?

4. What are you looking for in your next position that has been lacking in your previous positions?

Success in caring for patients is heavily dependent on proactive communication and collaborative problem solving. Asking the right questions is essential to assessing the candidate's ability to communicate and resolve issues. Using targeted, behavioral-based questions is likely to quickly reveal whether or not the candidate will be successful in the role and with the team.

Compensation, Benefits, and Pay for Performance

The main reasons employees leave their job are related to dissatisfaction with their supervisor, pay, or schedule. Contact your HR representative or compensation liaison to ask the following questions to gain a baseline understanding of compensation and benefits as they relate to your employees.

- *How is compensation determined?*

  Rationale: Understand how many years of experience residencies account for and how compensation varies for the bachelor degree versus the doctoral degree.

- *How often are compensation/salary surveys completed?*

  Rationale: Understand when the last survey was completed and the results; identify whether current salaries are competitive with the local market and both local and national roles that have the same job responsibilities.

- *When does health insurance commence for new employees?*

  Rationale: Commencement of health insurance varies from the first day of employment to completion of the first 90 days of employment. This may also depend if the position is exempt or nonexempt status. Knowing this information will help you recommend alternatives to potential candidates and prevent this from being a barrier to hiring a candidate.

- *What options are available for flexible schedules, telecommuting, and childcare?*

  Rationale: Employees today view these options as benefits that promote a better work–life balance. In 2013, 56% of pharmacists were women.[6] The majority of women in the workplace are working mothers and desire flexibility and childcare availability at their place of employment. Additionally, many fathers desire the same work–life balance opportunities.

- *What reimbursement is available for obtaining degrees and certifications (e.g., board-certified pharmacotherapy specialist and immunization administration certification)?*

  Rationale: Institutions vary from those that pay for certifications directly pertaining to the employee's job function to not paying for any certification. Additional educational degree reimbursement also varies across institutions.

- *How is performance assessed and rewarded at our institution?*

  Rationale: Many institutions are abandoning the traditional bell curve approach to performance management, which diminishes the value of high performers and pushes many middle-of-the-road performers into the bottom. Pay for performance in the context of the individual employee involves assessing the employee's annual performance and providing merit pay, an increase in base pay, which remains part of the employee's base salary for the rest of his or her tenure with the institution. Current trends in performance management include making behaviors and actions account for the majority of an employee's overall score and separating performance scores from compensation, thus engaging managers to provide continuous coaching and feedback to improve performance and compensating employees on results achieved.

Become a Self-Aware Leader

From the first day of pharmacy school, your focus has been on patients and serving their healthcare needs. Whether it was counseling an individual patient or implementing a drug-dosing service for your institution, patients have been at the center of your actions. This chapter indirectly focuses on impacting patient care by serving your employees' needs using Greenleaf's philosophy of servant leadership. A servant leader focuses primarily on the growth and well-being of people, while traditional leadership generally involves one person's accumulation and exercise of power at the top of the pyramid.[7] The servant leader empowers others by placing the needs of others first and helping them develop and perform as highly as possible. By choosing to implement the strategies described in this chapter, you will provide the necessary leadership resulting in more engaged and satisfied employees. Engaged employees provide better customer service to patients in addition to internal colleagues such as nurses, providers, and respiratory therapists. The outcome is increased patient satisfaction as well as internal satisfaction with the pharmacy department's services.[8]

"Know Thyself"—*Thales of Miletus, Greek Philosopher*

It is important that you identify your **emotional intelligence** as well as your strengths and weaknesses and understand how to apply them in your new role. Emotional intelligence involves self-awareness, management of emotions, empathy, people skills, and motivation.[9] Publications that can help you with this process include *Emotional Intelligence: Why It Can Matter More Than IQ*; *Now, Discover Your Strengths*; and *Strengthsfinder 2.0*.[10-12] You may already have 360-degree feedback or strength-finder objectives as part of your organization's performance management process. If not, consider asking a person in your organization with whom you worked closely and trust to provide honest feedback. Do not be offended if the feedback is brutally honest! Better yet, harness your emotion into becoming a better leader. Consider asking your employees what three characteristics they want to see in their formal leader. Common characteristics include being consistent, fair, and valuing the employee's perspective. Your success in leading your team hinges on your ability to exhibit these characteristics in your new role. Additionally, maintaining open communication and approaching situations with composure and integrity will build trust with employees.

Consider the Following Scenarios

A. You tend to become annoyed and short with your employees when they bring a problem to you. Thus, your employees avoid engaging you when they do have problems. However, you now receive panicked and frustrated emails and phone calls from nursing and physician leaders regarding pharmacy service issues.

B. You count to 10 in your head to avoid becoming angry when your employees bring problems to you. You ask your employees what solutions they have considered and discuss how to solve the problem. Nursing and physician leaders now express thanks to you for their pharmacist who helps resolve pharmacy-related concerns. Everyone wins—you, the employee, the pharmacy team, nurses, physicians, and the patient!

To find out more about how you respond to different stressors, refer to an excerpt of the first 10 questions from the Your Style Under Stress Test (**Figure 7-1**) from VitalSmarts. The full version of the assessment can be accessed at www.vitalsmarts.com.

After completing the assessment, you will be presented with a score that indicates how likely you are to move toward silence (masking, avoiding, or withdrawing) or violence (controlling, labeling, or attacking) during a **crucial conversation**. In *Crucial Conversations*, the authors explain that using these techniques is not a bad thing; it means we are human. Refer to *Crucial Conversations* for a list of tools to help avoid pitfalls and communicate more effectively and with confidence in the face of conflict.[13]

Set the Right Tone

Achieving better outcomes is the result of creating a culture that engages employees to perform at their best, promotes accountability for one's own behaviors and actions, and encourages an open and safe learning environment. Here are three practice tips you can implement immediately to begin building this type of culture:

1. Make introductions
2. Set ground rules
3. Lead by example

Introduce yourself and genuinely greet everyone. Learn their names and use their names when you see them. Meet with your direct reports individually to provide a brief background of yourself, express enthusiasm for the team, and ask three questions to promote a positive feeling about the future.

1. What is your favorite part of your role?
2. What keeps you working here as opposed to working for another institution?
3. What two things do you think our team/department does really well?

By establishing a positive personal connection initially, your employees are more likely to see you as approachable and seek your guidance.

When you start your new role, have your team participate in developing the ground rules. Your team will have a stake in defining the rules and will be more likely to uphold them. You can even use the following speech when you hold your first team meeting, "I understand and appreciate how passionate you are about what you do, and when we meet I expect to see you share new ideas and challenge each other to

FIGURE 7-1. Your Style Under Stress Test

T	F	I avoid situations that might bring me into contact with people I am having problems with.
T	F	I put off returning phone calls or emails because I simply do not want to deal with the person who sent them.
T	F	Sometimes when people bring up a touchy or awkward issue, I try to change the subject.
T	F	When it comes to dealing with awkward or stressful subjects, sometimes I hold back rather than give my full and candid opinion.
T	F	Rather than tell people exactly what I think, sometimes I rely on jokes, sarcasm, or snide remarks to let them know I am frustrated.
T	F	When I have something tough to bring up, sometimes I offer weak or insincere compliments to soften the blow.
T	F	To get my point across, I sometimes exaggerate my side of the argument.
T	F	If I seem to be losing control of a conversation, I might cut people off or change the subject to bring it back to where I think it should be.
T	F	When others make points that seem stupid to me, I sometimes let them know it without holding back.
T	F	When I am stunned by a comment, sometimes I say things that others might take as forceful or attacking—comments such as "Give me a break!" or "That's ridiculous!"
T	F	Sometimes when things get heated, I move from arguing against others' points to saying things that might hurt them personally.

Source: Reprinted with permission of VitalSmarts, LC., Provo, Utah (www.vitalsmarts.com). May not be further reproduced without the express written consent of VitalSmarts, LC.

help our department do better for our patients. With that said, we need to set some ground rules to maintain a healthy work environment and respect for each other."

Examples of Ground Rules

- No one should say "that is stupid" or "that will not work"; instead say "I am not clear on how that will work, can you explain further?"
- Do not interrupt the person speaking.
- If someone goes off on a tangent, tell them the idea will be placed in the "parking lot" (issues and topics to be discussed at a later date) and to stay on the current topic.
- Seek to understand; avoid assumptions.

You may recall a time where a fellow employee inquired about a decision you made regarding a patient's medication. Did the employee ask you in an open-ended, nonthreatening manner? Or was it asked in a more accusatorial "What did you do?" manner? You probably have experienced both scenarios in your career and prefer the open-ended, nonthreatening approach. As the formal leader, you want to disregard preconceived ideas or negative past experiences and focus on gathering the facts and understanding the situation before drawing conclusions.

Case Example 1

Gathering the Facts

You are contacted by Dr. Gibson, who is irate about his patient receiving two forms of pharmacological venous thromboembolism prophylaxis, subcutaneous heparin started on admission, and enoxaparin started 1 day after admission. He is very influential in your organization and tells you that your pharmacist is incompetent and asks how you could let an incompetent individual work in your department. You listen and reply that you will investigate it with the pharmacist involved and identify any action plans to prevent it from happening again. You ask if his patient is okay, to which he replies, "Yes, the patient is fine."

What Is Your Response?

A. *After investigating, you see that the pharmacist involved bypassed the duplicate anticoagulant alert when verifying orders. You are angry over this situation and the fact that Dr. Gibson took out his anger on you. Thus, you are not calm and raise your voice when discussing this event with the pharmacist involved. You also tell him that you will be forced to start the discipline process if this happens again.*

B. *Despite bypassing the duplicate anticoagulant alert, you assume positive intent and in a calm voice, you approach the pharmacist about the event. You ask him what happened and how this error may be avoided in the future.*

Response A reveals that Dr. Gibson transferred his anger to you, and now you are transferring your anger to the pharmacist involved. Disrespectful behaviors are all too common in healthcare, and they are detrimental to your ability to communicate and collaborate effectively with others.[14] This behavior disrupts the trust between you and your employee and prevents collaboration, communication, and teamwork.[15] The pharmacist involved now feels threatened and becomes defensive and angry. Thus, the communication line is severed, and you have not made any progress toward identifying the root cause of this event and developing an action plan to prevent it from recurring.

Response B shows that although this is very serious and the pharmacist may need performance improvement, you first want to understand the pharmacist's thought process before making a decision. During this discussion, the pharmacist says the duplicate anticoagulant alert was bypassed because this alert always fires when a patient is on a heparin infusion and is started on enoxaparin or warfarin for overlap therapy. The pharmacist asks if the alert

can be customized or somehow changed to only alert when it is clinically significant. Together, you determine that this action plan will need information technology support. In addition to a system change, you also discuss the importance of consistently following a process to carefully screen the profile for duplicate therapies when verifying orders. The pharmacist acknowledges the mistake and agrees to fully assess alerts rather than assuming the alert is not relevant. You document the conversation and guide the employee to submit a customized alert request to the clinical informatics team. Remember to close the loop by letting the provider (in this case, Dr. Gibson) know the action plan. In some situations, you can empower the pharmacist involved in the error to contact the provider to close the loop. This is an example of a crucial conversation, which is considered successful because you counseled the pharmacist in a nonthreatening and productive manner, keeping two-way communication intact and arriving at an action plan that will help prevent future errors.

When setting the right tone, aim to be consistent and objective when making decisions and have the conversation as soon as possible. The issue will only get worse if you do not address it immediately. It may be scary to you or make you very nervous to approach someone to have a crucial conversation, but if you do not you may miss an opportunity to enhance patient safety and lose the respect of the other employees (if they know about the situation). This will take practice, but with experience you will become more comfortable in knowing how to respond. Remember that your HR department is an excellent resource to assist you in resolving issues.

Case Example 2

Consistency and Objectivity

Janine asks you if she can work every fifth weekend instead of every fourth weekend because her husband now has to work weekends and she is having trouble finding childcare for her three children. She tells you how tough it is to raise three children when both parents work full time and one child has a learning disability.

First, if you have children you may empathize with how challenging it can be to juggle work and parenting responsibilities. If you do not have children, you may sympathize with the fact your employee is presented with a stressful personal challenge. Consider if any employees in Janine's peer group do not work weekends. If so, get the details to help guide your decision; if not, create a pros-and-cons list of Janine working weekends versus not working weekends.

■ **Option 1.** Janine continues to work weekends.

Pros—Maintain consistency among job responsibilities within Janine's peer group so staffing levels remain consistent.

Cons—Janine may be dissatisfied but understanding (best), disgruntled, or angry (worst).

■ **Option 2.** Janine does not work weekends.

Pros—Janine is satisfied.

Cons—Staffing levels may no longer be consistent on the weekends so you may have to pay overtime to cover the weekend opening or another pharmacist may have to work more weekends; inconsistency among the peer group as to how job requirements are applied; Janine's peers will see the inconsistency and may think it is unfair.

Early in your clinical coordinator role, it often helps to discuss your thought process and decisions with your supervisor so that you both develop trust and an understanding of how each other solves problems. Initially, this takes time, but in the long run it will prove valuable as your supervisor will trust you to make appropriate decisions independently.

What Is Your Decision?

A. You approve the request. Janine is going through a tough time; as a parent, you can understand the challenges and you want to help.

B. You do nothing. You listen to Janine and let her know that it might be an option, but you are not sure right now.

C. You deny the request. You tell Janine that all pharmacists work every fourth weekend, and it would not be consistent or fair to the group to change her to every fifth weekend.

Decision A will set a new precedent among your team. You can guarantee when the staff find out that her weekend schedule changed, they too will request changes. Then you will have to decide who to deny and who to allow. Even worse, what if you decide to deny employees who do not have children and they feel discriminated against because they do not have children? Decision B is your way to avoid making a decision that may not be favorable to either Janine or her colleagues. You realize that denying the request will upset Janine while approving the request will upset the team, so you choose not to make a decision. Your inaction is also a decision. If you choose to avoid these types of situations, you should question whether or not you are a good fit for a formal leadership role managing people. Decision C maintains objectivity and consistency; a crucial conversation is necessary with Janine. At the meeting, it is important to acknowledge that her situation sounds very stressful and recommend employee assistance or ask if she has a friend or relative who can help her during this time.

Now, adding to Janine's situation, consider what decision you would make if Janine was the highest-performing pharmacist on your team versus the lowest-performing pharmacist. You could easily be influenced to do everything possible to keep the highest-performing pharmacist, yet do nothing to keep the lowest one. If you uphold consistency and deny Janine's request, you should still offer help as mentioned above. It is also appropriate to encourage Janine to approach her peer group for ideas or suggestions. In a previous organization I encountered a situation where the peer group agreed to two pharmacists working every other weekend because it met their work–life balance needs and allowed them to work fewer weekends. As their leader, I agreed to their plan in addition to communicating and documenting that if either of the two pharmacists needed to switch back to every fourth weekend, the request would be granted because the baseline job requirement was to work every fourth weekend.

Here's another question to ask, "Am I applying the criteria consistently in an objective manner?" You can equate it to formulary decision making. Formulary decisions result from three primary criteria: efficacy, safety, and cost, which are rarely in perfect balance, so the pros and cons are weighed before arriving at a final decision. The three criteria used for personnel decisions can be how it impacts the institution, how it impacts pharmacy services, and how it impacts the team. Although you do not need to communicate your decision's rationale, it often helps the *team digest and more readily accept the impact of the decision.*

Case Example 3

Foster Teamwork

Valerie, the most junior team member identifies and reports medication errors related to the use of novel oral anticoagulants. She brings this to your attention along with literature supporting an idea to implement an anticoagulation stewardship. Valerie is not aware that two senior clinical pharmacists, Iesha and Dave, developed and proposed an anticoagulation stewardship program, which for the past 2 years was denied budget approval due to lack of financial support. Thus, additional resources were not provided, and Iesha and Dave are hesitant to accept new responsibilities to their current workload. You explain this to Valerie, and she replies that she wants to pilot only one aspect of the program, which is to perform a daily review of all patients prescribed novel oral anticoagulants. She will even look at the patients on the weekends during the pilot timeframe.

- **Option 1.** *You are excited to have Valerie who is enthusiastic and fresh compared to Iesha and Dave who have been in their roles for many years and do not show any interest in taking on new work. You give her approval to present her data in a month. Although you did not consciously realize it at the time, this decision may pit Valerie against Iesha and Dave and create competition. It could be healthy competition, but it could also divide the team and lead to unhealthy conflict.*

- **Option 2.** *You reiterate a team approach and ask Valerie to schedule a meeting to discuss pilot details with you, Iesha, and Dave. Valerie will bring new enthusiasm to the group. Iesha and Dave recognize the scope and bring their experience to the group. You meet, set expectations, and have the team agree on the pilot's three goals. Then you leave the team to work out the details of breaking the project into manageable components. At this point, you must assess the situation and give Valerie the opportunity to stand her ground with Iesha and Dave, who must realize that it is not an option to refuse change that could*

have a positive impact on patients. To help Iesha and Dave, ask them to list three tasks that could be completed by another staff member. Review the list and help them prioritize and shift responsibilities as necessary. For example, Dave is the pharmacy residency program director, so he has several administrative tasks. This is a great opportunity for a pharmacist interested in becoming a residency program director to gain experience. Now that Dave is not responsible for those tasks, he can focus on the pilot.

Case Example 4

Emotional Intelligence

Let's revisit emotional intelligence and how you can apply it in everyday situations. Just because you are now in a formal leadership role does not mean you must solve all problems. You must avoid taking on your employees' emotions and issues as your own.[16] For personal problems, often employees just need someone to listen, so let them talk. Remind them that work–life balance and being content with their personal life plays an important part in job satisfaction. Refer them to an employee assistance program, or encourage them to reach out to a trusted family member or friend for support. Get to know your employees. If a family member is sick or an employee took a personal day to attend a child's school celebration, then make sure to ask the employee about it. If this approach does not come naturally to you, then you must make a genuine effort to develop a personal repertoire with your team members. In the words of a former supervisor, "You do not have to be friends, but you do have to be friendly." This goes back to valuing your employees not only as pharmacists but as people too.

Sometimes, you are the one with emotions running high, so it is essential to be aware of how you express yourself when speaking with your employees. For example, you are about to take vacation leave and you just found out that an employee is going to be out unexpectedly, so you are rapidly trying to find coverage for openings in the schedule. You run out of options, so you contact another employee, Jeff, who is on leave because you want him to cover the next day's schedule. You explain what has happened and that you could really use extra help, but Jeff responds by saying he took these past few days off because his mother just had surgery, and he is helping to care for her. Because you are ultra-focused on covering those holes, you fail to recognize that Jeff is trying to tell you indirectly that he really cannot cover tomorrow. This scenario can end up going two ways: (1) Jeff uses more direct language and tells you, "No, I am not available tomorrow," or (2) Jeff feels he must work or you will hold it against him. This is intimidation although you never specifically told him he had to cover. Be mindful of the situation, and consider how you may feel if you were in the employee's shoes.

A leader's ability to laugh and lighten the mood when appropriate will relieve some of the workplace tension and will help your team to remain optimistic and continue their efforts. The time and effort you spend to set the right tone will reward you many times over in the future. Although problems arise and there is rarely one solution, establishing consistent ground rules, being approachable, and leading by example will empower your employees to address and resolve problems on their own. When employees are consistently exposed to this culture, they will know what you expect and have confidence to implement solutions independently.

"What You Allow Is What Will Continue"—Unknown

Accountability is part of setting the right tone. When beginning your new role, start building a culture of accountability immediately by holding yourself accountable for communicating expectations clearly and frequently. Work with your team to identify and agree on the best forms of communication. For example, they may send you long emails when you prefer to receive a page or text message and to follow up with a spoken conversation. You may prefer to send individual emails for different topics, whereas the team finds the numerous emails overwhelming and admits to not reading them. Two examples to facilitate timely and clear communication are 10-minute daily huddles and weekly huddle emails.

Collaborate with your operational pharmacy services colleague to communicate both clinical and operational information together. For example, drug shortages require clinicians to identify and recommend alternatives whereas the operational team executes the plan with the physical product. **Figure 7-2** describes the details of the 10-minute daily huddles. One crucial piece is to assign a timekeeper or bring a stop watch to adhere to the 10-minute timeframe. It is vital that time is respected for both the employee and the manager for two main reasons: (1) showing respect for your employees' time builds mutual respect among you and your direct reports; and (2) staying focused on the day's priorities and minimizing hour-long discussions about everything that is wrong or needs to be fixed. **Figure 7-3** is an example of a weekly huddle email where all pertinent information is copied into one email, and employees are directed to read this email weekly. Identify a person in your department, such as an administrative assistant, pharmacy resident, or pharmacist willing to take on the communicative responsibility to organize and send the weekly email. In the beginning, have the organizer submit the draft email to both you and your operations colleague to validate the information. This is a great way to identify inconsistencies. For example, a pharmacy technician submits a reminder on how to prepare the esomeprazole IV infusions. You recognize that your team recently recommended switching from intermittent infusions to IV push administration to better meet patient needs and nursing workflow; thus, the dilution and preparation process has changed. Upon following up, both you and your operations colleague identify and correct a gap in the education about this change. It is also important to identify what is emergent versus good to know that week. Emergent issues require timely face-to-face communication with employees.

Coaching While Rounding

Behaviors and actions are contagious. When your team sees you consistently rounding on individuals and reinforcing expectations and rewarding the right behaviors and actions, they will follow. This will help keep the right employees "on the bus," and allow you to reinforce accountability and take action when you encounter situations where performance improvement plans, disciplinary actions, and termination are necessary. Here are five questions to ask when rounding for outcomes[8]:

FIGURE 7-2. 10-Minute Daily Huddles

Why: *Quickly share crucial information for your shift*

Who: *All pharmacy staff*

What:

- **Are there any call-outs for the next 24 hours?**

    (e.g., call-out for evening shift, thus workload will transition to day shift restocking the IV room)

- **What shortages and resulting recommendations for the day?**

    (e.g., ketorolac IV—restrict IV formulation to those who absolutely cannot tolerate PO formulation; switch others to PO formulation. Although bioavailability of PO formulation is 100%, dosing of PO formulation is as follows and NOT EQUIVALENT to IV formulation. Route of PO formulation: 20 mg, followed by 10 mg q 4–6 hr prn; do not exceed 40 mg PO daily.)

- **Any significant actual/near-miss medication errors in the past 24 to 48 hours?**

    (e.g., wrong amount of PO furosemide dispensed, wrong concentration of isoproterenol dispensed)

- **Any patients with specific/atypical medication needs?**

    (e.g., Flolan patient on home pump currently in ED, oncology patient on extremely high doses of Dilaudid basal infusion and PCA demand dose)

When and Where: 0700 and 1500 daily in main pharmacy

ED = emergency department; IV = intravenous; PCA = patient-controlled analgesia; PO = by mouth, orally.

---

1. What is working well today?
2. Are there any individuals whom I should be recognizing?
3. Are there any physicians or ancillary services that I should be recognizing?
4. Is there anything we can do better?
5. Do you have the tools and equipment to do your job?

Bush and Walesh remind us that coaching is accomplished intermittently during the course of ongoing projects and activities. It is not a separate training activity or a scheduled meeting time; therefore, during daily duties watch for specific coaching opportunities that will take the employee up the "soft-side" skills learning curve.[17] Employees usually need to be told and shown by example how to blend clinical and soft-side abilities to achieve personal and organizational goals.[18]

Engaged Employees = Better Outcomes

Engaged employees are accountable and take ownership of their role and environment. Studies have shown that employee satisfaction is linked to increased positive outcomes.[19] Another study suggested employees who are not engaged are more likely to work around safety protocols, while highly engaged employees are not.[20] Contact your HR department about your organization's process for assessing and achieving high **employee engagement**. Once you have baseline data, you can begin the analysis and action-planning process. Below are two simple practice tips that improve engagement:

1. ***Listen.*** Use baseline data to develop open-ended questions to ask your team, then ask the questions and listen. Employees are more likely to provide feedback for action planning if they perceive their perspective is

FIGURE 7-3. Weekly Huddle Communications

January 5, 2016

People

Welcome new employees

Service

SBAR—What is it?

Situation, **b**ackground, **a**ssessment, and **r**ecommendation (SBAR) is a structured communication technique designed to convey information in a succinct and brief manner. This is important for patient safety, as we all have different styles of communication (varying by culture, profession, and gender). You will learn more about this communication method in the upcoming weeks.

Quality

Auto Stop Orders—Clarification of Interpretation and Education to Prescribers

Prescriber checks "reorder" if intending to reorder the medication.

If you know for how long, then also fill in the "duration," which would be the additional days from when it expires.

If you do not fill in the duration, then it would be a reorder and default to the pharmacy policy.

Discontinue would be from the last dose that is printed on the sheet unless otherwise specified (d/c now).

Practice Pearl: Tdap or DTaP?

DTaP (Daptacel) order received for an 11-year-old male patient in ED. What do you do?

A.   Verify order and dispense Daptacel.

B.   Contact prescriber to find that patient stepped on a rusty nail. Recommend Tdap (Adacel).

C.   Contact prescriber to find that patient stepped on a rusty nail. Recommend Td vaccine.

ISMP reports mix-ups between DTaP and Tdap resulting in inappropriate immunization. Daptacel is for active immunization in infants and children aged 6 weeks to 6 years. Adacel is indicated for active booster immunization as a single dose in persons aged 11 to 64 years. Per CDC, ACIP guidelines, and our institution antimicrobial stewardship team, Tdap should be recommended. The patient will get the needed tetanus component, and because there is a pertussis outbreak in the community, the patient will benefit from receiving pertussis as well. Recommend choice B, Tdap (Adacel), because the patient should receive a booster for both tetanus and pertussis based on his age and injury. Please contact antimicrobial stewardship pharmacist with questions. (CDC, ACIP recommendations, and ISMP Aug 24, 2006.)

Growth

Two new urgent care centers will open in late August. We will fill their medication totes on Mondays, Wednesdays, and Fridays.

Margin

Congratulations and thank you for everyone's efforts to minimize overtime this past week. We are slightly above our monthly budget due to recent hemophilia admission and high utilization of factor 7.

ACIP = Advisory Committee on Immunization Practices; CDC = Centers for Disease Control and Prevention; ED = emergency department; DTaP = diphtheria, tetanus, and acellular pertussis; ISMP = Institute for Safe Medication Practices; Td = tetanus and diphtheria; Tdap = tetanus, diphtheria, and pertussis.

genuinely valued.[21] Beware of speaking too much or interrupting employees as these actions are perceived as a lack of respect and caring, and employees may decide not to voice their ideas and opinions.

2. **Say "thank you."** Acknowledgment by management and among peers is the quickest way to build trust, restore strained relationships, and energize the workplace. Employees with supportive managers are 1.3 times more likely to stay with the company and are 67% more engaged.[22] Many organizations now provide stationery so leaders can handwrite thank-you notes. Set a goal to handwrite at least one thank-you note per week for a team member's action that exceeds expectations.

Conflict Can Be Productive

Creating a culture of engagement and accountability is the foundation to achieving positive outcomes across all pillars of excellence (people, service, quality, growth, and finance). Although you are doing the right thing in creating this culture, it will force change resulting in conflict. Conflict is simply the recognition and subsequent expression of differences in human relationships.[23] Conflict is uncomfortable, and the discomfort is normal. Be aware of how it impacts your own behaviors and actions. If you find that you have overwhelming fear, anxiety, or tendency to avoid addressing these situations with the employee involved, then ask a trusted colleague, mentor, supervisor, or HR representative for help. HR departments typically offer learning opportunities to help you build confidence in addressing conflict in a productive manner. Other helpful tools are books or journal articles, such as *Crucial Conversations* or "Conflict in the Healthcare Workplace."[9,13] One helpful exercise is to practice the crucial conversation with your supervisor or HR representative. Toby Clark, in his 2013 John W. Webb Lecture, reminded us "the greatest leadership sin is to remain passive in the face of challenges."[24] These challenges are positive conflicts on the road to a more engaged and accountable culture. Failing to address these challenges reinforces the wrong behaviors and halts progress, ultimately leaving both you and your staff frustrated and disengaged. To minimize conflict within a dynamic

environment, communicate clearly and often so expectations are known and fears of the unknown are minimized. You cannot control employees' actions and behaviors. Avoid setting unrealistic expectations of employees and yourself. Your role is to guide, influence, and hold employees accountable for their behavioral choices and actions. Remember, the employee is choosing—consciously or subconsciously—when to exhibit a specific behavior or action. Always discuss these matters in private with the employee involved and avoid any discussion about it with others. Confidentiality is vital to maintaining trust and integrity with your employees.

Case Example 5

Reinforce Expectations

Derek is late every day or does not respond in a timely manner. Ask Derek if everything is going okay. He will likely ask why you are asking. That is your opportunity to state the problem. If he does not ask, then state the following, "I'm glad to hear that everything is good. While reviewing attendance and tardiness, I noticed that you are coming in late, sometimes as much as 30 minutes, on a regular basis. What's going on?"

Derek may immediately state that he will arrive on time, or he may make excuses. If he makes excuses, then let him know that it is an excuse. For example, he may say that traffic is getting worse on his commute. Remind him that failing to arrive on time results in delays of the midnight pharmacists going home, patients may not receive timely care due to his tardiness, and it is his responsibility to leave early enough to arrive on time.

Regardless of how your employees answer, it is vital that you end the conversation by reminding them of your expectations, where they stand in the process, and the consequences if they choose to continue being tardy. Be extremely clear that this is a verbal counseling and that you will follow up with email documentation; if it is a written counseling, remind them that a copy will be sent to them and to HR. Contact your HR representative for specific guidance on your institution's policies and procedures regarding coaching, counseling, and documentation.

Case Example 6

Teach Employees to Fish

Remember the Chinese proverb: Give a man a fish and you feed him for a day. Teach a man to fish and you feed him for a lifetime. Sarah provides information and a recommendation that is not correct. Respond by asking, "Sarah, I'm following up on darbepoetin in a Jehovah's Witness patient in the medical intensive care unit. Can you help me understand what information you looked at and how you arrived at that dose?"

Sarah may or may not become defensive, but odds are that she will still accept your request to explain her thought process. This is your opportunity to identify where Sarah made an error. Ask her if she is aware of literature supporting use of a lower dose. If she is not, suggest reviewing the literature together so you can confirm that she understands what she should recommend in the future.

Case Example 7

Bad Behavior Increases Risk for Bad Outcome

Marcus is negative and unresponsive to others (colleagues, nurses, providers, and technicians). Engage Marcus in a conversation and let him know the following, "I'm glad things are going well today, but I'm concerned because I heard you snap at the technicians earlier today. Your comment about the technicians' laziness and inability to refill the automated dispensing machine correctly was rude and inappropriate. Why did you make that comment?" Or consider the example where the nurse manager contacts you about Marcus' comment to a nurse, "It was brought to my attention that you made a rude comment about a nurse being stupid for asking you how to administer an extended infusion antibiotic. What happened?"

Marcus may become defensive, so do not get drawn into the emotion and stick to the facts. Remind him that his inappropriate behavior impacts his working relationship with the nursing staff who often ask for his advice, and the behavior may dissuade the nurse from approaching him in the future, which could result in a medication error. What if she administers an incorrect dose that harms the patient? Marcus may recognize his mistake and verbalize his frustration with others. This is an opportunity to coach him about the importance of being approachable and how it impacts patient safety. In this case, you could suggest coping techniques that employees could use when frustrated, such as pausing and counting to 10 or identifying one positive outcome achieved on that day.

Case Example 8

Appreciate Different Perspectives

Carrie undermines fellow pharmacists. On four separate occasions she revised the aminoglycoside pharmacokinetic regimens left by her colleagues who covered her patients over the weekend. The regimens were correct based on our current protocol and the patient details. You ask her, "Can you help me understand why you revised them?

If Carrie states that the current protocol or policy is a problem, recommend that she highlight specific examples and propose revisions to the current protocol or policy. If she says her colleagues are not following the protocol correctly, ask her to provide specific examples so you can discuss it further. If she denies a problem, then continue asking questions to identify why she is making these changes. You may say, "Okay, so your colleagues are following the protocol and the recommendations are sound, can you see how the perception is that they are wrong and you are fixing it?"

Carrie may see only her perspective and approaches the solution one way; thus, she changes the regimens. She may also think that she needs to intervene to support her value to the team, despite the fact that the current regimen was appropriate. Explain that there is more than one way to achieve the same outcome and encourage her to consider the perspectives of her colleagues. If specific outcomes, such as time to achieve therapeutic level, are similar to outcomes based on regimens she chose, then she will see that her colleagues' perspectives and approaches produce the same outcome. On the other hand, Carrie may feel threatened by her colleagues; she may not verbalize this, but *you might sense it by how she answers questions. Remind her of the value she brings to patients and the department, as well as how beneficial it is to patients that all the pharmacists are competent in providing pharmacokinetic services.*

When high-quality pharmacokinetic services are provided, the patients win, the department wins, and team members feel confident in their team. Your goal is to help your employees recognize that everyone in the department can be successful without diminishing anyone's role on the team.

Case Example 9

Three Sides to Every Story: Yours, Mine, and the Truth—Robert Evans

Jacquelyn is an excellent pharmacist, but she does not get along with pharmacy technicians. Over the weekend, she told a technician he was lazy and she was going to report him to his supervisor. Immediately after the event, the technician emailed you, Jacquelyn's supervisor, detailing the conversation and highlighting her inappropriate behavior.

First, recognize that there are always two sides to every situation. The technician could have been watching television on his cell phone, and Jacquelyn witnessed the event and intervened. Although she called him lazy—not the appropriate course of action—he really was not working. Now consider the opposite, the technician could have been completing a work-related assignment on the computer, and Jacquelyn misinterpreted the situation.

Seek to understand the situation before judging or taking action. If there is a history of employee laziness, or in this case a pharmacist's inability to get along with technicians, then make sure to assume positive intent and avoid any preconceived notions. This will help you remain objective when speaking to employees. Whether they admit they acted unprofessionally or not, explain why such behavior is inappropriate, and end the conversation by confirming your expectations. If you encounter a situation that warrants formal disciplinary action, you should notify your HR representative as soon as possible. Your HR representative will assist you in communicating with the employee.

Recognize and Reward

Focus on the positive by recognizing both the individual and the team depending on the situation. One form of recognition is to ask employees to share their most recent wins during staff meetings and for you to share those wins with your supervisor or key leaders within the organization. Set a personal goal to recognize more than you counsel, correct, or discipline. An important aspect of recognition is understanding how each individual likes to be recognized. Consider having employees complete a questionnaire (**Figure 7-4**) detailing preferred methods of recognition. Some employees prefer public recognition while others prefer private recognition, such as a handwritten thank-you note or a small treat. For example, an employee faced challenges in completing a project and I was very appreciative that he was polite and persistent despite the unusual hardships. I bought him a small bag of his favorite potato chips and left it on his desk with a thank-you note. He asked how I knew those were his favorite chips so I pulled out his recognition questionnaire. It took only a small bag of chips and a simple thank-you for him to feel appreciated.

Also consider departmental and organizational opportunities for recognition within your institution, such as the "great catch" awards where an employee is recognized for preventing a potential medication error. In providing recognition, always be genuine and detailed. Let's consider two scenarios of recognizing an employee named Emmett by his manager at a staff meeting:

1. I want to thank Emmett for doing a great job with a warfarin patient. She needed help getting her warfarin and Emmett got it for her.

2. I want to thank Emmett for going above and beyond to help a warfarin patient by walking over to our retail pharmacy to pick up her newly prescribed warfarin. Her daughter was coming to take her home that night but could not get to the pharmacy before it closed. Emmett made it possible for them to go home that night with the medication and avoid having to come back the next day to pick it up.

FIGURE 7-4. How Do You Like to Be Recognized?

Name: _____   _____ Date: _____

15 Minutes of Fame!

Recognition matters. By filling out this form and providing information about your preferences, your manager will be able to recognize you in the way you wish to be recognized.

My Favorites

Snack/beverage: _____

Restaurant: _____

Hobbies/pastimes: _____

Stores: _____

Other: _____

I prefer to be recognized

_____ Publicly

_____ Privately

_____ As an individual

_____ As a team member

_____ Organizationally

_____ Within my department

I most appreciate recognition when given by

_____ Peers

_____ Patients/clients

_____ Staff reporting to me

_____ My manager or director

_____ Leadership team

I prefer the following type of recognition

_____ Ceremony/public meeting

_____ Certificate or plaque

_____ Formal letter

_____ Thank-you note

_____ Greeting card

_____ Gift certificate

_____ Flowers

_____ Lunch with manager or director

_____ Tickets to an event

I prefer to be recognized in a

_____ Novel and exciting way

_____ Quiet, dignified way

_____ No-nonsense way

_____ Professional development opportunity

I prefer recognition to be presented through

_____ Food

_____ Humor

_____ Personal stories

_____ List of achievements

_____ Historical data and facts

_____ Small gift for me

_____ Gift for my family

_____ Other (please specify)

_____

_____

Source: http://www.cdha.nshealth.ca/about-us/our-facilities/qeii-health-sciences-centre.

Scenario 1 is so general that everyone will wonder what is so special about Emmett. They will likely think this is exactly what they do every day. Scenario 2 provides the critical details as to what constitutes above-and-beyond actions. Can all the pharmacists on the team say that they would walk over to the retail pharmacy to pick up a patient's medication? This type of public recognition also serves to set expectations with your team that employees who exceed expectations take these kinds of actions.

Summary

Success in leading your team begins with your own self-awareness and building an accountable, engaging, and learning culture. Be intentional with your actions and words to establish the right tone. Invest in your own growth as a leader and recruit employees with the right behaviors and actions. For difficult or crucial conversations, make sure you have them sooner rather than later and work with your supervisor and HR representative if you need support on what to say. Lastly, build trusting collaborative relationships with your employees, reinforce expectations, recognize them, and empower them to achieve success together. In doing so, the outcome is an engaged, highly productive team.

PRACTICE TIPS

1. Become a better leader. Read and apply literature related to leadership. Reflect on yourself and have the courage to change your own behavior and actions to produce desired outcomes.

2. Overcommunicate. This involves regularly updating your team and continually reiterating expectations to keep the team focused and engaged.

3. Recognize and reward employees. No one ever says, "I'm recognized too much." Keep the recognition flowing for the right behaviors and actions.

4. Meet with your mentor. Discuss your leadership successes and failures with someone you respect and trust.

References

1. Fair Labor Standards Act of 1938, 29 C.F.R. § 541.

2. Family Medical Leave Act, 29 C.F.R. § 825 (1993).

3. Society for Human Resource Management. *FMLA and Its Impact on Organizations: A Survey report by the Society for Human Resource Management.* Alexandria, VA: SHRM; 2007.

4. The Predictive Index. http://piworldwide.com. Accessed January 3, 2015

5. American Society of Health-System Pharmacists. ASHP guidelines on the recruitment, selection, and retention of pharmacy personnel. *Am J Health-Syst Pharm.* 2003;60(6):587-593.

6. US Department of Labor, Bureau of Labor Statistics. Labor force statistics from the current population survey. http://www.bls. gov/cps/cpsaat11.htm. Accessed February 26, 2014.

7. Greenleaf RK. *The Servant as Leader.* Westfield, IN: Robert K. Greenleaf Center; 1982.

8. Studer Q. *Hardwiring Excellence: Purpose Worthwhile Work Making a Difference.* Baltimore, MD: Fire Starter Pub; 2004.

9. Ramsay MA. Conflict in the health care workplace. *Proc (Bayl Univ Med Cent).* 2001;14(2):138-139.

10. Goleman D. *Emotional Intelligence: Why It Can Matter More Than IQ.* London, England: Bloomsbury Publishing; 1995.

11. Buckingham M, Clifton DO. *Now, Discover Your Strengths.* New York, NY: Free Press; 2001.

12. Rath T. *Strengthsfinder 2.0.* New York, NY: Gallup Press; 2007.

13. Patterson K, Grenny J, McMillan R, et al. *Crucial Conversations: Tools for Talking When Stakes Are High.* 2nd ed. New York, NY: McGraw-Hill; 2002.

14. Institute for Safe Medication Practices. ISMP Medication Safety Alert. Disrespectful behavior in healthcare...have we made any progress In the last decade? https://www.ismp.org/newsletters/acutecare/showarticle.aspx?id=52. Accessed June 15, 2015.

15. The Joint Commission. Sentinel Event Alert. Behaviors that undermine a culture of safety. http://www.jointcommission.org/assets/1/18/sea_40.pdf. Accessed April 18, 2015.

16. Crowley K, Elster K. *Working with You is Killing Me: Freeing Yourself from Emotional Traps at Work.* New York, NY: Warner Business Books; 2006.

17. Bush PW, Walesh SG. *Managing & Leading: 44 Lessons Learned for Pharmacists.* Bethesda, MD: American Society of Health-System Pharmacists; 2008.

18. Berg R. *The Soft Side of Operations: Why Good Management Skills Matter.* Fort Worth, TX; Perr & Knight; 2009. http://www.perrknight.com/2009/11/the-soft-side-of-operations-why-good-management-skills-matter/. Accessed May 2, 2015.

19. Harter JK, Schmidt FL, Hayes TL. Business-unit level relationship between employee satisfaction, employee engagement, and business outcomes: a meta-analysis. *J Appl Psychol.* 2002;87(2):268-279.

20. Halbesleben JR, Savage GT, Wakefield DS, et al. Rework and workarounds in nurse medication administration process: implications for work processes and patient safety. *Health Care Manage Rev* 2010;35(2):124-133.

21. Campbell U, Arrowood S, Kelm M. Positive work culture: a catalyst for improving employee commitment. *Am J Health-Syst Pharm*. 2013;70(19):1657, 1659.

22. Eisenhauer T. 10 simple secrets you need to know to increase employee engagement. *Entrepreneur.* http://www.entrepreneur.com/author/tim-eisenhauer. Accessed May 29, 2015

23. Porter-O'Grady T. Constructing a conflict resolution program for health care. *Health Care Manage Rev.* 2004;29(4):278-283.

24. Clark T. Leading healers to exceed. *Am J Health-Syst Pharm.* 2013;70(7):625-631.

Staff Development—
10 Factors to Guide Performance

Jean B. Douglas

KEY TERMS

Academic Professional Record (APR)—A document used to record professional activities of preceptors of the ASHP-accredited residency programs.

Adult Learning Theory—Assumptions made by Malcolm Knowles showing how adults learn differently than children. Adults prefer to learn with self-directedness and to pull information immediately with a problem-oriented approach.

Career Development—The lifelong psychological and behavioral processes shaping one's career over the life span. Career development includes how jobs fit together into a career pattern; how decisions are made leading to career choices; and how job, life, and family roles play into one's work history.

CIPE (Continuing Interprofessional Education)—Education strategies to develop collaborative teams and provide education for patients in today's changing healthcare system.

DiSC Personality and Behavioral Testing—A leading personal assessment tool to improve work productivity, teamwork, and communication. It provides a common language to better understand and to adapt behaviors with others.

Myers-Briggs Type Indicator—An instrument to measure one's personality type based on four preferences (focus on world, information, decision, and structure). From these, 16 personality types have been defined to help understand and to explain differences between people.

Personalized Learning—The tailoring of curriculum and learning environments to meet the needs and aspiration of individual learners.

Quality Improvement Pharmacist Teams—Pharmacists working to improve practice by meeting at least monthly for process improvement, staff and resident education, research support, and conducting medication-use reviews.

SMART (specific, measureable, attainable, realistic, and timely)—Objectives that lead to positive results.

Introduction

The primary role of the clinical coordinator is to build and manage a strong team of caring, clinical pharmacists who practice using sound principles. With meticulous follow-up, they seek solutions to problems and effectively guide patient therapy. Every pharmacist needs to be a patient-centered team player, interacting with pharmacy colleagues and other health professionals. The pharmacist team needs to work well together and establish a high degree of trust. The clinical coordinator in facilitating this high-performing team must be flexible to meet the needs of the individual and the team. Because people are the primary asset for a strong clinical pharmacy program, coaching for performance and developing the individuals on your team should take at least 40% of your time. The remainder of the time may be spent developing new programs and delegating projects to staff members to build their skills, confidence, practice depth, teaching prowess, and recognition.

The clinical coordinator may pattern his or her approach like a sports team coach or a symphony conductor.

- In the coach scenario, think of your responsibility as the person who knows the owner/manager's team goals and the person who defines the strategy for the offense/defense/special teams to meet these goals. You must have the necessary clinical skills and know-how to train your players to work cohesively to meet the goals consistently.

- As the symphony conductor, your role is leading the various instrumental sections to play in time and rhythm to produce music that is pleasing to the ear. The conductor makes sure everyone is playing in harmony and is on the same page.

Either of the above descriptions should give you a sense of the creativity and discipline needed to help your employees achieve or exceed goals through your direction, planning, and attention to detail. The satisfaction that comes from developing your pharmacists and technicians will more than make up for the patient care specialist duties that you may be used to. Your impact will be felt by many in the role as clinical coordinator, and the pharmacy department will flourish through your coaching to achieve patient and departmental goals.

Developing the Clinical Pharmacist Team: Getting Started

The clinical coordinator, whether new in the role or having served in this capacity for a few years, should do a staff assessment periodically to determine what skills need to be developed. Understanding the mission, vision, and values of the institution and the pharmacy department will help you identify the goals on which to focus. Align and assign the important goals to your employees, making certain that these are in line with those of the institution and the pharmacy department.

- ***Review the pharmacy practice model to determine if existing resources are being used effectively to meet service outcomes.*** A recent national review of practice models identified many new strategies to improve professionalism of pharmacists and technicians as well as an assessment tool to identify areas of discussion and work.[1] An integrated clinical and distributive practice model allows pharmacists to employ their skills to meet patient outcomes in an effective manner. The practice model affects morale, efficiency, teamwork, satisfaction, and growth opportunities. As health-system departments are working together on patient-centered teams, your pharmacists will want to have the same opportunities to collaborate and excel as employees in other departments.

- ***Evaluate medication management of clinical pharmacy services and medication services.*** You need to be aware if problems occur with medication distribution. The pharmacist review is a clinical function that is a safety factor for patients. Work on issues together with the pharmacy operations coordinator. Be aware that you may need to assist in both areas at times.

- ***Review clinical pharmacist practice guidelines, protocols, and prescriptive authority responsibilities.*** Verify that caregivers have access to read and act on these services using the electronic medical record. Recommendations must be documented so the team knows what the pharmacist has done.

- **Review clinical workload assignments.** Look for equitable pharmacist workload, transitions of care, transfer patterns, etc. If patients are seen efficiently, time may open up for more precepting and pharmacist development. Knowing the number of patients assigned to each pharmacist will allow you to determine if additional resources are needed to meet the workload. Also, make certain there is a definite plan detailing staff members and time that transferred patients will be seen. Regulatory agencies have focused much attention on hand-offs, so it is essential that information is shared between the pharmacists at transfer and shift change.

- **Review service standards.** Reviewing core measures, meaningful-use metrics, response times, and other dashboard numbers are important to meet the goals for The Joint Commission (TJC) and Centers for Medicare & Medicaid Services (CMS) accreditation. Review these metrics at least weekly and update specifics as needed. Implement improvement processes as necessary based on the recorded data. If this information is not readily available, seek assistance from information systems and your departmental leadership.

Next, you should develop a structure or checklist to help the team members improve their performance (see **Appendix 8-A**). This "score card" for each of your pharmacists will help with coaching and performing performance appraisals. Some options are below:

- **Human resource electronic programs, such as Halogen, that allow the manager to track goals and progress of direct reports.** Notes of recognition, praise, and concern can be placed in this electronic program for review before preparing and evaluating progress on assigned goals for the quarterly and annual performance evaluations. Employees can also record their comments, recognition received from others, and action plans in this program.

- **Paper file/folder in a secure file cabinet or hard drive.** Each employee should have a folder in a locked file cabinet or secure hard drive with all documents. Confidentiality is expected.

At least twice weekly you should document meetings with the new pharmacist, initial daily meetings with the pharmacist and trainer, and who you assign to train the new hires. You might uncover something that has been missed or find a miscommunication between the trainer and the new pharmacist. Include the trainer in the conversations or touch base at least weekly to reinforce what is needed or how things are going. Set a standing meeting time. Summarize new training plans in an email to the three of you for clarity and accountability.

The more advanced long-term employee will not need the same type of coaching as the newer employee. Alter what you offer employees based on each person's practice and aspirations. As your employees become more trained and confident, assign them more responsibility for skills development. Delegating will allow you to spend more time with the newer employees, develop new programs and quality improvement activities, and communicate/problem-solve with other professionals within the organization. Coaching and delegating will enable you to develop problem-solving skills.

After reviewing and completing these steps, you will have a good idea of your priorities to build a stronger clinical pharmacy team. You will also gain important insight. The knowledge gained in the above process will enable you to plan the future direction of clinical pharmacy services and achieve your goals. Write out your goals and review them often.

10 Factors to Improve Pharmacist Team Performance

There are variables or factors that relate to performance to address proactively or when the need arises. These 10 performance dynamics factors are pieces of the pie tied integrally to morale, character, integrity, honesty, etc., and if managed well, will lead to a successful career (**Figure 8-1**). A successful career comprises making job decisions, life needs, and satisfaction.[2] In working with new employees or seasoned staff members, use the suggested time or percentage spent initially with each factor as a guide only. The time spent on each factor moves dynamically as one changes position, job, life events, etc. When the employee consistently achieves these "pieces of the pie," both of you should identify how you can further assist in the employee's job performance and career. A nonpharmacist mentor within the institution may be considered to help a high-performing pharmacist move to the next level.

Below are 10 performance factors for a successful practice:

1. Performance and skill development to become a high-level clinical pharmacist

2. Effective communication skills, listening and informing to the level of understanding

3. Professional goals with quarterly and annual feedback to facilitate growth and improvement

4. Having a mentor and also serving as a mentor/buddy to help foster confidence and identify change

5. Continuing education (CE) plan to become a lifelong learner

6. Work–life balance for energy and satisfaction

7. Ongoing review of practice outcomes and accomplishments to know how your decisions affect patients and the team

8. Active participation in a pharmacy professional organization to learn advocacy, leadership, and networking

9. Poster presentations and publications describing innovation and solutions to practice issues that will advance the science of pharmacy practice

10. Teamwork for a rewarding practice environment

FIGURE 8-1. 10 Performance Factors

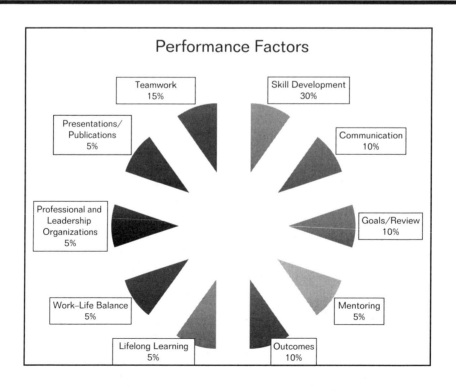

Each of these 10 factors will be addressed from a clinical coordinator's perspective, with tips for helping the pharmacist learn and become a great practitioner.

1. Performance and Skill Development: 30%

New Hires

Pharmacists are well educated in the science and practice of pharmacy by school curriculum, rotations, and residency programs. Time spent with academic preceptors is limited, so more in-depth goal planning and modelling are needed when they are hired. A skills assessment should be the initial step followed by a training plan. Over the first 90 days, a new pharmacist will receive training necessary to successfully practice on the team. Engage the pharmacist in the process of learning, observing, and then performing to build the needed skills with confidence and satisfaction.

After the training is completed, blend the pharmacist into the pharmacy team by assigning specific responsibilities in addition to routine assignments. These might include asking the pharmacist to identify a clinical pharmacy service to serve as a preceptor for students and residents, joining a **quality improvement pharmacist team** to address practice issues, and picking which new drug to present to the pharmacy and therapeutics (P&T) committee within the next year.[3,4] These are examples to help the pharmacist begin networking and learn how the team makes decisions. It is also important to help the pharmacist learn about nonpharmacy staff. As clinical coordinator, encourage the pharmacist to ask questions of the physician or nurse seeing a patient on the unit and introduce themselves, etc. Inform the physician or nurse ahead of time that a new pharmacist would like to ask questions and discuss what they value about pharmacy services. This exercise will help the pharmacist become familiar with the different providers seeing patients on the units.

Finally, ask the pharmacist to attend a meeting with you so he or she can see how to interact with and get involved in making decisions for programs and patients. Help the pharmacist get involved in multidisciplinary functions to represent the department.

Case Example 1

*A new pharmacist who attended our stroke team meeting heard discussion for improving response times for **tissue plasminogen activator** (tPA) administration and shared his experience from his previous hospital. The stroke team incorporated the new suggestions into their plan. The new pharmacist quickly became recognized for his knowledge, ability to communicate, and became a sought-out member of the team. This was a big positive for pharmacy and the new pharmacist.*

Ongoing Training Staff for High-Level Practice (Information, Feedback, Major Work Activities)

The clinical coordinator should present information at pharmacist staff meetings that will improve practice for the pharmacist team. Although educational topics and speakers are a great way to learn new information, a hands-on or skills workshop will better meet the adult learner's need to grasp and retain information. **Adult learning theory** includes some of the following tactics: KISS (**k**eep **i**t **s**imple **s**tupid), weekly emails with reminders, a case of the week with a prize for the correct answer, a practice pearl email or comment on a clinical conundrum, patient huddles, workshops with a demonstration of learning, interdisciplinary huddles, and short case presentations.[5] New TJC training guidelines suggest that clinical training be performed with the whole multidisciplinary team to allow team accountability.[6] It is best to utilize a variety of methods to educate staff and to seek feedback, as well as topics that staff want to learn more about.

Note: If you ask a colleague in another department to give a presentation to your staff, do not be surprised if you are asked to present a topic to them in return. This is a bonus—both departments and staff will learn how to work together better. It is even suggested to have periodic joint clinical meetings with departments such as nutrition, medical teaching service, and the hematology laboratory. If skills or important information is provided, document it to meet competency guidelines. There will be times when the institution will initiate new programs or hire a special expert to develop a patient care service. Even if this is not directly related to what a pharmacist does, education and knowing about new health-system services/programs should be covered at staff meetings. Some staff members may not realize why they need to know this, but as the hospital becomes more of an environment without boundaries, providers need to know about patient services to make adequate referrals, answer patient questions, etc. You will have to inform the doubters why this information is important to their practice.

Plan educational activities with the following facts in mind:

- Most recall just 10% of what they hear and just 20% of what is read.
- Visuals with an oral presentation adds 30% retention.
- Observation of an action along with explanation gives 50% retention.
- Doing the task provides 90% retention of information.

A fun and game-like atmosphere helps some learn better, such as Jeopardy questions and answers with team points. Provide structured learning in an efficient manner.

Accomplish group learning of new programs and services in an efficient manner:

- Put training lectures with case discussions on YouTube.
- Ask academic colleagues to sponsor monthly hour-long CE sessions with the Accreditation Council for Pharmacy Education for staff to attend over lunch. Grad Forum is an excellent way for clinical staff to present project work; residents to meet a residency objective; and administrative staff to update on new healthcare changes, such as payer changes, accountable care organizations, etc.
- Define one theme of the year for all staff to implement to achieve better outcomes. Examples include the following:
  - Stroke guidelines, including tPA dosing in interventional radiology
  - Core measures with detailed specifics of what the pharma-

cist should know and do to see that these are met routinely on patients (Videos, workgroups, defined documentation, and review of the metrics should be shared.)

- Magnet components, such as exemplary practice, transformational leadership, outcomes measurement, etc.

Feedback

A role of the clinical coordinator is to provide feedback to pharmacists. When pharmacist trainers work with pharmacists being trained in a new area, they are usually uncomfortable with giving feedback. They expect the clinical coordinator to give this feedback, especially if it is negative. Even if you encourage this, it often is not performed in the manner you would prefer. You need to listen to what is being said and what is not being said. Provide both positive and negative feedback. Identify a way that you are comfortable with to give feedback such as the show-and-tell method, the discussion method (the situation is described and the result is addressed), and the "sandwich technique" (state a positive, deliver the negative, and close with a positive comment). The most effective method is for you to look the pharmacist in the eye and state that behaviors must change or there will be consequences. Giving feedback can be difficult, but the team will not be strong if feedback is not shared and performance improved. A weak link in a chain (i.e., team) will make the chain break. The clinical coordinator must keep the chain strong and effective in providing patient care outcomes.

For exemplary accomplishments, you should see that recognition is given to the pharmacist in an appropriate way, such as an announcement in a hospital newsletter, local newspaper, or department meeting; a handwritten letter; or lunch with the leadership team. Research has shown that money is not the biggest motivator. Recognition is what most people really care about. Suggestions include plaques, paper weights, certificates, party, meeting with CEO, etc. Recognition for work accomplished leads to retention and the individuals wanting to achieve even more success.

Major Work Activities

To reward performance, department leadership develops major work activities (MWAs) for each position and assigns a percentage of importance to it, equaling 100% (see **Table 8-1**). This process will give the pharmacist a good description of what is important to be done and how much time should be spent doing it. Oftentimes, extra definitions are provided so that one will know if the MWA has been mastered to the expectation of the manager/coordinator. Performance descriptions of high, solid, and inconsistent help the employees know what needs additional work. This process makes up the basis of the annual merit performance system. However, this same process can be used outside of the MWAs. You can add other projects or work activities and list what is expected to achieve a high, solid, or inconsistent performance for these special projects. For example, if a pharmacist who has mastered the MWAs at a high level wants to keep learning and growing, the coordinator could write a goal to be worked on over the next year, discussed often, and evaluated at the next performance appraisal.

Under each MWA, examples of the level of expertise and skill needed to achieve a rating of top decile performance, solid performance, and inconsistent performance are provided. For example, for the third MWA in Table 8-1, this might appear as seen in the left column in **Table 8-2**. An example of an assignment to improve skills to enable the pharmacist to achieve the top decile rating the next year might look like the right column. As clinical coordinator, define the major steps that will need to be accomplished to achieve the goal. The pharmacist can use this as a checklist or the steps to achieve the goal.

If you are not involved in seeing patients daily or do not have time to spend on the floors/clinics often, making rounds with each pharmacist periodically on a day or service is recommended. Staff members want to know that their leaders can dive in and do what they are doing. It is hard for the clinical coordinator to be an expert on everything, but knowing the department's routine protocols is expected. This is not usually a problem because the clinical coordinator is involved in writing the protocols and getting them approved by P&T committees, etc. Often, clinical decision-making skills can be applied to give insight to the pharmacists so they can expand their skill set. Working with staff online will also help identify new protocols or revisions of procedures and protocols, which will improve patient outcomes. Stay involved in patient care and rounds.

2. Communication: 10%

Communication, which is part of every activity, is important in accomplishing duties as a clinical coordinator and pharmacist. Saying what you mean, hearing what is being said, picking up when something is not clear and miscom-

Table 8-1. Clinical Pharmacist Major Work Activities in an Integrated Practice Model

Major Work Activity	Percentage
Analyzes and promotes optimal medication therapies	20%
Supervises and evaluates the activities of pharmacy technicians in filling medication orders for inpatient and outpatient services	20%
Provides and monitors drug utilization and medication-related information to healthcare professionals, patients, and the public	20%
Utilizes drug dosing protocols, medication reviews, and consultations on physician request	20%
Serves as a preceptor and role model for all pharmacy staff including students, fellows, residents, and pharmacists	20%

Source: Courtesy of Cone Health, Greensboro, North Carolina, © 2015.

Table 8-2. Example of Writing a Goal with Specific Steps to Achieve an MWA

Major Work Activity	Assignment for Skill Improvement
Provides and monitors drug utilization and medication-related information to healthcare professionals, patients, and the public.	*Develop a dosing protocol based on primary literature and guidelines to improve patient care; get P&T committee approval; collect patient data to see if patient care is improved and, if so, prepare presentations for professional meetings and/or publication*
Top Decile Performance	
■ Develops, promotes and monitors practice changes based on literature and clinical data, which results in improved patient care and safety ■ Recognizes practice changes on a state and/or national level ■ Develops presentations, publications, and participates in professional meetings	■ Seek input from clinicians, literature, national guidelines, etc., where patient care improvement is needed (i.e., mortality and morbidity from anticoagulated patients with head injury) ■ Write a pharmacist dosing protocol utilizing ED collaboration, with prompt response and resources available; present to various committees for input and support; take to P&T committee for support to begin data collection
Solid Performance	
■ Monitors drug utilization and recommends changes where appropriate ■ Effectively communicates information to medical staff and other healthcare professionals ■ Utilizes drug usage evaluation information to alter medication therapies effectively ■ Provides educational presentations to pharmacy staff, students, other healthcare professionals, and the public	■ Develop paperwork, orders in computer system, data extraction, outcome measurement processes, etc., and begin staff education ■ Evaluate care with each patient to make certain that no excess risk is seen; tabulate patient data and discuss with project group ■ Prepare PowerPoint presentations for same groups who helped guide the protocol and total outcomes achieved ■ Submit for presentation to national or state meeting
Inconsistent Performance	
■ Avoids or does incomplete collection of data for department MUE initiatives ■ Monitors drug utilization and recommends medication changes not appropriate ■ Inconsistently communicates appropriate medication therapies to healthcare professionals including poorly written notes/communication forms ■ Does not meet performance expectations although issues have been identified and discussed during the year	

ED = emergency department; MUE = medication-use evaluations; P&T = pharmacy and therapeutics.

Source: Courtesy of Cone Health, Greensboro, North Carolina, © 2015.

municated, and knowing the expectations for how to communicate lead to success. Pharmacists are trained to know how to communicate drug-related problems to prescribers and nurses. Oftentimes, orders do not appear to be correct or are missing essential information, or the nurse questions an order and this leads to further investigation. The computer system may fire an alert, but the severity may be hard to determine in the individual patient. In all of these situations, communication is needed to resolve the concerns. Having the persistence and courage to find the facts is hard without positive communication, especially when workload is high. All questions that could lead to harm in a patient should be given priority regardless of who is asking. Remember, the best way to answer your concern is to ask for clarity. This is a nonthreatening way to say that the order or communication is not clear and you are requesting more information so as to avoid an error. When speaking with a patient or employee who is resistant to what you are saying, ask them to repeat what you are telling them in their own words. Then ask them to state what will happen if poor communication continues, such as patient misadventures, mistrust, etc. When one can individualize the situation's importance, understanding can begin to happen. Staff members expect the clinical coordinator to communicate with anyone who has a problem or is rude to other staff members. It is best to gather all the facts, speak with the person in private, and discuss how others perceive the behavior. Discussion topics could include how no one intends to make an error, how to avoid errors, and how to build trust, which is important for a good working relationship. Seek to find solutions and, if necessary, ask that an apology be made to your staff member. Keep channels of communication open and strive for healthy relationships among coworkers.

Inform each pharmacist of your preference on how to contact you and speak with you. An open door policy gives one the opportunity to discuss issues when things happen. Try to see staff in the pharmacy area/units in the morning or afternoons and ask how the day is going. Make it easy for staff to speak with you by making yourself accessible. If something needs discussion, ask to set up a separate meeting to guarantee privacy and a time where no interruptions should occur. Should there be a problem with the meeting time or meeting your commitment, communicate with the staff member and make a new plan. Impress on the pharmacist how important it is to meet commitments.

SBAR (**s**ituation, **b**ackground, **a**ssessment, and **r**ecommendation), a structured template for healthcare workers to communicate clearly, was developed by the U.S. Navy and is now recommended by TJC.[7] It is a particularly helpful tool for communicating patient information or asking questions because the information is presented in a consistent format, allowing ease of understanding.

Much of the pharmacist's work involves being signed onto a computer or laptop, and such tools as instant messaging, Lync, and Spark, which allow pharmacists to send questions to each other, facilitate communication with staff. Spark displays messages and those who are currently online in a small box on the screen. This feature allows communication without having to call on a phone or page someone. A new hire can type out a question and send it to his or her trainer who may be seeing patients or entering orders in another area.

It is important to practice good communication techniques so that staff can learn from your example. The following guidelines will facilitate good communication:

- ***Be professional and show a genuine interest in those around you.*** Introduce yourself and others in a way to "build them up," especially around patients and coworkers. You should show your confidence in their abilities and that you appreciate what they do.

- ***At meetings, educate others on your departmental projects.*** Explain what you and your staff are doing so they can relate similar projects for increased traction.

- ***Know your strengths and weaknesses.*** If, for example, you are invited to a planning meeting to set up a new service that will include clinical and distribution services, ask a coworker who is strong in the distribution side of things to go with you. Or, if you are more right-brain oriented, ask a left-brain pharmacist to attend with you. That way, all key points will be covered and addressed easily.

- ***Keep important information short and brief, especially in emails.*** It is hard to determine how much information to share in explaining why something needs to be done a certain way; but, if the email is too complicated, it will not be read. Most will put the email in a folder with plans to read it later. The information will not be learned, and they will not know how to handle the situation when it occurs. Use bullets and examples to aid in memory retention. Then repeat the information, such as in sending another email later with slightly different content (e.g., a case example). It may take several times to have someone remember what they need to know.

- ***Remain positive with staff.*** No matter how frustrated things are getting, stay the course. If you need to vent and you have a good relationship with your supervisor, talk with him or her. If not, find another member of the leadership team. However, be certain that they understand their role is to help redirect you and to provide guidance to you. Do not join in with staff complaining and negative discussions.

- ***Develop a relationship with your staff.*** Get to know how they think and process information. Ask your training department or human resources to administer the **Myers-Briggs Type Indicator** personality test to your team.[8] This does take a little time to explain what the results mean, but understanding one's personality type does help in relating to colleagues. The test identifies if you have a tendency for extroversion or introversion, sensing or intuition, thinking or feeling, and judging or perceiving. For example, if you need to deliver information that will require change in work details to an ISTJ (introversion, sensing, thinking, and judging) pharmacist, it is best to just go tell the person and then leave. Return in about an hour after they have had time to process the information and then have the discussion. Many pharmacists test as either ISTJ or INTP with few scoring as EFNP or ESTJ—the exact opposite. Knowing a person's score can help improve communication. Another method to help staff members understand their differences and needs is the **DiSC** (**d**ominance, **i**nfluence, **s**teadiness, and **c**onscientiousness) personality and behavioral style assessment.[9] *Dominance* is how assertive and results-focused you are, *influence* pertains to how sociable and people-focused you are; *steadiness* is how reliable and team-focused you are; and *conscientiousness* is how analytical and accuracy-focused you are. All four descriptors capture the personality traits found in most people. It would be helpful to know your style and your supervisor's style in one or both of these tests so you can tailor your messages.

3. Professional Goals with Quarterly and Annual Feedback: 10%

Every employee should have goals to work on. It has been suggested that three is the optimum number that can be accomplished over a short period of time. Goals should be written in a format known as **SMART** (**s**pecific, **m**easureable, **a**ttainable, **r**ealistic, and **t**imely).[10] Match the pharmacists' goals with departmental goals and show the pharmacists how their goals fit in with what is expected of the department.

Case Example 2

Complete the reading and practice requirements to pass the ACLS (advanced cardiovascular life support) certification and become a trainer for the department before the next renewal date (7 months). Offer information on how to proceed to accomplish the goal. If the pharmacist is experienced, then you may just need to give the pharmacist boundaries of money and time restraints, etc. If the pharmacist is newer to practice, then some coaching and educating will be necessary. Be certain that the pharmacist can accomplish the goal. If the pharmacist responds, "why don't you just do the goal," then you know that the pharmacist has not bought-in and is not empowered on the team. At this time, further counseling and discussion are needed.

Goals may be selected from departmental projects, outcome data from service and drug protocols when dosing drug-level mismatches occur, medication-use evaluations (MUEs) to study high-risk drugs, new therapies needing proof of benefit to patients, etc. Encourage pharmacists to document their skills by adding the completed goal/project to their resume. If your institution has its own pharmacy residency program, ask to include these in the **academic professional record** (APR) each year at performance appraisal time. This document is reviewed for each preceptor during an ASHP residency accreditation (visit http://www.ashp.org/DocLibrary/Accreditation/FAQResidencyAccreditation.aspx).[11]

Continuous professional development (CPD) is encouraged by boards of pharmacy as a means of CE. This process allows the pharmacist to reflect on practice needs and to develop a plan for training needed to improve practice and patient care. Most state boards have a template for pharmacists to write their goals down and to record their educational activities each year. Credit is given for activities such as the learning that occurs when taking care of patients and extensive literature searches.[12] You have the flexibility to choose learning activities to meet your professional and patient-related goals. It can include many different tools to learn and improve competency such as giving drug therapy lectures, counting drug information responses, developing a new protocol that improves patient outcomes, precepting students and residents, or providing medication management consistently to improve patient outcomes. The benefit of CPD is the ability to select specific practice-learning activities that will count as required CE and allow a **personalized learning** plan.[13]

Encourage team members on the importance of defining the steps to accomplish each goal. Although most people know what needs to be done, taking action to get started is hard. Share examples to motivate staff members to get started on their goals, projects, etc. One helpful example that usually requires little explanation is the parable of the boiled frog in Peter Senge's *The Fifth Discipline*.[14] The parable shows the importance of gradual change instead of rapid change. If you place a frog in a boiling pot of water, it will try to jump out because it senses danger. If you place a frog in a lukewarm pot of water and gradually turn up the temperature, the frog will adjust to the temperature and not sense the danger of being boiled to death. Working gradually will accomplish something; waiting until the water is dangerously hot shortens your progress and success. If you wait to jump into the project at the last minute, you will not get as much accomplished.

The old saying, "Keep the monkey off your back," has such a true meaning.[15] If someone brings a problem to you and you decide to solve it yourself, you lose valuable time as the team's coach/conductor and you deny the pharmacist the opportunity to find a solution and learn new skills. Tell the person to solve the problem and assist only as needed.

4. Having a Mentor and Serving as a Mentor/Buddy/Preceptor to Help Foster Confidence and Accept Change: 5%

Most of us have had professors who took an interest in us, and we responded by doing our best to meet their expectations and often asked them for advice. After graduation, many of us forget about needing or retaining mentors. Pharmacy residents and new pharmacy staff should identify a mentor within the first 2 months of their residency or new position. New staff members may want their initial mentor to be their pharmacist trainer or the clinical coordinator. Over time, relationships will dictate which colleagues have similar interests and practice styles. The mentor should be comfortable sharing confidential concerns and personal feelings. The pharmacist should respect and value the mentor's opinion. Most times, no special meetings are needed because conversations happen naturally and spontaneously. The mentor can also be someone outside of the department, such as in nursing or medicine. To be successful, the relationship should be nourished over time—the outcome is directly related to what you put into the relationship. So, both the clinical coordinator and staff members need mentors to help propel performance and development.

Case Example 3

A pharmacist could not understand why she did not get chosen to work on certain project teams. The clinical coordinator knew she needed help with her people skills. After identifying a gifted department head in another department to privately help with her people skills, the clinical coordinator arranged for them to work together. The pharmacist could see that this person had outstanding people skills but did not understand the differences in the two departments to merit benefit. Even though this was explained and a nonpharmacy mentor was selected for privacy, the pharmacist just could not get outside the pharmacy "box." If this happens, select a mentor for the pharmacist within the pharmacy system at another hospital or consider a member of the leadership team other than yourself.

As you mentor the pharmacist, review what the pharmacist does well and consider if the pharmacist's current position is the best fit. Oftentimes, after working in a position for 4 to 5 years, a pharmacist may want to move in another direction of pharmacy practice. Within the profession, there are many parallel tracks to practice pharmacy successfully. As a mentor, you should help differentiate these tracks for possible future growth. Explain what additional education and training may be required for some of the higher level or specialized positions when mentoring staff (see **Figure 8-2**).

Encourage your pharmacists to keep their curriculum vitae or resume updated. This is important if they are asked to be a speaker on a program or serve as a preceptor for the university, etc. If your practice site has a residency program, ask that the APR be updated at least annually. Additionally, having an updated resume keeps people from feeling trapped in their current job. You want your team to *want* to be on your team. If they are unhappy, an updated resume will allow them to seek other opportunities or find out that they have a great place to work compared to others.

5. Continuing Education Plan to Be a Lifelong Learner: 5%

Practice excellence is dependent on getting education after one gets a university degree and a state license to practice pharmacy. CE is more than just facts about drugs and disease states. Today's pharmacist needs to know how to apply the information in patients who may have multiple diseases, in patients aged from 1 day to more than 100 years; know if the drug is gender and/or race specific; and have allergies that may interfere with the prescribed medication. It is also expected that the pharmacist not only know the pharmacology, but also goes one step further to prevent any drug-related misadventures due to various unique patient conditions. Because a practicing pharmacist needs expanded skills, there is a trend toward CPD for learning and **CIPE (continuing interprofessional education)** for team-based skills development. Below are examples of multidisciplinary team learning:

- Focus on care delivery process
- Professional and interprofessional competency development
- Describing changes in individual and/or team-based practice performance
- Knowledge sharing—case presentation (i.e., rolling case discussion) with panel discussion with various professions
- Self-reflection, self-assessment, identity theory, and interactive learning

FIGURE 8-2. Basic Career Options for Pharmacists

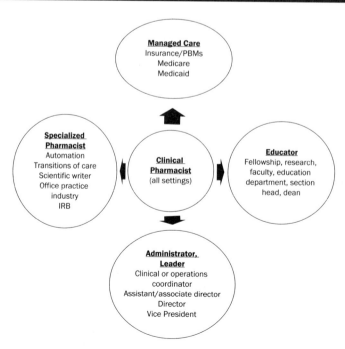

IRB = institutional review board; PBM = pharmacy benefit manager.

(learning about, with, and from other health professionals)

- Best practices evaluations (i e., and analyze *why*)
- Room of errors (i.e., note as many errors as possible)
- Assessment of core competencies and improved team function/clinical outcomes

To perform at a high-practice level in a team environment, staying proficient in drug knowledge, and having good communication skills are important for pharmacists. Theodore Roosevelt said it best, "Nobody cares how much you know, until they know how much you care."[16] Each state sets different CE requirements to maintain practice privileges, and the number of required hours will vary among staff. It is the pharmacist's responsibility to maintain a current license to practice. Make verification of the required hours for license renewal part of each annual review, tying specific educational programs to match what the pharmacist needs for his or her practice site and state. The pharmacist should maintain documentation of completed activities for license renewal, which is also kept in the employee's educational file.

Encourage every pharmacist to read literature from pharmacy and other disciplines to learn about new trends, new technology, results of national trials, emerging changes in healthcare and reimbursements, and national guidelines that will affect practice per TJC and CMS. Staying current will help with communication and problem solving. Ask each pharmacist to make a list of five to seven key journals and websites to read each month and check them off when read. Encourage sharing innovative research and helpful review articles with colleagues to advance knowledge and develop better communication skills. The clinical coordinator may need to jump start this by making key articles available or emailing them for staff to read. Journal clubs are also helpful, but interest waxes and wanes, so a personal checklist will be more accountable.

You should plan learning activities/teaching moments as part of doing routine activities whenever possible. For example, build in alerts for intravenous (IV) to oral administration, renal function for pediatric dosing, and medication and laboratory testing into the order verification process. These alerts will help the pharmacist learn new information and prevent misadventures from occurring in patients. Encourage systemwide culture and care initiatives woven into meetings, presentations, and huddles, using storytelling and sharing. This will help you incorporate these values into your staff's practice.

6. *Work–Life Balance for Energy and Satisfaction: 5%*

Everyone has the same number of hours in the day. The difference is how one balances the time in the work and life sectors by time management and prioritization. Although work is important to fund the life portion, family must come first. To accomplish this, good planning is a necessity. You can't do everything. What you can't do, find or hire someone to help you. Prioritize what needs to be done and stick to that plan. Technology such as smartphones for quick phone calls, text messages, and appointment setting can improve your time management. Investigate the features to see which will add value to your daily life at home and work. Many institutions are offering concierge services for employees to help with their work–life balance. Consideration of outside assistance can allow focus on what is important. Keep in mind that *life is not a dress rehearsal*. Take this saying to heart and spend time doing what is important to have a meaningful life.

As a clinical coordinator, when you see an employee struggling to deal with issues at home and not completing expected tasks, it is time to discuss work–life balance issues. A referral to the performance manager or employee assistance program should be offered. Do not become too involved in helping to solve the employee's personal problems but provide feedback and input concerning the employee's work performance. All employees should meet their performance expectations so the team will value them as team members. If they slack off, their coworkers will not be supportive, and their reputation on the team will be negatively impacted.

Below are some suggestions for using time wisely and evaluating what you accomplish:

- Read email only 2 or 3 times a day.
- Include mentoring moments on your calendar.

- Schedule priorities early in the day when productivity is highest.
- Ask support staff to set up meetings, record minutes, plan celebrations, etc.
- Schedule time to accomplish goals throughout the year to reduce procrastination.
- Break down projects into tiny pieces and then schedule each piece in a time sequence that will allow the project to be completed.

7. Review of Practice Outcomes and Accomplishments: 10%

Data are essential in decision making. With most steps in providing patient care being automated, more data are available to the pharmacist and manager. With economic reimbursement changes, efficiency is crucial to stay in business. Interpreting data supplied by information systems shows if goals are being met. Using the data, a better workflow, staffing arrangement, or pharmacist assignment schema can be developed to meet established goals. Pharmacists should know TJC standards for medication quality and assist each other in meeting them as they perform their job responsibilities. Many quality indicators are tied with a time metric to when therapy (i.e., the first dose) should be given for improved patient outcomes. For example, a patient who is septic in the emergency department (ED) should receive the first antibiotic dose within 4 hours to meet the metric.[17] CMS also has core measures to receive maximum reimbursement. A drug-related example in the stroke core measures is for tPA to be administered to a stroke patient in a timely manner. Therefore, strategies, such as informing the pharmacist via beeper and a technician taking the prepared drug to the ED, should be clearly defined. Encourage pharmacists to verify if the measures are met and, if not met, make an intervention. Use various means to help pharmacists remember these measures, such as including them in the electronic medical record, defining them in the clinical decision-support alerting tool used by pharmacists, defining a template to pop up when certain conditions are met, etc.

The interventions should be recorded for use as a story for the Magnet Writing Committee to use as documentation for recertification if your institution is a Magnet hospital, as well as for the pharmacist intervention log. Pharmacists should be involved in each of the mandated national set of core measures. Scores should be shared with staff, and procedures to meet the standards should be reviewed often. Timed practice runs for tPA delivery and other tactics should be considered. Place pharmacy core measures on the dashboard and review with staff members often. As clinical coordinator, educate and reward appropriately. Also, remember to review how transferred patients are handed off and if valuable information is shared with the next pharmacist at shift communication.

8. Professional Organization Membership to Learn Advocacy, Leadership, and Networking: 5%

One of the best opportunities for **career development** is active membership in professional pharmacy organizations, which have a mission, vision statement, and goal setting (i.e., strategic plan to accomplish collective goals and practice advances). With every discussion to solve problems and seek opportunities for improvement, one learns new information, which could be factual and hands-on or demonstrated leadership techniques. You can observe professionalism, learn the importance of motivation, and direct the future of the profession. The key professional pharmacy organizations include ASHP, the American College of Clinical Pharmacy, The American Pharmaceutical Association, and the Academy of Managed Care Pharmacy. Each of these organizations has excellent websites for accessing information about their products and services. Encourage pharmacists to read the newsletters, participate on the email listserves, and attend meetings. Networking and meeting other pharmacists in similar positions across the state/country encourages communication on perplexing patient care issues or new service implementations.

Because professional organizations serve as an excellent opportunity to develop leadership skills, encourage skilled staff with an administrative flair to accept committee leadership positions to develop problem-solving and communication skills. Many Baby Boomer pharmacists nearing retirement may not be as interested in leadership positions as the younger Millennials or Generation Xers, so determine who is interested in making broad changes in the profession and encourage them to participate in professional organizations. Younger pharmacists want to change things for the better and see this as their purpose in life. If a pharmacist is selected to serve in this leadership capacity, arrange coverage for the pharmacist to have time from work to attend the meetings or teleconferences. In times of economic crunch, attending outside professional meetings may not be feasible. In that case, expand opportunities for pharmacists to participate in group purchasing meetings (supported by the institution), interdisciplinary planning sessions, and community service projects sponsored by the hospital or company.

If staff members are interested in leadership development, investigate other options below:

- **Engage colleagues on your leadership team to assist them.** This will be a positive indication of your own leadership and relationship with them.

- **Expand growth internally for leadership assignments and/or outside committee work.** Examples include asking pharmacists to inform high school students about pharmacy careers, lead brown-bag sessions during pharmacy week, deliver information clips on radio and television, etc.

- **Educate about the importance of professional organizations.** Relate how organized pharmacy has initiated changes, such as provider status, immunization care provision, and medication-therapy management. Many pharmacists do not realize that practice opportunities result from negotiations within legislative bodies at the state and national levels. What most understand is the pharmacy organizations' quality of publications and up-to-date meeting content.

9. Poster Presentations and Publications: 5%

The ability to analyze data to determine if improvements are needed to achieve better outcomes is important to your professional growth as a pharmacist practitioner. In a

way, this is like an ongoing research project. The data collected on dosing services can be analyzed to see if the target endpoints are met. If not, the dosing strategies can be restudied and changed. Once a new method has improved dosing outcomes, it should be shared and presented as a poster and/or a publication. If you share the poster with the TJC or Magnet teams when they are onsite, it will lead to a better understanding of the quality of your team's practice. Presentation at state and national meetings will also help other pharmacists improve their practice of pharmacy.

Case Example 4

One pharmacist colleague developed flow sheets (or monitoring sheets) for drug-specific parameters to be recorded on each patient each day for rounds. These flow sheets included the time the drug was given and the resulting changes in physiologic response. Doses given were recorded, and drug levels were also documented in the timeline of drug effect. This quick view of how the drug was working allowed the pharmacist to know when changes were needed or when the drug had achieved the therapeutic marker. The data would be tabulated to identify if the dosing strategies were successful or changes were needed and submitted for poster presentation or publication. This team practice expanded research and allowed recognition for team members.

Another good way to build outcomes measurement into one's practice is having students and residents gather data and ask pharmacists to serve as advisors to guide the research. A learning cycle develops, leading to new knowledge to apply to patient care. Another smart approach is to have pharmacists document kinetic parameters in their notes and have the data pulled from the electronic medical record into a table for review. When the project is completed, it can be reviewed to determine if recommendations are sound enough to implement into practice. Ask pharmacists who completed a project to share their work at various institutional committees where this information should be known. For example, if a pharmacist documents the value of anti-Xa levels in reaching therapeutic heparin levels sooner, presenting this research will provide valuable experience and recognition. Also, request a poster be submitted to a state and/or national meeting in the appropriate category. This process will give pharmacists experience in writing a paper, reading feedback, editing, designing a poster, talking to others who are interested in their work or want to challenge their work, and submitting the paper for publication. The presenters at a poster learn from the questions and comments shared by attendees. The pharmacist will establish an area of expertise and meet other experts in the field. This is a real growth opportunity! As clinical coordinator, you may need to identify a statistician and/or researcher to assist in the writing of the paper. If you do not have one on staff, most institutions have relationships with university statisticians.

10. Teamwork for a Rewarding Practice Environment: 15%

Team management is a trend that is finally emerging at quantum speed due to healthcare access and affordability. Growth has been promising in patient-centered medical homes with multidisciplinary teams working seamlessly with defined care plans on and off campus. At the macro level, these changes are producing some amazing results. At the individual pharmacist level, health disciplines are beginning to respect and realize that the expertise of all those involved with a patient should be counted on to perform in a timely and responsible manner. Communication is improving, and each discipline can read, document, and access the electronic medical record. This has improved efficiency and allows quicker decision making. New guidelines for CE call for multidisciplinary education to help teams become more accountable in the care arena. Some believe the teamwork management trend will take the high costs out of our healthcare system and help us regain our position as one of the world's quality healthcare nations.

It must be noted that each team member needs access to others on the team; thus, electronic devices, such as secure smartphones and iPads for patient information, are a must. With the new emphasis on teams, pharmacists should be comfortable and accountable for taking charge of medication-related care. As clinical coordinator, your top priorities are team building and helping your pharmacists function well on interdisciplinary teams.

Inexpensive ideas and tools to help keep the team positive include the following:

1. Share exemplary performance and feedback with team members inside and outside of the department so that conversations and positive words can be said.

2. Ask staff to share incidents of superlative teamwork and performance with others by writing the essence of the good work on a card and tacking it on a highly visible wall for viewing. The cards should be removed each month and one drawn at random for a gift certificate and celebration by the department.

3. Ask pharmacists on a multidisciplinary team to invite a team colleague to present a case or new topic to the pharmacist staff meeting.

4. Ask pharmacists to send a pharmacy email when they observe a colleague making a significant intervention with a "catch of the day" and share this with all pharmacy staff. Ask department managers to share the intervention specifics with the upper hospital leadership team.

5. Post publications and posters in the department so that staff can review work presented at offsite meetings.

6. Form a team to develop recognition strategies for Pharmacy Week and other special events, such as completion of a training class or graduation of the residents.

7. Host showers and parties for team members to celebrate weddings, baby announcements, graduation from advanced education degrees, promotions, acceptance to graduate programs, etc.

8. Plan an outside lunch for a team that worked hard to achieve their goals, etc.

9. Send gift cards to express appreciation for good teamwork.

Teamwork is also important for daily departmental functioning. It is impossible to determine exactly how long patient care interventions will take; thus, when assigning the number of patients to a pharmacist's daily workload, it is not known if the number of patients fills up or exceeds the hours scheduled to work. When a strong team ethic is present and work is completed, pharmacists should help those still seeing patients, making interventions to meet core measures, precepting students/residents, etc. When a team works together, no one is stressed, and the work gets completed in a professional fashion without hints of anger or resentment.

The problem arises when some team members are consistently slower than others or rush through their patients not taking the time to find potential problems. The faster pharmacists think they should spend their extra time working on their special projects instead of constantly helping the slower pharmacists catch up on their work assignments. The slower pharmacists who take the time to educate each patient and solve potential problems before discharge are frustrated that others do not practice with the necessary depth. This is a tricky problem to address. Everyone works at a different pace and has different organizational skills. In these situations, you should look at the workload reports to help pharmacists see the number of patients on each work assignment, have pharmacists rotate work assignments, or schedule a slower pharmacist to work with a faster pharmacist to learn organizational approaches.

If you work in an integrated team environment and these options fail, then this may become an issue where the leadership team has to decide if the slower pharmacist meets the team's expectations and retains a position on staff or if the speedy pharmacist makes appropriate interventions consistently. If patient outcomes can be tabulated for each pharmacist, this will be the best option to resolve such a situation. If the slower pharmacist's patient outcomes are superior to the fast pharmacist, then a discussion can be better directed where it needs to be. Great patient outcomes with reduced readmissions are important in today's healthcare environment. Speed does not determine who the highest performing pharmacist is in today's environment.

The more your team works together, socializes together, and generally respects each other, the better the teamwork should be. However, when a problem is noted, the clinical coordinator must take action quickly to resolve this as soon as possible.

Case Example 5

On morning rounds, the coordinator observed a pharmacy resident to be unprofessionally dressed. The resident was asked to go home and not return until he was dressed in a professional manner. What was the problem? The resident had on a shirt that was excessively wrinkled. Staff immediately heard about this, and everyone's dress improved. Sometimes, taking the time to help someone become better instills pride for the whole team.

Teamwork Primer

A must read for a clinical coordinator is *The Five Dysfunctions of a Team* by Patrick Lencioni.[18] This leadership fable discusses teams and their importance to achieving success. The author identifies five practices needed for an effective team and lists five dysfunctions that cause teams to fail. The factors for a successful team are trust, comfort to debate, making a commitment, being accountable, and achieving results. Lencioni lists the five dysfunctions in a pyramid (most important on the bottom) and describes the results of not having the five dysfunctions present in your team (see **Table 8-3**). The clinical coordinator should proactively monitor each member of the team and help each work better together. The pharmacy team must build on its mission, vision, and values to create a sense of importance around pharmacy care and the people providing this care. Focus should be on building trust, engaging in good conflict, committing to common goals, holding each other accountable, and measuring and celebrating the team's results.

Case Example 6

Cone Health is a six-hospital, health-system pharmacy that saw the economic pressures of reimbursement limiting the opportunities of pharmacists and technicians to expand patient-specific services. Cone Health decided to take a proactive approach that involved team building. This approach followed in sync with what was happening in other disciplines and complemented these changes well. Formalized service teams were being developed, such as stroke teams, STEMI (ST segment elevation myocardial infarction) teams, and sepsis teams where

Table 8-3. Summary of Lencioni's Five Dysfunctions of a Team

Dysfunctions/Problems	Barriers Seen from Dysfunction	Practices of Effective Teams
1. Absence of trust	Invulnerability	Team members open up, accept feedback, believe in each other's strengths No cliques or talking behind backs, etc.
2. Fear of conflict	Artificial harmony	Teams engage in open and constructive conflict (not holding back on opinion and concerns) to improve results
3. Lack of commitment (failure to buy-in to decisions)	Ambiguity	Team members are committed to goals Each member's ideas are heard and discussed
4. Avoidance of accountability	Low standards	Team members desire high standards for their work
5. Inattention to results; lack of commitment (failure to buy-in to decisions)	Status and ego (i.e., superstars) Ambiguity	Team members are focused on results Team members are committed to goals Each member's ideas are heard and discussed

trained staff members knew their role and could provide up-to-date care to accomplish outcomes set by national accrediting bodies. These teams were mainly based in the units where the patients were treated. Specialization seemed to be the way to differentiate excellence and meet patient and payer expectations. At this time, pharmacists were assigned to attend these team meetings and to learn and participate in the specialized care. However, they were not in the driver's seat. So, in an effort to allow pharmacists to drive medication therapy in clinical services, quality improvement pharmacist teams were formed. Several core teams were initiated with oversight by clinical coordinators, and a staff clinical pharmacist led each team (rotated every 2 years). Meetings were to be held monthly, during shift overlap, and assignments were accepted and reported at the next meeting. Decision making was made by democratic process. Staffing resources were adjusted to allow time for pharmacists to work on projects, etc. Coordinators/managers supported and mentored the pharmacist leaders and assisted with communication needs.

On the infectious disease team from the first year, there were 11 pharmacists and pharmacy resi-

dents from across the system who met monthly to decide on clinical projects that would improve the triple aim of quality, service, and cost. Some key practice improvements implemented over the first year included a pharmacist protocol for all pregnant HIV+ patients to receive IV zidovudine at the start of labor. Antibiotic dosing in continuous ambulatory peritoneal dialysis and a pediatric protocol for once-daily aminoglycosides were also approved, built into the computer and evaluated for quality. Three MUEs were completed, and these included sepsis protocol, extended piperacillin/tazobactam, and Pseudomonas isolate susceptibility study for patients in the system.

The teams were successful in engaging staff to become accountable and to drive decisions to take care of patients. Additionally, decisions were based on evidence, and if no or limited research existed, research projects were designed for residents, MUEs were designed to show what was actually being done, and topics for staff and resident education were generated from the work of the teams. However, the biggest outcome of the quality improvement pharmacist teams was generating pharmacists from the six hospitals to work together as a team and to get recognition from physicians, nurses, and hospital administration for the quality work that enhanced the patient care. The mission of pharmacists directing medication therapy was being accomplished. In terms of developing staff and your team, a quality improvement initiative that improves practice and elevates pharmacist value within the organization should be considered. Twelve quality teams have been formed within the pharmacy systemwide, and major accomplishments have come from the team contributions, causing positive impact on patient care for the health system. In fact, these quality teams have been the second most positive force in the history of the pharmacy department (after the pharmacy residency program).

Summary

The clinical coordinator holds the team together by keeping everyone on the same page, moving in the same direction, and producing an outstanding performance. A clinical pharmacist is more involved in direct patient care and multidisciplinary team functions. The pharmacy director and assistant directors are more involved in setting direction, maintaining budgets, aligning the department with the organization, and making key decisions for the department. The role of the clinical coordinator is satisfying because you maintain patient care and define service/protocols to improve patient outcomes. If you can step aside from a front-line position and use your abilities to direct the pharmacist team to excel with strong patient outcomes and improve the use of pharmacotherapy, then this role is for you. You are the coach that sets up the plays, defines the playbook, and gets satisfaction when the game (i.e., patient care) is recognized by patients and medical and nursing staffs. As readmissions rates and other mandates are becoming measures of patient and financial success, the clinical coordinator who can direct a team of outstanding clinical pharmacists will become invaluable for the department and organization. What an exciting challenge!

PRACTICE TIPS

1. Embrace technology and tools that are available for your use, such as hardwiring orders, processes, etc. Offer templates on how to document patient care and seek consistency in practice by your team. Reinforce learning by reviewing what your staff members are doing and identifying how things could be improved.

2. Encourage staff members to give you feedback so that you can improve. Ask staff to complete your competency assessment and to give you feedback. Listen and improve. Also, admit when you were short-sighted or did not understand what was meant during a discussion. Thank staff members when they help you grow.

3. Be willing to help when workload gets busy or when a complicated situation arises. Staff members need to know that you are willing to step in to help resolve problems. This can be difficult if you personally are working on something that is time-dependent. In that case, find a way to identify someone to help resolve the problem. If you do not personally assist and when you complete what you had to do, follow up to see how you can assist if additional resources are needed.

4. Be fair, consistent, transparent, timely, and honest about what should be done. Show respect and discuss sensitive issues in private. Create an atmosphere of fun in meetings. Treat your team like you would like to be treated.

5. Take up the baton and lead your clinical pharmacists to new levels of performance. Be aware that your position is more than being a great clinical pharmacist. It is to lead staff so patient outcomes are achieved and staff members enjoy providing outstanding clinical pharmacy services.

References

1. Herr EL, Cramer SH. *Career Guidance and Counseling Through the Lifespan: Systematic Approaches.* 6th ed. New York, NY: Pearson; 2003.

2. http://www.profilesinternational.com/employee-assessment-products-overview/profiles-performance-indicator-employee-performance-test/. Accessed November 28, 2014.

3. Hasspacher JB, Roh JM, Absher R. *Get on the Bus: Pharmacist Teams Drive Quality.* Submitted for ASHP Best Practices Award. 2008.

4. Collins J. *Good to Great: Why Some Companies Make The Leap....and Others Don't.* New York, NY: HarperBusiness; 2001.

5. Knowles MS. *The Adult Learner: A Neglected Species.* 4th ed. Houston, TX: Gulf Publishing Company; 1990:119.

6. Lake D. CIPE—New Way of Thinking, Teaching, Coaching. Presented at the NC AHEC Continuing Interprofessional Education Summit. Friday Center, University of North Carolina, Chapel Hill, NC. November 11, 2014.

7. http://www.ihi.org/resources/Pages/Tools/SBARToolkit.aspx. Accessed November 28, 2014.

8. http://www.myersbriggs.org. Accessed November 22, 2014.

9. https://www.discprofile.com/what-is-disc/overview/. Accessed November 22, 2014.

10. https://en.wikipedia.org/wiki/SMART_criteria. Accessed November 26, 2014.

11. http://www.ashp.org/menu/Residency/Residency-Resources. Accessed November 28, 2014.

12. http://www.acpe-accredit.org/pharmacists/CPD.asp. Accessed November 25, 2014.

13. http://www.talentlms.com/blog/elearning-trends-follow-2015-infographic/. eLearning trends to follow in 2015. Accessed November 22, 2014.

14. Senge P. *The Fifth Discipline.* New York, NY: Currency Doubleday; 1990:22-23.

15. Oncken W Jr, Wass D. Management time: who's got the monkey? *Harv Bus Rev.* 1974;52(6):75-80.

16. http://www.brainyquote.com/quotes/quotes/t/theodorero140484.html. Accessed November 25, 2014.

17. http://www.jointcommission.org/core_measure_sets.aspx. Accessed November 25, 2014.

18. Lencioni P. *The Five Dysfunctions of a Team.* San Francisco, CA: Jossey-Bass; 2002.

Suggested Reading

Herr EL, Cramer SH, Niles SG. *Career Guidance and Counseling Through the Lifespan: Systematic Approaches.* 6th ed. New York, NY: Pearson; 2003.

Niles SG, Harris-Bowlesbey JE. *Career Development Interventions in the 21st Century.* 4th ed. New York, NY: Pearson; 2002:7.

Appendix 8-A

Checklist for Administrative Decision Making

Administration, Management, and Leadership Checklist

	Explained Discussed (RPh/Date)	Demonstrated Proficiency (RPh/Date)
(Director of Pharmacy Operations and Technology, Cone Health)		

■ Technology and systems, including timeline for new technologies
  ■ Cone HealthLink
  ■ Barcoding of medications
  ■ Talyst and automation for accuracy and safety
  ■ Pyxis Enterprise plans across the system
■ Drug philosophies and policies
■ Utilization strategies as it relates to formulary management
■ Buying groups, wholesaler specifics and contracts
■ Roles of business manager, 340B manager, inventory specialist, information system analyst, and data support technician
■ 340B program
■ System reports (nonformulary, expensive drugs, etc., and why these are run)
■ How we interact within information systems pharmacists and their roles with automation implementation and maintenance		

(Senior Clinical Coordinator and Director of Pharmacy Residency, MCH)		
■ ASHP-accredited pharmacy practice PGY1 and PGY2 residencies; selection processes, training guidelines, and requirements ■ Quality improvement pharmacist teams and expected participation/resultant outcomes ■ Schedule specifics ■ Cardiology services/center of excellence structure and teams ■ Precepting expectations and what makes a good preceptor, residency goals and how best to work with our residents ■ Decision making on who attends meetings outside health system ■ Laptops/iPads/Lexicomp subscriptions ■ Research protocols, projects, and practice decisions ■ Institutional review board (IRB) ■ Cone Health Research Institute		

Appendix 8-A, continued

Checklist for Administrative Decision Making

Administration, Management, and Leadership Checklist

	Explained Discussed (RPh/Date)	Demonstrated Proficiency (RPh/Date)
(MC Pharmacy Director)		
■ Pharmacy mission, vision, and standards ■ Triple aim: service, quality, and cost; dashboards ■ Job descriptions in pharmacy ■ Support staff guideline, duties of office manager, administrative assistant, departmental secretary, and financial audit coordinator ■ Role of pharmacist supervisor, technician supervisors, role of area supervisor ■ Role of technician IIIs and career ladder program ■ P&T committee (systemwide) and guidelines for topics ■ Pharmacy departmental staff meetings ■ Service recovery/complaint management ■ Disaster plan, worker's comp, infectious disease prevention, etc. ■ Indigent accounts and role of pharmacist ■ Communication tips and email tips ■ Shared governance for nursing and pharmacy ■ Medical committees and services ■ Six Sigma and CPI teams; Lean Six Sigma methodology for continuous improvement; Black Belts versus Green Belts ■ Continuous professional development—license renewal ■ Schools of pharmacy in state; Area Health Education Centers ■ Magnet and other honorable designations ■ Core measures ■ Hospital dashboard: PSIs and never events ■ Performance appraisal process/journaling ■ Environment of learning and CBLs ■ Working with other departments to achieve mission and vision ■ Hiring and training plans for all learners and need for documentation for TJC		
(Executive Director of Pharmacy Services, Cone Health)		
■ Communicating with the C-Suite ■ Six pharmacy departments = Cone Health Pharmacy Services ■ Mission and goals of the Cone Health Pharmacy Services ■ Getting the most value from drug representatives/status blue ■ Aligning pharmacy mission and goals with health network vision, mission, and goals ■ Tips for succeeding at Cone Health ■ Using data to make points for decision making ■ Planning and project management		

Administration, Management, and Leadership Checklist

	Explained Discussed (RPh/Date)	Demonstrated Proficiency (RPh/Date)
(IV/Manufacturing Coordinator, MCH)		
▪ USP Chapter <797> compliance ▪ IV/manufacturing supervision; services provided, workflow, etc. ▪ TNA-dispensing specifics ▪ IV policies (KCl, etc.) ▪ Patient care specifics in IV issues ▪ How department serves as support section for whole department ▪ Drug shortage management ▪ Conflict resolution ▪ Coordination of services with other pharmacies in system ▪ Role IV—manufacturing therapy technician III		
(Manager of Medication Safety and Quality, Cone Health)		
▪ Role of manager of medication safety and quality ▪ SZP and why it is important to complete these in a timely manner ▪ How SZP data are used to make improvements ▪ VigiLanz and how this has been implemented to improve patient safety and pharmacist workflow/documentation ▪ Amalga and how this tool has helped in identifying patient data ▪ IV pumps/Alaris library ▪ How behaviors are changed to improve medication safety (+ examples); just culture versus reckless behavior ▪ Protocols and other ways to "hardwire" for safety ▪ Pharmacy clinical and operational quality improvement teams ▪ Structure of quality at Cone Health remaining TJC-ready ▪ FDA medication safety alerts and what Cone Health does with this information		
Items Requiring Knowledge of Skills/Understanding and Where to Find Information		
▪ Need to adhere to state and federal laws		
▪ Privacy policy (HIPAA)		
▪ Hospital disaster procedure		
▪ Security for department and safety for employees (combination locks, name badge)		
▪ Location of fire extinguishers and sprinklers/showers		
▪ Workers' compensation procedures		
▪ Maintaining cleanliness in the worksite		
▪ Strategies for managing stress/teamwork in the workplace		
▪ Duties of area supervisor in work environment		
▪ Accountability and follow-through		

Appendix 8-A, continued

Checklist for Administrative Decision Making

Administration, Management, and Leadership Checklist

	Explained Discussed (RPh/Date)	Demonstrated Proficiency (RPh/Date)
■ Culture of timeliness and attendance policy specifics		
■ Emergency codes (red, orange, yellow, triage, black, pink, gray)		
■ Items requiring participation		
■ Complete CBLs that are required and document (print transcript)		
■ Aseptic technique (CBL transcript)		
■ Control numbers, combination locks, passwords, security		
■ Attend a CPI meeting (Meeting and date:)		
■ Attend a P&T committee meeting (Date:)		
■ Attend a pharmacist staff meeting (Date:)		
■ Attend a pharmacy technician staff meeting (Date:)		
■ Attend a Graduate Forum (Date and Topic:)		
■ Observe medication administration process/documentation (Date:)		
■ Meet with care manager to understand discharge role (Date:)		
■ Attend cardiac rehab class for 30 minutes (Date:)		
■ Visit the rapid response lab (Date:)		
■ Medical team rounding—pediatrics and CCM (Date:)		
■ Documentation in the medical record		

ASHP = American Society of Health-System Pharmacists; CBL = case-based learning; CCM = critical care medicine; CPI = continuous process improvement; C-Suite = senior executives; FDA = Food and Drug Administration; HIPAA = Health Insurance Portability and Accountability Act; IV = intravenous; KCl = potassium chloride; MCH = Moses Cone Hospital; PGY1 = postgraduate year 1; PGY2 = postgraduate year 2; PSIs = patient safety indicators; P&T = pharmacy and therapeutics; RPh = registered pharmacist; SZP = safety zone portals; TJC = The Joint Commission; TNA = total nutrient admixtures; USP = U.S. Pharmacopeial Convention.

Source: Courtesy of Cone Health, Greensboro, North Carolina, ©2015.

CHAPTER 9

Development and Assessment of Competency

Lynn Eschenbacher and Rhonda Zillmer

KEY TERMS

Audience Response—Incorporating audience members into the presentation by asking questions and getting responses via raised hands, text messages, or official technology system.

Balanced Scorecard (BSC)—A strategic planning and management document to align all of the activities within your department to the vision and strategy of the senior leaders and the organization's board of directors.

Educational Needs Assessment—A question-and-answer process (paper or electronic-based) that determines the current level of knowledge on a topic.

Flipped Classroom—A method where students learn content on their own prior to class (e.g., recorded lecture and completed activities) and then apply that information during student-centered learning activities in class.

Introduction

Ensuring that your staff is prepared and competent is essential for a clinical coordinator. If you want to implement a new service, continue to advance practice, or adhere to your strategic plan, the pharmacists and technicians must be prepared, knowledgeable of the process and essential elements, and able to apply their knowledge in the clinical and operational setting to achieve the intended outcomes. Competency is more than just signing off on a new process or completing a checklist. If your organization currently has an annual process of a packet of papers for the pharmacists to sign, then perhaps you do not have a robust competency process to support your endeavors to provide positive patient outcomes. Becoming competent in any area is a journey; training and education are the cornerstones of competency. We describe in this chapter how to identify the competencies required, develop a competency education plan, assess your employees' competency, and, finally, implement an ongoing process.

Starting Your Competency Plan: Alignment and Value

The first part of developing your organization's competency plan is to know what you want to focus on for the current and coming years. This is where strategic planning is important. You need to know what pharmacy services are value-added to the organization. Use the value equation that **Value is equal to Quality plus Service divided by Cost** to determine in each of these categories how pharmacy can increase quality or decrease cost.

$$\text{Value} = \frac{\text{Quality} + \text{Service}}{\text{Cost}}$$

Although cost is the denominator in the equation and could easily be all you focus on to reduce costs, it is important to understand and communicate how increases in quality and service also increase value. A focus on increasing quality and/or service is how clinical pharmacy services bring value to the patient experience. It is always important to monitor and be aware of cost and incorporate ways to eliminate waste and cost in your processes.

To determine what your organization considers patient quality and value, seek out senior leadership's **balanced scorecard** (BSC) or other dashboard of priorities set for the organization. A BSC is a strategic planning and management document to align your department's activities to the vision and strategy of the organization's senior leaders and the board of directors. Having all of the information in one document or tool helps to ensure that the priorities are clearly stated for the organization and serves as a monitor of organizational performance against the strategic goals (see **Figure 9-1**). How does pharmacy fit into these goals or advance these goals? How can you use them to identify which services you want to start or expand? (For more details on how to conduct a strategic plan, see Chapter 10: Strategic Planning and Project Management). It is important to start with the desired outcome—what you want your staff members to know—and then work backward, developing the competencies, how you will teach it, and how you will know that they fully understand and can apply the information. This process is called *reverse engineering*.

Identification of Baseline Knowledge and Annual Education Plan Development

Once you know your strategic direction and the value-added services for your organization, you should determine your staff's baseline knowledge specific to that initiative. In addition, there are foundational competencies including knowledge of sterile compounding; control substance rules and regulations; special patient population areas such as neonatal, pediatrics, geriatrics, and oncology/chemotherapy; and other high-risk medications or processes. These might not be new clinical services or value-added programs, but they are core to your organization, and competency must be performed on a regular basis or annually.

Is your staff ready? Do they have the skills and knowledge that they need to be successful and lead the way to positive patient outcomes? Which initiatives are you going to implement this year? Which initiatives will be implemented over the next few years that you need to develop the foundational knowledge with your staff now so that you can continue to

FIGURE 9-1. Department of Pharmacy FY15 Strategic Goals

Pharmacy Goal for FY15	Corporate Measures Alignment	Pharmacy Activities to Meet Goal	Tips to Meet Goal	Resources/ References
Improve patient transition of care, reduce preventable readmissions, and improve hospital HCAHPS scores	■ Quality experiences	Achieve 500 documented heart failure/MI/stroke and transitions of care interventions	■ Review discharge medications for core measures, accuracy, home medication discrepancies, etc. ■ Document interventions in TheraDoc with appropriate intervention types	Discharge medications packet
Operate within budgeted expenses (salary, revenue)	■ Financial stewardship	Identify and evaluate medication usage unsupported by organization formulary, clinical guidelines, etc.	■ Identify inappropriate and/or unnecessary medication-use practice and suggest completion of an MUE ■ Provide feedback to coordinators on specific medications to review based on prescribing practice or frontline issues	SharePoint Systemwide folder, P&T collaboration, MUEs folder
Provide comprehensive medication therapy management	■ Empower and partner with healthcare team	Perform prospective patient profile review and make interventions as needed Achieve 1,150 documented interventions	■ Participate in rounding opportunities such as SIBR and medication teaching rounds (pediatrics and adults) to discuss potential interventions with physicians ■ Strive to meet profile review expectations in nonrounding areas such as ED ■ Streamline and improve workflow to allow profile review for patients not on rounding teams ■ Document interventions in TheraDoc with the appropriate intervention types	SIBR document
Provide education and competency assessment opportunities to all pharmacists	■ Leadership in safety, innovation, education	Develop and adhere to pharmacist education plan Provide 20 hr/month of pharmacist education	■ Participate in learning activities and peer review ■ Practice knowledge on daily basis ■ Consult with content experts when questions arise ■ Complete annual competencies	Pharmacist education plan
Increase patient awareness of inpatient pharmacy services	■ Foster trust and transparency	Achieve 20 documented pharmacist or pharmacy student introductions to patients	■ Familiarize yourself on the steps to determine who needs a pharmacy introduction on your patient care unit ■ Ensure documentation of the pharmacy introduction service in the EMR	Pharmacist/ pharmacy student introduction handout
Partner with university and schools of pharmacy	■ Partner with others who value our culture	Precept 120 students from local schools of pharmacy	■ Become primary preceptors and/or assist with student activities ■ Participate in preceptor development activities to enhance precepting skills ■ Develop practice environment that encourages teaching and learning	Preceptor development opportunities in Microsoft Outlook Student calendar

ED = emergency department; EMR = electronic medical record; HCAHPS = Hospital Consumer Assessment of Healthcare Providers and Systems; MI = myocardial infarction; MUE = medication-use evaluation; P&T = pharmacy and therapeutics; SIBR = structured interdisciplinary bedside rounds.

expand and reinforce that knowledge? Even if the initiatives will not be implemented this year, you should begin developing that knowledge now because the information might be difficult to learn or very new to the staff members. They may need to focus on it several times before implementation to ensure they can apply the information successfully. It important to clearly state to the staff what your focus will be this year and upcoming years. This could be a combined strategic plan with the associated educational/competency developmental plan (**Figure 9-2**). Your transparency with staff members will ensure better understanding and their successful acceptance of proposed changes. Review the document and plan at staff meetings, post a physical copy in the pharmacy department as well as electronically online, and place a copy in the decentralized notebook (electronic or hardcopy). Talk about the plan and what staff members will be required to learn prior to the implementation. They will then realize you have provided ample preparation before implementing the change. Being transparent is also important to determine their current knowledge base on the subject. If you are able to offer continuing education credit for any of the educational topics, your staff will appreciate that as well.

Analyzing the current knowledge base to determine which competencies and skills must be developed should not be overlooked. It might be easy to just jump straight into education, but if you do not know what to focus on, you will either provide information that is too basic or not provide adequate foundation to tie in the information. Humans are more successful at retaining and applying information if they have a neural pathway to tie in the information when processing the new information. Every time you learn something, neural circuits are altered in your brain. When you learn something new, your brain creates new connections between neurons. To learn this new process or fact, you have to repeat it several times to strengthen the connections. To remember the new process or fact days or years later, you will have to successfully reactivate these same neural circuits. The new pathways become stronger the more they are used, causing the likelihood of new long-term connections and memories. To determine baseline knowledge, you can conduct an **educational needs assessment**.

This could be a written or oral assessment, or it could be a direct observation. There are ASHP assessment tools for competency assessment, or you can develop it internally.[1] If you internally develop your tool, you need to validate it. Working with a local school of pharmacy or other expert resources available to you are ways to effectively validate your needs assessment. The assessment method will depend on your time and available resources. For the decentralization of our department's pharmacy services, we needed to conduct an overall assessment of the general knowledge in areas such as antimicrobial management, cardiology, intravenous (IV) to oral medication conversion, identification of drug therapy interventions, hypertension, stroke, anticonvulsants, diabetes, pain management, drug information, heart failure, anticoagulation, and pediatrics. Because pharmacy services were moving from the central pharmacy to the patient care areas, we had to determine what skills and competencies our staff needed to be successful. We developed an educational needs assessment tool that was a case-based, short-answer, multiple-choice, and true/false written assessment (see **Figure 9-3** for sample questions in an educational needs assessment). The pharmacists were given 4 hours of time during work (their staffing assignments were covered) to complete the assessment. We had all staff members complete the assessment and used the information to create an educational plan over the next year using the acronym SHAPE (**s**troke, **h**ypertension, **a**nticoagulation, **p**ain management, and **e**ducation). We shared this plan with the staff members and promoted it to help them know our focus and how it would be taught over the year. By carefully assessing staff knowledge, you can modify your education plan to determine what needs to be covered only a few times or repeated many times so they will retain the information.

There might be times that it is not necessary to understand the staff's baseline knowledge, for example, implementing a new computer system or a completely new service. As a clinical coordinator, you should have a strategy when to get baseline information and when it is not required. Staff members may be resistant at first to being tested on what they know. However, if you are transparent with your department's goals and the plans to get them

FIGURE 9-2. Educational/Competency Developmental Plan

January–February

Pharmacy skills day

January preceptor development: Assessments that improve outcome

February preceptor development: Creating residency projects that make a difference

March–April

Pyxis ES

ADA guideline update

Aminoglycoside small group discussions starting March 24

March preceptor development: Improve preceptor assessment of student clinical skills

April preceptor development: Innovative residency applicant screening and interview strategies

May–June

Anticoagulation: Factor products

JNC 8 update

May preceptor development: Residency QA session and strategic planning

June preceptor development: Incorporating residents and students into pharmacy practice

July–August

July preceptor development: Professionalism

August pharmacy grand rounds: HIV

August preceptor development: Managing multiple residents with incongruent personalities

September–October

Phenytoin small group discussions starting September 18

September pharmacy grand rounds: Organ donation

October pharmacy grand rounds: Aortic and mitral stenosis and TAVR

September preceptor development: Practice management training in PGY1 residency year

October preceptor development: Role of the student pharmacist

November–December

EPIC training from November 2014 to January 2015

November pharmacy grand rounds: Cutaneous mucormycosis

December pharmacy grand rounds: Digoxin in atrial fibrillation and heart failure

November/December preceptor development: Learning taxonomy and level

---

ADA = American Diabetes Association; ES = enterprise server; HIV = human immunodeficiency virus; QA = questions and answers; PGYI = postgraduate year one; TAVR = transcatheter aortic valve replacement.

FIGURE 9-3. Sample Questions for an Educational Needs Assessment

1. Please give an example of an appropriate empiric regimen for community-acquired pneumonia in a hospitalized patient.

2. Which of the following is an appropriate empiric regimen for aspiration pneumonia in a hospitalized patient?
   a. Piperacillin/tazobactam
   b. Doxycycline
   c. Dicloxacillin
   d. Clarithromycin

3. Which of the following criteria may indicate that a patient is not appropriate for an intravenous to oral switch?
   a. Improvement in temperature curve
   b. Infection site signs and symptoms improving
   c. Decline in ANC
   d. Hypotension resolving

4. The higher the MIC, the more susceptible the pathogen is to the antibiotic.
   True
   False

5. M. J. is a 55-year-old male who presents to the ED at 1300 with slurred speech and hemiplegia. He woke up with these symptoms at 0800 this morning after falling asleep on his couch as usual last night. His current blood pressure is 190/100, and his heart rate is 105 bpm. He has a PMH significant for DM and hyperlipidemia. Home medications include ASA 81 mg daily, lisinopril 10 mg daily, and metformin 500 mg bid.

   Is M. J. a candidate for tPA therapy? Why or why not?

   The next day the medicine teaching team decides to start drug therapy for secondary stroke prevention. Please list two possible antiplatelet therapy options for M. J., and list pros and cons for each option.

   Therapy options: _____
   _____

   Pros: _____
   _____

   Cons: _____
   _____

FIGURE 9-3. Sample Questions for an Educational Needs Assessment, continued

6. Please review the following questions and match them with the most appropriate resource for finding the answer (letters may be used more than once):
   a. *Drug Facts and Comparisons*
   b. *Micromedex*
   c. *UptoDate*
   d. *Appropriate Treatment Guidelines*
   e. *Handbook on Injectable Drugs, Sanford Guide*

   _____ Does rifampin cover *Staphylococcus epidermidis*?
   _____ Does ceftriaxone need to be renally dosed?
   _____ What is the recommended therapy for a copperhead snake bite, and who should be treated?
   _____ Can you run ampicillin and heparin through the same line?
   _____ How long should patients take warfarin after their first unprovoked DVT?
   _____ What is the recommended empiric treatment regimen for community-acquired pneumonia?
   _____ Which drugs are most commonly implicated in causing pancreatitis?
   _____ Does methotrexate contain red dye #3?

7. A. B. is a 65-year-old female admitted with community-acquired pneumonia. Which of the following is the most appropriate empiric regimen for treatment? (Assume there is no renal insufficiency.)
   a. Levofloxacin 750 mg PO daily
   b. Amoxicillin 500 mg PO tid
   c. Primaxin 1 g IV q 6 hr
   d. Cefotaxime 1 g IV q 8 hr

8. A Gram stain that shows gram-positive organisms could be indicative of all of the following *except* _____
   a. *Staphylococcus* spp.
   b. *Enterococcus* spp.
   c. *Enterobacter*
   d. *Streptococcus* spp.

9. Which of the following *is not* considered an anaerobic organism?
   a. *Clostridium*
   b. *Bacteroides* spp.
   c. *Pseudomonas aeruginosa*
   d. *Actinomyces* spp.

10. A neonate is defined as newborn less than 6 months old.
    True
    False

FIGURE 9-3. Sample Questions for an Educational Needs Assessment, continued

11. Which of the following medication orders must be clarified?
    a.   Septra suspension 5 mL PO bid
    b.   Baclofen suspension 4 mL PO tid
    c.   APAP 120 mg/codeine 12 mg/5 mL: take 7.5 mL PO q 4 hr prn pain
    d.   None of the above need to be rewritten

12. What is the infusion rate (mL/hr) required to administer dopamine 5 mcg/kg/min when it is mixed 200 mg/50 mL NS. The patient's weight is 22 kg.

ANC = absolute neutrophil count; APAP = acetaminophen; ASA = acetylsalicylic acid; bid = two times a day; bpm = beats per minute; DM = diabetes mellitus; DVT = deep vein thrombosis; ED = emergency department; hr = hour; IV = intravenous; MIC = minimum inhibitory concentration; NS = normal saline; PO = orally; PMH = past medical history; prn = as needed; q = every; tid = three times a day; tPA = tissue plasminogen activator.

---

ready, they will more easily accept the assessment. If you assure them it is not related to a raise or job security, and it is only focused on improving their knowledge and skills, they are usually more receptive and accepting. As a coordinator, take the lead and discuss why this is important and how you will work as a team to positively impact patients.

There are many different methods for education: didactic, **audience response**, patient cases, one-on-ones, peer teaching, small groups, and the **flipped classroom**. Each of these techniques has pros and cons. As a coordinator, you need to determine which method or methods will work best for the material and develop your personal tool kit with these methods. There might be times when you only need one method and other times when you will need several. You can mix and match the styles and present the same or variations of the information in different formats over time.

Competency Development

Didactic

The *didactic* method is the educational method that you are probably most familiar with. The format is the traditional lecture where someone either just speaks or uses a PowerPoint presentation to share information about a topic. This is very one-sided and mostly involves telling the audience about the topic. There might be questions or cases to help apply the informa-

tion during the presentation. However, even the cases in a didactic lecture are not truly active learning. The audience members are not required to answer, and there is no feedback regarding the accuracy of their answers. It is important to find more active methods to help the staff retain and apply the information.

Pros

- Large groups
- First time to introduce the topic and overview of the topic
- Easy to prepare
- Not too time-consuming
- No advance preparation by the audience

Cons

- Not active learning
- Passive
- Not well retained
- No application of knowledge
- Does not develop critical thinking

Audience Response

The second educational method is incorporation of audience response methods into a traditionally didactic lecture. *Audience response* can be done by either having staff members raise their hands for a low technical option or use their mobile devices to answer questions in the presentation. To use their mobile devices there are many options—some free and some subscription—available on the Internet. An example would be polleverywhere.com. Another option would be independent technology that is specific to an audience response system. However, such technology is expensive and if your staff members have their own mobile devices, they can just use their own devices. Medical and pharmacy schools often require students to purchase audience response pads. You could contact those at pharmacy schools or other professional organizations and ask if you can borrow them. During the presentation, the speaker incorporates cases or questions, and the staff members either raise their hands or use the response key pad to answer via their mobile device or independent audience response key pad. Some examples of how to use this technique could be with antimicrobial stewardship and a focus on gram-positive cocci in clusters, gram-positive cocci in pairs and chains, and gram-negative rods with extended-spectrum beta-lactamase and *Pseudomonas*. You can teach the material, and during the lecture, ask the audience questions to see if they understand the material and have retained the information. Incorporation of audience response is a low-cost technique that provides better outcomes in learning the material than traditional didactic lecture.

Pros

- Some active learning
- Better if answers are typed and hidden until all have submitted their answers rather than raising hands to reduce bias from observing how other participants answer
- Immediate feedback and ability to modify presentation based on responses and knowledge (if several people answer incorrectly, the presenter can go over the material again; if everyone gets it correct, the presenter can move to the next topic)
- Large groups
- Presenter can see a counter of the number of responses and can keep the question open until all have responded
- Identification of future educational opportunities if certain answers are incorrect; can determine if a future focused learning session on those topics might be required

Cons

- Possible that some do not answer
- Cannot know which participants do not understand because answers are anonymous; not individualized or customized by person
- Not well retained
- Little application of knowledge
- Answers may be biased based on responses by others in the group if the responses are not hidden until all answers are submitted
- Possible that someone is a good guesser in answering and does not really know the material

Patient Cases and Scenarios

The next option for education is *patient cases* and *scenarios*. Patient cases can be done by collecting real patient cases that the staff performed either correctly or incorrectly. Another option is to create your own patient cases or find examples from an ASHP reference or Koda-Kimble and Young's *Applied Therapeutics: The Clinical Use of Drugs*.[2] The patient cases can focus on one disease state or across various disease states. One example we used was a packet that contained 25 different pharmacokinetic cases for vancomycin, aminoglycosides, and phenytoin (see **Figure 9-4**). The cases contained our daily monitoring sheets with all pertinent laboratory values and daily monitoring notes with specific questions associated with each case. We also created a packet of 20 different anticoagulation cases for warfarin dosing and monitoring, heparin dosing and monitoring, and other newer oral anticoagulants and options for reversal. For this packet, the staff members should work through the packet, answer the questions (showing their work), and include progress notes. They decide the appropriate dose, when to get levels, and how to communicate their recommendation and progress notes. Then the clinical coordinator and/or clinical specialists can review the answers to determine what is correct or not. The important next step is to meet with staff members individually to review the packets and discuss the answers.

FIGURE 9-4. Sample Pharmacokinetic Questions

Kinetics Patient Cases

For each case, please answer the questions below. In addition, please fill out the monitoring sheet (progress notes section and lab sheet when indicated) and write a progress note for each of the cases.

1. **Vancomycin and CRRT**

   When did the patient start CRRT?

   Vancomycin started. What is your initial and maintenance dose of vancomycin?

   Vancomycin level was drawn the next day. Why was the level drawn?

   How would your dose change, if at all, in reaction to the level?

   Five days later, CRRT was discontinued. How, if at all, would your vancomycin dose change?

2. **Tobramycin**

   Why is the patient on tobramycin?

   What is the target peak/trough?

   Why did we not initiate once-daily dosing in this patient?

   Based on the levels, how should we have adjusted the tobramycin dose?

3. **Vancomycin and Doripenem with CRRT**

   What should our doses be for these medications?

   When should we draw levels?

   Would the dosing change when they transition to hemodialysis? If so, what should the new dosing be?

4. **Vancomycin and Gentamicin**

   What should the initial doses of vancomycin and gentamicin be for this patient?

   When should we draw levels?

   Blood cultures came back growing MRSA MIC = 1. Would this guide your dosing at all? What would you recommend? What if his MIC was 2?

5. **Vancomycin and Gentamicin MRSA Endocarditis**

   Why is the patient on gentamicin?

   What is the goal peak/trough for gentamicin?

   When should we draw gentamicin levels for this patient?

   What should our initial gentamicin dose be for this patient?

   Later the patient's vancomycin level came back at 22.3. Would you change the dose? If so, what would you change the dose to?

   How long should this patient receive vancomycin and gentamicin?

6. **Phenytoin**

   This patient had a free phenytoin level of 0.5 mcg/mL. What would you recommend to change the dose to?

   You increased the dose and the level came back at 0.4 mcg/mL. What could be some reasons for this? What would you do now?

7. **Vancomycin**

   Vancomycin trough level was 33.3 mg/L. How do you respond to this information?

FIGURE 9-4. Sample Pharmacokinetic Questions, continued

8. **Vancomycin**

   Patient's trough level was 23.7 mg/L. What could have caused this increase without a change in dose?

   Would you adjust the dose? If so, what would you change the regimen to?

   When would you draw the next trough?

9. **Phenytoin**

   The patient started on phenytoin with a 2-g load and then started on 200 mg IV bid. Total phenytoin level was 15.3 mg/L. The patient's physician changed the dose to 100 mg PO tid. Patient had no active seizures, and albumin is normal; however, the patient still had slurred speech and dizziness. How do you respond?

10. **Phenytoin**

    The patient started phenytoin for postoperative craniotomy. The patient received a 1-g load in the OR. What would your initial phenytoin dose be for this patient?

    Based on the free level of 1.5, what, if any, changes would you make?

    When would you draw another level?

   _____

   bid = two times a day; CRRT = continuous renal replacement therapy; IV = intravenous; MIC = minimum inhibitory concentration; MRSA = methicillin-resistant *Staphylococcus aureus*; OR = operating room; PO = by mouth, orally; tid = three times a day.

There are a lot of gray areas in medicine, but there are standards for your organization on how to dose certain medications, write notes, and provide feedback to your staff. You can decide if you let the staff members take these cases home or if they need to do them at work. If a staff member is working and takes 2 hours to do a case that should ideally be done in 5 minutes, it might not be a fair assessment. However, if the staff member does not get the correct answer after an extended period of time working on the case, then it might indicate areas that need improvement. Patient cases are a great way for staff members to apply their knowledge while giving you time to review their answers and provide feedback. A slight variation on the packet of cases described above would be for staff members to collect their own patient cases that you can review with them. Another option would be for you to pick several patient cases. Depending on if you capture this information using daily documentation on paper or electronically, you could select several vancomycin, gentamicin, phenytoin, warfarin, etc., cases that the employee worked on and then individually discuss them.

Patient scenarios or "what would you do" situations are another approach we have utilized formally and informally with our pharmacy residents (see **Figure 9-5**). These patient, operational, and leadership scenarios are presented to the residents at our regular clinical specialist, coordinators, and residents meetings. The scenarios are real examples from patient care submitted by the specialists, and our clinical coordinators and other department leaders submit operational and leadership examples. The topics have included managing a request for an orphan drug and European drugs; handling an unexpected drug recall; and managing specific patient care such as a drug overdose, suspected public health emergency, and responding to a medication error. The residents are asked to describe what they would do in the situation, and then the specialists and coordinators provide immediate feedback or insight as to how they handled the situation. We also utilize these types of questions in our pharmacist interview process to help provide a clear picture of what the residents or candidates know or do not know about specific medications or situations as well as to observe their critical thinking and response skills.

FIGURE 9-5. What Would You Do?

1. A physician sends you an email asking about IV acetaminophen use for neonatal patients and the cost of IV acetaminophen. What do you tell him?

    a. After the initial email, you learn it is for PDA closure refractory to NeoProfen and pain management. What are your thoughts? What information do you need to know? What do you do?

    b. Before it is resolved, the physician orders IV acetaminophen on two babies. What do you do?

2. Dexamethasone injection product is pulled up on the nursing unit and given orally in the ED. Does this concern you? What would you do to investigate other options? What are the other options?

3. A septic patient has single-lumen PICC, and phenylephrine and dopamine are infusing. The patient is also receiving acyclovir and meropenem for mucosal HSV and pneumonia, respectively. The antibiotics are incompatible with phenylephrine and dopamine. The patient's doctor wants to run carrier fluid to dilute out the drugs and then run incompatible things together. What would you do?

4. How do you dispense enoxaparin for a 2-year-old in outpatient therapy? Dose is 16 mg SC q 12 hr.

5. A patient is in complete circulatory arrest in the OR and is cooled to 18°C. The OR needs dosing on pentobarbital. List the dose, rate of infusion, and how to dilute.

6. Norepinephrine is in shortage, and the only way to get it is from the gray market. What do you do?

7. Lorazepam can be used up to 90 days out of the refrigerator. Another brand has 30 days, but it is on shortage. What do you do?

ED = emergency department; hr = hour; HSV = herpes simplex virus; IV = intravenous; PDA = patent ductus arteriosus; PICC = peripherally inserted central catheter; OR = operating room; q = every; SC = subcutaneous.

Pros

- Active learning
- Individualized and customized when you meet with each employee to review the cases and provide feedback
- Real patient cases and scenarios
- Application of knowledge
- Development of critical thinking
- Patient care is not directly impacted because these are historical cases and not real cases that need answers the day they are being completed.
- Opportunity to set and reinforce expectations

Cons

- Not real time; usually completed in a more controlled environment
- Time to have the employees complete the scenarios
- Time to "grade" the cases and then to meet individually with each employee to provide feedback on what was done well and what needs improvement
- If using multiple preceptors, could have variability in review and feedback, unless you have a standardized tool
- Remembering to save cases and keep the cases contemporary

One-on-Ones

A fourth option for education is individual *one-on-ones* with the staff. The goal of this method is modeling, shadowing, and coaching each individual employee. One-on-ones allow for the maximum amount of customization and individualization in real-life scenarios in patient care areas. For this method, the clinical coordinator (or clinical manager or specialist) divides the staff and works with staff members individually. This could be done for any period—

concentrated into 1 week or spread out over several months to a year. It is best not to use other decentralized staff for this because it may be perceived as awkward to have a peer shadowing and coaching. One approach to the one-on-one would be for the pharmacist to complete his or her daily work. Then at a specified time, the clinical coordinator would meet with the pharmacist to review the patient cases and discuss evidence-based practice and opportunities for improvement. Another approach is to have the clinical coordinator work up the same patients, suggest how he or she would have reviewed the patients, describe interventions, and then provide feedback and coaching. However, because pharmacists may share only the cases they feel confident about, the clinical coordinator could shadow on rounds or work in close proximity to the pharmacist. Although this method takes more of the coordinator's time during the day and may be more intimidating to the pharmacist, it is the best way to gather real-time information about what pharmacists are doing during shifts.

It is important for all clinical coordinators to use a guide to ensure standardization of the one-on-ones. The grid can contain training topics, training objectives, date taught/reviewed, competency assessed, and any comments (see **Figure 9-6**). The clinical coordinator can fill this out for each employee and use it as a learning plan. Some areas used for one-on-ones are pharmacokinetics, therapeutic drug monitoring, and anticoagulation management. Working daily with the employee allows for robust discussions about disease states, products to dispense, transitioning patients to the next level of care, and ensures a sound pharmaceutical plan.

Clinical coordinators are extremely busy with their clinical services, students, residents, and other clinical responsibilities, so adding more can be a challenge. Also, if you decide to conduct one-on-ones, week-at-a-time scheduling might be difficult, especially for 12-hour or part-time employees. The final disadvantage might be staff perception. Many staff members have done residencies and are board certified and might take offense to someone checking in on them or shadowing them. Again, being transparent as to why you are doing this and showing them examples of opportunities for improvement can help open the conversation. We focused

on how we invest in them and give them time to grow in a customized and individualized manner. Once we began the process, many staff members were thankful for the time to discuss recent journal articles, evidence-based practice, and patient cases. It is important to keep talking about this at staff meetings and provide updates and feedback about how the process is going.

Pros

- Highly individualized and customized
- Real time while caring for patients; real-world situation with support and coaching as needed
- Development of critical thinking
- Application of knowledge
- Real-time feedback
- Demonstrates how much you value the staff members and want to invest in their learning and development
- Whole-patient approach rather than focused on one aspect of care (e.g., if you did a patient case that was only on anticoagulation)

Cons

- Time (amount of time depends on if shadowing during a shift or meeting at the end of the shift)
- Variability of feedback if using multiple preceptors (evaluation tool can help mitigate some of this); however, different clinical knowledge and interpersonal skills sets
- Staff hesitancy and uneasiness
- Scheduling

Small Groups

A fifth option for education is *small group discussions*, which are sessions facilitated by an expert, and the participants prepare prior to coming to the discussion. Having a smaller group helps the staff feel more comfortable to openly discuss issues, and the facilitator can ensure that all members are participating. Larger groups allow for staff members who are less confident in their answers or have wrong answers the ability to hide and not be noticed that they lack the knowledge or competency. Small groups allow for individualized atten-

FIGURE 9-6. One-on-One/Observational/Side-by-Side Assessment

Clinical Staff Pharmacist

Name _____

Training Topics	Training Objectives	Date Reviewed/ Initials	Comments
Anticoagulation	Verify appropriateness of dose for each anticoagulant order		
	Verify appropriateness of indication for each anticoagulant order		
	Verify appropriateness of duration for each anticoagulant order		
	Identify the appropriate therapy goal for each patient with an anticoagulant order		
	Identify and manage major drug–drug interactions involving anticoagulants		
	Appropriately manage supratherapeutic levels of anticoagulants		

Training Topics	Training Objectives	Date Reviewed/ Initials	Comments
Therapeutic drug monitoring	Identify the appropriate reference range for all drugs with levels to be monitored		
	Verify appropriateness of indication for drugs with levels to be monitored		
	Identify the potential consequences of subtherapeutic/supratherapeutic levels		
	Appropriately manage subtherapeutic/ supratherapeutic levels		

Preceptor signature _____

Date _____

tion. The group size should be four or five staff members with the facilitator who is the subject matter expert. The staff members can prepare by reading a journal article or other literature and then completing patient cases. The small group discussion would then focus on reviewing the cases in depth and answering the questions associated with the cases. You can either have the staff members turn in their work at the beginning of the session for the facilitator's review, or make a copy to see how they did prior to discussion. Then during the session, staff members can use their completed patient cases for the discussion. If you are not the facilitator, make sure the facilitator keeps a record of the accuracy of the participants' answers. As a coordinator, you can follow up with those individuals who were not getting the right answers to remediate and develop an action plan to ensure they know the material and can apply it to make clinically sound decisions for patient care. You also need to have a content expert to successfully facilitate the session.

We completed a study on the knowledge retained using this method and the satisfaction of this method. The pharmacists performed better on an assessment and with the patient cases using the small group method versus the didactic lecture method. In addition, the pharmacists preferred this method because they could ask all the questions they wanted and did not feel intimidated or nervous to discuss the information in detail.

Pros

- Not as time-consuming as other methods
- Individualized feedback
- Comfort in a smaller group
- Active learning
- Knowledge is better retained due to required preparation as well as discussion of cases during the session
- Critical thinking development
- Facilitator can ensure member participation

Cons

- Time for the subject matter expert to hold several sessions

- Time for the staff members to prepare prior to the session
- Scheduling (patient care comes first, and staff members might need to miss the session)

Flipped Classroom

A sixth option for education is the *flipped classroom*. There has been a recent shift in curricula of pharmacy professional programs in the direction of active learning, which involves activities such as case studies, teamwork, and debates to engage the learner at a higher level. The flipped classroom method involves the students learning content on their own prior to class (e.g., recorded lecture and completed activities) and then applying that information during student-centered learning class activities. This can be easily applied in the workplace for your pharmacists, technicians, and even students who are on rotation at your site. For the flipped classroom, you can develop a PowerPoint presentation, complete the voice recording, and post the presentation on your organization's Intranet or another site on your network. Then, require the pharmacists to review this prior to the session. You can have an online assessment through Google docs, SurveyMonkey, or another form that records their answers to confirm that they have prepared in advance. You can also have them complete patient cases prior to the classroom session. Then, during the classroom session, you can do case studies or have a pros-and-cons debate on the topics so that the pharmacists better apply and retain the information. Overall, this method is the method of the future, and you should become familiar with the style and determine if there are opportunities for you to implement this within your organization.

Pros

- Active learning with robust, in-depth discussions
- Application of knowledge
- Critical thinking development
- Many interactions with the materials to build the neural pathways by preparing before session and then active learning during the session

- Learning from peers during case discussion
- Generation of new ideas during the discussion and future opportunities for education based on needs heard in the sessions

Cons

- Time to prepare and change from didactic presentation to what should be flipped (should be one time to get program started)
- Time to post articles or record presentation (should be one time to get program started)
- Scheduling (patient care comes first and staff members might need to miss the session)
- Time for staff to prepare

Peer Teaching

A final option for education is *peer teaching*, which allows for participation and engagement by your entire team. Once you determine the focus area, you can divide the topics among the staff to prepare the information and present to the team. You can either assign the topics or have the staff select topics. The staff member who prepares each topic should become the content expert on that topic. If you have the expertise, you or the clinical specialist should review what the staff member has prepared to ensure accuracy. You should also set deadlines and prepare a calendar for scheduled presentations to the staff. Some possible topics are anticoagulation in pregnancy, pediatric hypertension, sickle cell disease, and skin and soft tissue infections. Staff members should use active-learning techniques in their presentations. They should have audience response questions, small groups, or flipped classrooms. You should record the staff members' presentations so they can be used in orientations or for those who missed the live presentation. One inexpensive method to record the presentation is to use PowerPoint and the voice-over function. Then you can save the series of presentations to a shared site or Intranet. These modules should be reviewed on a regular basis and updated as new information is available. In addition, with the presentations you can have preassessments, postassessments, and annual assessments. This will allow you to determine

the retention of the information, and, if the assessment is constructed properly, it can also assess the application of the knowledge.

Pros

- Entire team involved, not just one person responsible for preparing all sessions
- Staff members become the subject matter experts
- Need to incorporate active-learning methods listed above
- If recording staff presentations, then they are available for new hire orientation

Cons

- Variability of staff knowledge (use specialist or coordinator to review the material to mitigate)
- If active-learning methods are not incorporated with a didactic method, then staff members may not retain information
- Time to record the presentation (one-time issue)

Competency Assessment

As licensed pharmacists, we demonstrated a specific level of competency on graduation from pharmacy school and successful completion of board exams. We also are required to maintain our education by completing hours for continuing education. There are various job descriptions for different types of pharmacists; each description should include the skills required for position competency. For example, clinical staff pharmacist competency requirements are different than those of a coordinator or manager. A competent pharmacist is one who can independently perform the expected and required duties of the position.

The required elements and expectations of the specific position should be reviewed during the hiring phase and then at orientation. The pharmacist's competency must be assessed and discussed regularly to ensure that once the orientation phase is completed, the pharmacist is prepared to meet expectations.

Once a specific area of knowledge or skill set is identified, you should select a method to assess or document competency. An ideal assessment method

- accurately measures the quality of performance,
- indicates how well the pharmacist will perform similar tasks,
- and reflects what the pharmacist will do in general practice.[1]

If your organization is utilizing an annual sign-off or has an annual competency packet that contains the same content every year, then there is definite room for improvement. An annual checklist may meet requirements from regulatory or accreditation organizations, but a static list does not help your staff grow and develop. Our department utilizes an annual checklist, but the contents change annually and are tailored to match the department's strategic goals and the various competencies and assessments we conduct each year (see **Figure 9-7**). As we developed various educational methods for competencies, we also transitioned from process-oriented assessments such as checklists and tests to methods that focus on outcomes and accountability for a specific knowledge or skill. To be successful, all pharmacists in the hospital setting must have a broad range of clinical and operational knowledge as well as critical thinking and interpersonal skills. As you develop competency plans, it is important to determine the appropriate method of verification or assessment for the skill being developed. We will review the following competency assessment methods: written tests, observational/side-by-side reviews, case studies, demonstration of skill, self-reflection, presentations, simulation, and quality improvement monitoring.

Written Tests

Written tests typically measure cognitive skills or knowledge. But, in our experience, written tests typically fall short in demonstrating how people think or arrive at their answers or decisions. We continue to utilize them in a variety of settings specifically if the competency is process-oriented, such as understanding the contents of a new chemotherapy policy or procedures or understanding specific calculations to determine an IV solution osmolality.

Observational/Side-by-Side Reviews

Observation of staff performing a specific skill provides a method to view and analyze performance in real time. We have utilized side-by-side observation on patient care rounds to assess the pharmacists' critical thinking skills. On rounds, the observer can review a pharmacist's clinical reasoning, problem-solving, and interpersonal skills, such as communication, listening, speaking, and collaboration with the healthcare team and patients. Challenges of observational assessments are the time the observer is required to spend and the possibility that the pharmacist will not be comfortable being "watched." Also, you need to consider the Hawthorne effect—watched individuals perform differently and often better than they would normally if not being watched. When completing the assessments, the observer should have a checklist or a rubric for the specific skills assessed. We utilized a format that was directly tied to the pharmacist's job description. Observational/side by side reviews or one-on-ones can be used for teaching the information as well as evaluating the competency (see Figure 9-6). Another option for observational assessment is reviewing the pharmacist's performance when communicating via the phone. Although many of our pharmacists are decentralized, we still make many of our interventions and recommendations via non–face-to-face communications. Verification of phone etiquette can assess clinical and operational skills, and it is necessary to ensure these types of communications are as effective as possible. Phone reviews can be completed side-by-side or via recorded phone conversations if available in your department. If your department does not currently have a recording system in place, consider checking with your organization's telecommunication department to see if a recording and playback system is available.

Case Studies

Case studies can be used to demonstrate critical thinking skills, teach materials, and evaluate competency. They can be created from your patient population examples or obtained from textbooks or websites designed by pharmacy organizations, such as www.ashp. org. *Competence Assessment Tools for Health-*

FIGURE 9-7. Annual Competency Checklist

JOB-SPECIFIC & POPULATION-SPECIFIC ANNUAL COMPETENCY CHECKLIST
Jan 2016–Dec 2016

Department Name: **Pharmacy**
Job Title:
Evaluator's Name:
Evaluator's Title:
Employee Name:
Employee #:
Staff
Classification
(mark one):

Employee: __X__   Volunteer: _____   Contract Worker: _____

Employee Signature:

Date:

Patient Populations Served: (mark as applicable) Infants √ Children √ Adolescents √ Adults √ Geriatrics √

CODE KEYS:
Assessment Method: O = Observation; W = Written Test; S = Self-reported; V = Verbal Test; D = Documentation
Assessment Outcome: S = Satisfactory; U = Unsatisfactory; N = No opportunity to demonstrate; Blank = not applicable

	Required Competencies (skills/knowledge/abilities—note: age-specific competencies must be skills; if age-related, it means that it is a skill where technique varies when performed with different age groups) * = High-risk/low volume; n = new skill	NOT AGE RELATED	INFANTS	TODDLERS	CHILDREN	ADOLESCENTS	ADULTS	GERIATRICS	Assessment Method	Date Assessed or Assessment Period	Evaluator Initials	Action to Be Taken	Date of Next Assessment
	A. Job Specific Competencies												
New Skill	Pharmacy Skills Day	√							O,W,D	3/1/14	KC		
New Skill	Pyxis ES	√							D,W	12/15/14	KC		
New Skill	Factor replacement products	√							D	12/15/14	KC		
New Skill	Aminoglycosides small group discussion	√							D	12/15/14	KC		
New Skill	Phenytoin small group discussion	√							D	12/15/14	KC		
New Skill	Pass medications (Google doc)	√							W	12/15/14	KC		
New Skill	Neonatal starter lipids (peds and IV only)	√							W	9/1/14	KC		
New Skill	Opioid safety	√							W	10/8/14	KC		
New Skill	Peripheral artery disease guideline update	√							W	10/8/14	KC		
New Skill	Basic life support renewal	√							W,D	12/15/14	KC		
	B. Job Specific Competencies—Population-specific												
High Risk	Pediatric competency (Google doc)		√	√	√	√			W	12/15/14	KC		
High Risk	Chemotherapy update (Google doc)	√							W	12/15/14	KC		

IV = intravenous.

System Pharmacies, which is filled with educational materials to teach your staff members and assess their competency. You can upload pages from the book or CD (request permission from ASHP) to your online learning system.[1] We have employed case studies in conjunction with small group discussions for specific topics such as fosphenytoin or phenytoin and aminoglycoside management. Case studies were distributed prior to scheduled small group discussions, and the pharmacists' competency was assessed based on the level of readiness and participation in the small group discussion. We have also utilized case studies as a stand-alone method of verification of a specific skill. We distributed a vancomycin patient case to pharmacists who were instructed to complete it and return it within 30 minutes. We assessed the time management of staff in efficiently completing a drug-level review, determined a recommendation or plan, and completed the required written documentation. The specific answers to the vancomycin case study were reviewed at staff meetings or directly with the individuals if the coordinator deemed necessary.

Demonstration of Skill

At our hospitals, nurses have utilized educational days called *blitz* or *skills day* as a method to teach and verify competency of a variety of skills. We recently implemented a pharmacy skills day focused on staff demonstrating specific competencies. We utilized the method-of-return demonstration of several common operational or technical skills as well as some clinical skills. Specifically, pharmacists demonstrated proper technique for checking a crash cart prepared by a technician, proper verification of the Baxa Compounder utilized for preparation of parenteral nutrition, as well as accurate completion of paperwork for when patients utilized their personal (home) supply of controlled medications at the hospital because the hospital does not carry the specific controlled substance. In addition, a clinical case of vancomycin dosing and progress notes were included. The demonstrated skills are specific tasks pharmacists are expected to know and complete in an accurate manner. The skills selected are also common tasks that are performed regularly. The supervisor observed each skill demonstration; if any deficiency was identified, there was immediate corrective education. The pharmacists then completed the demonstration and signed off. The pharmacy skills day is an annual activity for our department. The activities are changed each time to keep it fresh and ensure a variety of operational skills are measured (see **Figure 9-8**).

Self-Reflection

Our pharmacists complete *self-reflections* as part of their trimester reviews. The written reviews serve as a framework for organizing and achieving daily activities. Typically, the pharmacist describes either a clinical scenario in which an intervention based on the patient's clinical status or laboratory results led to a change in medication therapy, or how a review of a patient's profile prior to discharge ensured a patient was released on the proper medications for home. The pharmacist's written description allows the coordinator to observe critical thinking skills, clinical knowledge, and interpersonal communications while providing documentation for the pharmacist to highlight his or her daily accomplishments. During the trimester reviews between the pharmacist and coordinator, the coordinator can use the self-reflections to highlight areas where a pharmacist is excelling or areas where there is opportunity for improvement.

Presentations

Another method of competency verification is for the pharmacist to do a *presentation* on a specific topic. This method is useful to demonstrate understanding of a topic, the ability to teach others, and the ability to answer questions and evaluate the pharmacist's comprehension. We use this approach with our pediatric core competency lectures. Each pharmacist is assigned a topic from a preselected list of common disease states, and then he or she prepares a 30-minute presentation. The goal is to expand the core competency of the entire team while at the same time developing an area of expertise for each pharmacist. After the initial presentation, the pharmacist continues to develop his or her knowledge by leading topic discussions or presenting to students or residents who were completing their pediatric rotations each month. Although presentations may not be a

FIGURE 9-8. Annual Skills Day Competency Checklist

ANNUAL SKILLS DAY COMPETENCY CHECKLIST

Jan 2016

Department Name: .... Pharmacy
Job Title: ....
Evaluator's Name: ....
Evaluator's Title: ....
Employee Name: ....
Employee #: ....
Staff Classification
(mark one):

Employee: X   Volunteer: _____   Contract Worker: _____

Employee Signature:

Date:

CODE KEYS:

Assessment Method: O = Observation;   W = Written Test;   S = Self-reported;   V = Verbal Test;   D = Documentation
Assessment Outcome: S = Satisfactory; U = Unsatisfactory; N = No opportunity to demonstrate; Blank = not applicable

		Required Competencies (skills/knowledge/abilities; note: age-specific competencies must be skills; if age-related, it means that it is a skill where technique varies when performed with different age groups)	Location	Assess-ment Method	Date Assessed or Assess-ment Period	Evaluator Initials	If Unsatisfactory	
							Action to Be Taken	Date of Next Assess-ment
		A. Job-Specific Competencies (not population-specific)						
		All Staff						
		Crash cart checking	Crash cart room	O				
		Expiration date tracking	Packaging room	O				
		Home medication process	PCR	O				
		Baxa compounder set-up (IV room staff only)	PCR	O				
		Medication checking	Packaging room	O				
		Technicians Only						
		Math test	Central pharmacy	W				
		Pharmacists Only						
		Code stroke	PCR	O, W				
		Vancomycin case	Central pharmacy	W				

IV = intravenous; PCR = pharmacy conference room.

traditional method to assess a competency, we think it is useful to demonstrate specific areas of knowledge and allow a coordinator another way to evaluate and document a pharmacist's competency.

Simulation

At our medical facility, we are fortunate to have access to a high-fidelity *simulation* classroom. We have incorporated simulation-based competency and assessment with our pharmacists who respond to code blues, traumas, and code stroke. For each specific scenario, the pharmacists completed a didactic course with a written assessment. The pharmacists then moved on to participate in a recorded multidisciplinary simulation scenario in the hospital's simulation classroom. The pharmacy clinical specialist assessed the pharmacists' performance, which was reviewed individually. Once a pharmacist had completed a variety of simulation scenarios, he or she then participated in live scenarios with a preceptor; after completing a specific number of these events, the pharmacist was signed off as a member of the code team.

This method of competency assessment is complex and time-consuming. It requires clinical expertise and knowledge in the areas being taught; time to design, validate, and implement the simulation scenarios; and coordination between disciplines to provide an environment most similar to what the pharmacists will encounter in the real-life settings. We used simulation when implementing our pharmacists' formal role on our code blue team as well as simulation on a smaller scale for code stroke. For code stroke, the emergency department (ED) clinical coordinator designed a specific process for the pharmacists to respond and prepare tissue plasminogen activator (tPA) for a patient in the ED. She did not utilize the simulation classroom but provided the scenario verbally to the pharmacists and had them simulate response by completing the necessary calculations and preparation of the tPA for administration to the patient. The implementation of simulation provides coordinators with a method to verify complete competency for complex operational and clinical tasks, critical thinking, and interpersonal communications.

Quality Improvement Monitoring

Recently we began integrating the hospital's quality improvement committee's feedback into our competency assessment program. Specifically, we review medication errors or near misses that are reported as a "great catch" to document pharmacists' competency to assess a situation and make an intervention (clinical and critical thinking skills). We then share these with the pharmacy staff at staff meetings as a way to acknowledge the pharmacists' work as well as to raise awareness of problems and encourage discussion of ways to improve processes or individual knowledge. The benefit of utilizing data from the quality improvement committee is that it allows synergy of information serving to document performance and assess areas of opportunity.

Documentation

Accreditation requirements include orientation documentation, job description, performance evaluations, initial and annual competencies, and licensure verification. We maintain a paper file for each employee with these documents in the pharmacy department, which could also be kept electronically as long as it can be readily produced when requested. An example of an annual competency checklist can be seen in Figure 9-7. Annual competency is extremely important, and you should use this chapter to develop a robust program to not only meet the minimal requirement, but also to advance your services to provide optimal patient outcomes.

Ongoing Process

First, you determined how pharmacy would add value, and then you determined your required competencies and methodologies to educate and assess the competencies needed to hardwire this process so it occurs each year. Maybe you have an annual strategic planning session that includes the education and competency plan. Or maybe when the annual evaluations are completed, you share the competency plan for the next year with your staff. Whatever your approach, make sure this is not a one-time competency plan that is blindly repeated each year with no thought as to what you are really trying to develop with your staff. Remind yourself every year to follow all of the steps outlined in this chapter.

Summary

Developing competencies and assessment of competencies for pharmacists and technicians is an important role of the clinical coordinator. The areas of competency and methods to assess must be dynamic enough to meet the department's needs and align with strategic goals and direction as well as robust enough to meet the regulatory requirements from organizations such as the Joint Commission, Occupational Safety and Health Administration, and state regulatory agencies. Various methods to assess competency are available. The method of verification must demonstrate the specific knowledge or skill set for a delivered competency.

As clinical coordinators, we have worked to incorporate personal accountability into our competency assessment program by including pharmacists in strategic planning sessions to determine goals and areas of focus. Early in the development process, sessions are held with the staff for feedback on concepts and goals. The coordinators are responsible to develop the educational and assessment plan and communicate the plan to the pharmacists. Then each employee is accountable as part of his or her job descriptions to complete trimester reviews and competency activities. The clinical coordinators are accountable for organizing and developing the competencies, selecting the appropriate assessment methods, and providing an environment that supports the pharmacists in achieving the plan. Documenting the activities of competency assessments and communicating the ongoing progress to the management team and the front-line staff on a continual basis are also a coordinator's responsibility. The open communication of the competency plan will help to identify future areas of growth and development on a continual basis.

PRACTICE TIPS

1. Know where you want to go and what you want to do to ensure the pharmacy provides value to your organization.

2. Determine the baseline understanding of staff.

3. Use active learning, repetition, and customization to teach the information.

4. Assess the competency to ensure the information is being retained and applied.

5. Develop a process and plan to ensure its occurrence on a regular basis.

6. Be open and transparent with your staff members so they know you are thinking of their best interest as well as their patients' best interest.

References

1. Murdaugh LB. *Competence Assessment Tools for Health-System Pharmacies.* 5th ed. Bethesda, MD: ASHP; 2015.

2. Koda-Kimble MA, Young LY. *Applied Therapeutics: The Clinical Use of Drugs.* Baltimore, MD: Lippincott Williams & Wilkins; 2012.

CHAPTER 10

Strategic Planning and Project Management

Jennifer M. Schultz

KEY TERMS

Charter—A statement of the scope, objectives, and participants in a project; a critical document to ensure that everyone involved in the project is aware of its purpose and objectives.

Project Scope—The part of project planning that involves determining and documenting a list of specific project goals, deliverables, tasks, and deadlines.

Of all the things I've done, the most vital is coordinating the talents of those who work for us and pointing them towards a certain goal.

—Walt Disney

Introduction

A clinical coordinator is in a unique position within the pharmacy department, serving as a bridge between pharmacy staff and management. You represent the organization's clinical pharmacy programs, serve along with your peers as part of the clinical pharmacist staff, and have additional responsibilities to ensure your pharmacists have the appropriate resources and competencies to function in their clinical roles. Not only do you find yourself juggling leadership and management responsibilities on top of staffing a clinical position, you will find that you are integral in many operationally-based projects. To be successful as a clinical coordinator, you must have strong project management skills, delegate effectively, be proficient in time management, and have strong interpersonal communication skills.

It is important for you, as the clinical coordinator, to understand how a healthcare system develops organizational priorities and the importance of departments within the organization that contribute to those initiatives. Once you understand this process, you will realize the importance of prioritizing resources within your pharmacy department to focus your work on the issues that have the most impact for your organization. This chapter presents an overview of strategic planning on organizational and departmental levels, and the components of project management are discussed, including utilizing a strategic plan, developing project teams, using facilitation methods, communicating, applying conflict resolution, and measuring project progression.

Strategic Planning

The purpose of *strategic planning* is to develop a blueprint for the organization's future. This blueprint will determine the organization's direction over the next few years, how it's going to get there, and if the goals have been met. The way that a strategic plan is developed depends on various factors including the nature of the

leadership, culture and size of the organization, and the complexity of the organization's environment. Strategic planning is a critical step to help an organization be more productive in guiding the allocation of resources to achieve targeted goals and objectives.

Strategic Planning Overview

The strategic plan is the long-range view of the organization's blueprint for a defined period of time, usually a period of 2 to 5 years. In healthcare, strategic plans are usually generated by the health system's executive team with guidance and approval from their board of trustees. The organization first conducts an environmental assessment based on competitive advantages and disadvantages, future conditions forecast, and an initial list of critical issues. Based on this assessment, the organization determines the organizational direction (mission, vision, strategy, and values) to develop a strategy formulation based on goals, objectives, and major initiatives. Once this is completed, then the strategic plan is presented to other leaders within the organization for input on implementation planning. This results in the creation of action plans, approval processes, and timelines for progress updates.

Key Elements of the Strategic Plan

To create a strategic plan, the organization first needs to have values that define the organization's basic philosophy, principles, and ideals. Once these are confirmed, the first element of a strategic plan is to define the organization's mission answering these key questions:

- Why do we exist?
- What do we want to be in the future?
- How will we achieve the vision?

Strategic planning includes an environmental assessment known as a SWOT (**s**trengths, **w**eaknesses, **o**pportunities, and **t**hreats) analysis, which is a popular tool used to complete this assessment (**Figure 10-1**). The SWOT analysis enables you to create an organized list of your company's greatest strengths, weaknesses, opportunities, and threats. Strengths and weaknesses are internal to your health system (reputation, services offered, location). You can change them over time but not without some

FIGURE 10-1. Environmental Assessment

Strategic Planning Worksheet: Where Are We Now?

Strengths/competitive advantages:	Opportunities/competitive disadvantages:
Future conditions forecast for your business segment:	Potential threats of changes needed:

Initial list of critical issues/areas of importance:	What will be the principal strategic purpose of the department/service line over the next 3 years?	What can we do to positively impact patient experience?

work. Opportunities and threats are external (suppliers, competitors, prices). They are out there in the market, happening whether you like it or not, and you can't change them.

Once the SWOT analysis is complete, the next step is to critically evaluate the areas of focus specific to the health system over the next several years. The health system's board of trustees helps the executive team in determining these areas of focus. Are there service lines that need to grow or be developed? Are there changes that need to happen to positively impact the patient experience or financials? When the strategic plan is done, it is distributed to the department leaders throughout the organization for their department-directed initiatives. Strategic plans for nonprofit health systems are usually focused on quality/safety, people, service, finance and growth, and

community benefit. An example of a health system's strategic plan is shared in **Table 10-1**.

Strategic Planning—Pharmacy Department

Your organization's strategic plan is your guide for focusing your pharmacy initiatives and resources. How does pharmacy fit into this large picture? It is important that the pharmacy department leadership team is evaluating how it can both contribute to the organization's defined strategic plan *and* be proactive in continuously feeding initiatives in the strategic planning process up through administration. Aspects from the strategic plan that can help the organization meet its goals and objectives must be clearly outlined to the C-Suite (senior executives) to gain proper resources (people, tools, etc.).

Table 10-1. Organization Strategic Plan

Strategic Plan for 3-Year Timeframe		
Mission: To improve community health and quality of life **Vision:** To be a leading integrated health system ranked in the top 10% in the nation **Anchor Strategies:** How will we achieve the vision? 1. Be a high-reliability healthcare organization 2. Achieve maximum value enhancement		
Goal Area	**Goal**	**Objectives**
Quality/safety	Demonstrate consistent excellence in quality and safety across all services, which is maintained over long periods of time	■ Safety: Reduce preventable harm rate by 80% by end of fiscal year ■ Quality inpatient: Achieve a VBP score for quality and outcome components in the top quartile based on four quarters of data reported in fiscal year
People	Increase employee, medical staff, and volunteer engagement	■ Achieve an overall score greater than 0.015 above the most recent employee engagement survey score ■ Achieve 5% increase over most recent year's employee participation in philanthropy
Service	Provide an excellent customer experience	■ Clinics: Achieve top 10% score in the CGCAHPS survey for "Would you recommend?" by end of the fiscal year ■ Inpatient: Achieve a patient experience VBP component score in the top quartile based on four quarters of data reported in fiscal year
Finance and growth	Demonstrate value, enhancement, affordability, access, and efficiency Expand and maintain a competitive regional market presence	■ Achieve finance scorecard targets by end of fiscal year ■ Inpatient: Achieve efficiency measure VBP component score in the top quartile based on four quarters of data reported in fiscal year ■ Identify, define, and evaluate value components of regional affiliations by end of fiscal year ■ Achieve market share and community attitude scorecard targets
Community benefit and collaboration	In collaboration with community partners, help meet healthcare needs and promote population health	■ Achieve community benefit implementation plan targets by end of fiscal year ■ Advance medical and health sciences education in our community

CGCAHPS = Clinician and Group Consumer Assessment of Healthcare Providers and Systems; VBP = value-based purchasing.

The pharmacy department leadership team should create or revise a department-specific strategic plan that outlines goals for the next 2 to 5 years, following the same format as the organization. The team should also meet as a group—no matter how large or small the team is—to complete this activity together to create a meaningful and achievable product. First, from the organization's strategic plan, how can pharmacy contribute to help achieve the organizational priorities? These should be drivers for the department and have the highest potential to obtain needed resources and attention. With these goals, pharmacy has an opportunity to demonstrate to senior leadership the value that pharmacists have in organizational outcomes. How can the pharmacy department assist in preventing readmissions, complying with core measures, meeting patient safety goal targets, and improving HCAHPS (Hospital Consumer Assessment of Healthcare Providers and Systems) scores? Here, list the goal and objectives, and then break down the objectives to specific tasks that must be completed to achieve that objective. Also, it is critical within your strategic plan to assign a responsible staff member for each objective, along with an anticipated completion date.

Besides the organization's priorities, it is also important for the pharmacy leadership team to have goals and objectives specific to the pharmacy department that are (1) organized into the same categories as the organization's strategic plan (quality/safety, people, service, finance and growth, community benefit and collaboration, etc.), and (2) more personal to the pharmacy staff. As a clinical coordinator, it is your role to ensure clinical performance improvement initiatives are built into your strategic plan. Are there new clinical guidelines to be created or modified, staff development opportunities, quality indicators of practice that pharmacy may be actively involved with, practice model changes to standardize the provision of patient care, or new tools/resources for clinical staff to effectively practice? There are plentiful resources that can be useful for the pharmacy leadership team in planning strategic initiatives. The annually updated report, *Pharmacy Forecast 2013–2017: Strategic Planning Advice for Pharmacy Departments in Hospitals and Health Systems* describes trends in healthcare that may have an impact on pharmacy.[1] The ASHP Pharmacy Practice Model Initiative (PPMI) and the ASHP Ambulatory Care Pharmacy Practice Model Initiative may also serve as a guide to help drive practice initiatives.[2,3] The ASHP PPMI website hosts both a hospital self-assessment tool and an AmCare self-assessment tool that has an online survey you can complete and then compare your organization compliance with the PPMI recommendations to results from other sites.[4] These resources help you to create a gap analysis of the areas where you may need to focus efforts by providing you comparable data from similar-sized organizations or geographical locations. Another resource to guide your department's initiatives is the annually published *AJHP* article, *National Trends in Prescription Drug Expenditures and Projections*, which outlines trends affecting drug spending in the inpatient and ambulatory settings.[5] This information will help you plan budget and practice initiatives including targeted medication class reviews, medication utilization activities, or disease-state treatment guidelines. As a clinical coordinator, you should be reviewing

these resources and strategically targeting activities that would benefit your department. Examples of pharmacy department strategic plans are shared in **Table 10-2**.

Involvement of the Front-Line Staff

It is essential to communicate the organization's strategic plan to the pharmacy staff. It is also important to involve your staff in the development of the pharmacy department's strategic plan. The more you engage your staff members in developing the department's goals and objectives, the more ownership you will nourish within them. There are different ways to involve your staff members in this process. One method is to have smaller groups called *sensing sessions* to present ideas and obtain their ideas and feedback. Then you can incorporate these ideas into the leadership team sessions. In my experience, the method that works best is to ask for input after the pharmacy leadership team presents its initial strategic plan to the pharmacy staff. At this time you may also ask if any staff members are interested in volunteering for specific project teams related to your defined goals.

The process for engaging staff in the department planning process can be accomplished during a department retreat, a staff meeting, or daily huddle. The department's strategic plan should be a living document that should be referred to often and posted in a prominent place in both hard copy form and electronically. Metrics should be updated monthly so staff members can see their progress in achieving goals.

Project Management

Project management is important to you as a clinical coordinator to accomplish your department's strategic plan goals. An effective clinical coordinator utilizes the skills and expertise of others as appropriate to advance projects. Because there will be several people working on multiple projects, you need to develop a project management system to oversee all of these projects.

Project management is a complicated process. Many large companies even employ personnel as project managers. These people have specific skill sets in project planning, training, facilitation methods, conflict resolu-

Table 10-2. Pharmacy Department Strategic Plan 2014–2016

Goal	Objectives	Tasks	Responsible Person(s)	Timeline	Progress
Quality/safety: Demonstrate consistent excellence in quality/safety	**Safety:** Reduce preventable harm by 80% by end of 2015 **Quality:** Improve VBP scores in relation to core measures	■ Redesign order-entry area to reduce number of distractions ■ Implement tech-check-tech program ■ Incorporate transition-of-care pharmacist into team to ● Provide discharge medication reconciliation ● Assess adherence to medication requirements for CMS core measure patients	Operations manager Operations manager Clinical coordinator	■ 4th quarter 2015 ■ 1st quarter 2016 ■ 3rd quarter 2016	
People: Support professional growth	Identify, define, and develop a process for professional growth and development to improve pharmacist satisfaction		Clinical coordinator		
Service: Provide an excellent customer experience	Improve HCAHPS score related to medication education by 20% by end of 2016	■ Identify target patients for medication teaching by pharmacists ■ Create system for educating patients on medications ■ Create documentation tool for education activities ■ Education to pharmacists/nurses on process ■ Implement program ■ Monitor progress ■ Staff feedback ■ HCAHPS scores	Clinical coordinator Clinical coordinator/ project team	■ 1st quarter 2015 ■ 1st quarter 2015 ■ 1st quarter 2015 ■ End of 1st quarter 2015 ■ Begin 2nd quarter 2015 ■ 4th quarter 2015	

CMS = Centers for Medicare & Medicaid Services; HCAHPS = Hospital Consumer Assessment of Healthcare Providers and Systems; VBP = value-based purchasing.

tion, and interpersonal communications. As a clinical coordinator, project management is one component of your responsibilities. You manage your own projects as well as the clinical projects within your department. The following sections will provide some insight into the different areas of project management to help you in this process.

Prioritization of Projects

Prioritization of projects is essential to effectively assign resources. Refer to your department's strategic plan to develop your project timelines. You should develop a timeline based on the length of the projects, anticipated time for completion, and urgency. High-urgency projects, such as patient safety issues or new clinical guidelines not originally in the strategic plan, may develop, which must be prioritized with other projects and worked into your timeline.

In my experience, the most effective use of project management tracking occurs when the pharmacy leadership team has regularly scheduled meetings (whether weekly or monthly) and actively utilizes the department's strategic plan as a guide for the meetings. These meetings help answer the ongoing questions: How are we progressing toward our goals? What are new struggles or barriers, and how do we address them? Do we need to reprioritize any projects based on current demands? The strategic plan becomes a living document and a measure of progress.

There are always more projects that you and your staff would like to accomplish than are included within your strategic plan. It is a good idea to send out a document every year to your staff with a running list of projects. Consider sending it in late spring every year (hint: prior to July 1 when new pharmacy residents start) and ask that staff review it and add any other project ideas to the list (see **Table 10-3** for an example). This list should be posted on your department's shared network drive and accessible for staff members when they want to consider a project for themselves, a student on rotation, or a pharmacy resident. These projects are not critical enough to be included in the project plan, so they do not have any projected completion timelines until they are chosen to be worked on.

Projects that originate from your strategic plan will generally need a formal project team and outlined completion plan. There will also be many smaller issues that arise on a daily basis that require process changes or decisions to be made. These items may not need a formal team to make a change but should have staff input to make sure the strongest decision is implemented. If you approach these smaller issues the same as a larger project team—but on a smaller scale and more urgent basis—you can be confident that the majority of the change ramifications will be addressed. Every leader has been involved with making a quick decision and realizing later that important details were missed. This usually involves reworking the solution to implement a process that works for everyone involved. Utilizing the skills and expertise of your staff earlier in the process will help you make a sound decision.

Developing the Project Team

When pulling together project teams, it is important to pick the right players. Who has the ability to effectively lead the project? You need at least one leader on your team who demonstrates the enthusiasm, optimism, and support to move others in line with the project goals. You want the person serving as project lead to have some project management or performance improvement training or experience, if possible. This type of training may be available within your organization or may be found in online continuing education programming or through professional association conferences. Because it is critical to have an effective project leader, you may find that you are the one leading the project teams initially. Over time, it is important to identify other pharmacists and pharmacy technicians within your department who may have natural leadership qualities and help them develop into effective leaders with additional training. ASHP has numerous online resources through the Practice Managers Leadership Development Tools webpage. There are also resources through the ASHP Foundation that can serve as formal leadership programs to develop both you and targeted staff members.

Once you have chosen the appropriate team leader(s), you then need to pick content or process experts who can contribute value in moving the project forward. These are important team members as they usually are the people

Table 10-3. Pharmacy Project List[a]

Major Projects			
Project	**Responsible Party**	**Goals**	**Timeline**
Transition of care	Betsy	■ Determine a system of identifying patients at high risk of medication-related issues postdischarge ■ Determine a system of effectively transferring discharge medication information to the health group clinic ■ Pilot the system with before and after measurements for improved capture of accurate discharge medication getting into patient's outpatient EMR *or* focus on some specific clinical outcome	■ Completed—October 2014
Development of pharmacy service for inpatient dialysis patients	Shaundra	■ Develop medication guidelines ■ Review dialysis patients and medication utilization/timing ■ Implement pharmacist review and monitoring system for appropriate dosing	
Development of an infectious disease pharmacy monitoring program	**Nicole/Alexa**	■ **Education sessions held** ■ **Antimicrobial rounds started** ■ **Clinical tracking of interventions** ■ **Competency testing needs to be completed**	**In progress**
Review and modification of our diabetes glycemic control program	**Jen**	■ **Revision of adult DKA order set** ■ **Insulin drip adjustments** ■ **KCl and Na bicarbonate replacement recs** ■ **Monitoring recs** ■ **Parameters to discontinue insulin drip and start SC insulin**	**In progress—June 2015**
Stroke alert/stroke kit	Amanda	■ Assess time to IV tPA following implementation of stroke alert process (door to needle) ■ Assess time to IV tPA following implementation of stroke kit in the ED (order to administration)	In progress
Medication Utilization Reviews			
Project	**Responsible Party**	**Goals**	**Timeline**
Xarelto/warfarin complication rates postsurgery ■ Bleeds ■ PE/DVT	Cody		
Ketamine use for pain control in the ED	Amanda		
Exparel use for orthopedic surgeries	Cody	Determine if our Exparel use is appropriate and reduce the number of pain medications utilized or time of discharge	Completed—2015
Entereg opioid reversal for GI motility to prevent SBO postoperation			

Table 10-3. Pharmacy Project List[a], continued

Quality Projects			
Project	**Responsible Party**	**Goals**	**Timeline**
Prospective order verification process in the ED	Amanda		
Pharmacist clinical intervention tracking	Jen		Awaiting RX productivity consultant July 2015 IVents in EPIC December 2015
Allergy performance improvement project	**Jen** **Medication management team**	**Educate nurses, differences between allergies/adverse reactions/intolerances** **Re-evaluate arm-banding process to conform with national standards (nursing)** **Educate physicians, nurses, and pharmacy staff on penicillin allergies and cross-reactivity to cephalosporins**	
Monographs			
Project	**Responsible Party**	**Goals**	**Timeline**
Novel anticoagulant class review	Cody/Alexa		Completed— June 2015

[a]Shading: light gray = completed; dark gray = in progress; white = up for grabs!

DKA = diabetic ketoacidosis; DVT = deep vein thrombosis; ED = emergency department; EMR = electronic medical record; EPIC = electronic patient information chart; GI = gastrointestinal; IV = intravenous; IVents = intervention tracking process; PE = pulmonary embolism; RX = drug prescription; SBO = small bowel obstruction; SC = subcutaneous; tPA = tissue plasminogen activator.

doing the work on a daily basis and dealing with the ramifications of system changes. Project goals should be clearly defined to the team and focused enough to outline specific measurable goals, available resources, and timeline for completion. The team should be given the autonomy to work within these parameters to achieve the project goals. The project team needs appropriate resources, which—depending on the scope of the project—may include specific training, references, financial assistance, and time.

The structure of project teams can be set up in many different ways. The team can be a focused group pulled together for a specific project, or the team may have ongoing responsibilities and different projects throughout the continuum. These teams can also be mandatory or volunteer-based. Each team should have

a project leader to direct the responsibilities of the group. This person should have some experience or training with group facilitation and/or project management. These programs may exist internally within your organization through the human resources department or other disciplines. The nursing department commonly offers leadership development programs and may be willing to open up the opportunity for some pharmacy staff to participate in these programs as well. It is important to pick a strong leader for this role (see **Table 10-4** for leader characteristics). The pharmacy leadership may assign or the pharmacy staff may nominate the group's leader. Having an appointed leader with expertise and interest in a certain area is recommended for designated project opportunities, whereas it may be better to nominate or elect a leader from the majority of the staff for an ongoing committee or group.

Table 10-4. Characteristics of Our Leaders

Personal Qualities

- Positive attitude
  - Zero tolerance for negativity
  - No complaining, whining, blaming, or gossiping
- Diligent and hardworking
- Energetic and enthusiastic
- Flexible
- Honest and trustworthy
- Thoughtful and caring
  - Cares about the patient, their coworkers, and their job
- Respectful of all
- Sense of humor
- Good listener and understanding
- Patient
- Friendly
- Mature

Professional Qualities

- Strong communication skills
- Organized and efficient in care
- Time management skills
  - On time to work
  - Accomplish work in a timely manner
  - Ability to accurately prioritize
- Self-directed
  - Independent
  - Confident
  - Assertive
  - Motivated
- Lifelong learner
  - Able to take constructive criticism
  - Learns from mistakes
- Calm
  - Follows through with calm demeanor in stressful situations

Practice Qualities

- Knowledgeable
- Critical thinker
- Competent
  - Delivers evidence-based care
  - Skillful and current in practice
  - Careful with aseptic technique
- Thorough
  - In delivered care
  - In documentation of care
- Lifelong learner
  - Continuous learning and educating of self
  - Investigates best practice
  - Researches nursing practice
  - Confident to question own care
  - Changes and grows with profession
  - Values and seeks educational activities

Leadership

- Leadership
  - Resource for others
  - Mentors others
  - Shares knowledge
  - Takes leadership responsibilities
- Fiscally responsible

Teamwork Qualities

- Team player
  - Works well with others
  - Fully present
  - Helps others without being asked
  - Goes the extra mile
  - Willing to help others out
- Collaborator
  - Someone you can confer with in a collegial and collaborative way
  - Shares responsibility
- Loyal to coworkers, department, and organization
  - Pulls their own weight
  - Fully engaged and present
  - Wants to be at work
  - Comes to work and fully immerses self with patient and their family
  - Likes their job and their work
- Responsible and dependable
  - Someone who backs you up
  - A person you can count on
  - Someone you can lean on

Patient and Family Qualities

- Compassionate
  - Cares for the patient as if the patient was their loved one
- Patient-focused
  - Loves caring for people
- Patient-centered
  - Patients are the #1 reason for being at work
  - Always does what is in the best interest of the patient
  - Immerses self with patient and family
  - Listens to patient and family
  - Engages with patient
- Patient advocate
  - Nonjudgmental attitude toward the patient
  - Motivates the patient to improve
  - Always advocates for what is in the best interest of the patient
- Customer service focus

Professional Appearance Qualities

- Professional behavior
  - Consistently acts in a professionally responsible manner
- Professional appearance
  - Consistently dresses in a manner nonoffensive to the patient and coworkers

The team's meeting schedule should be predetermined. For focused projects, there should be a defined timeline for meetings and project step completion. There also should be a standard process for holding a meeting, whether on a large or small scale. In my organization, our pharmacy councils refer to *A Chair's How-To-Guide: Running an Effective Meeting* that our nursing governance created (**Table 10-5**). Meetings should be scheduled in advance staff so staff can make the appropriate accommodations to attend. This is one of the most difficult aspects in moving projects forward with staff members. It is essential in a busy work environment to find some free time for staff to work on these projects. This may mean building project time into the schedule with paid workdays; reorganizing staff workflow to accommodate for meeting times; or covering the workload to allow staff members to participate. Giving individuals time to spend on specific projects is vital to overall success and motivation to move the project forward. It also creates ownership into the process and, therefore, employee engagement!

Defining Clear Roles and Responsibilities of Project Team Members

It is essential to have roles and responsibilities defined for your project team members. You can have a basic team structure for any of your ongoing or ad hoc project teams. These responsibilities may be formal or informal depending on the scope of the project. It is crucial that you have designated a project manager to lead the team who clearly understands the goals. You also will have project team members who need to understand their role in helping to achieve the goal(s) outlined. It is a good idea to have these roles and responsibilities outlined in a document that you can present to the team at the initial meeting (see **Table 10-6**). You may decide to add additional roles and responsibilities to the document including scribe, facilitator, or another designated role.

Case Example 1

Jane's hospital recognized that there was a need to add an additional pharmacist shift on the weekends. It was determined that this new shift would be a swing shift into the evening, but because many find it dissatisfying to work weekends and evening shifts, this decision had been delayed as long as possible. When pharmacy management determined that it was time to move forward with this new shift for the benefit of patient safety, the clinical coordinator met with the staff and asked for a group of volunteers to help redefine the roles and responsibilities of all the weekend pharmacist shifts. Jane's two newest employees stepped up to the plate to offer their help. As a supervisor, she knew she needed to get representation from pharmacists who had been employed at the hospital longer. She stressed the importance with her staff of having a mixture of seasoned staff and new people to be on this team to make the best decisions about shift responsibilities. Jane was able to recruit three more volunteers from the tenured employees. Once she had the team established, she found a time on the schedule, organized a meeting place, and pulled together all of the pharmacist shift documents for them to review. She began the meeting by discussing the ground rules and expectations with the group. These included listening to and respecting everyone's ideas, establishing priorities for the new shift to aid in completing current workload requirements, identifying additional clinical opportunities for the new shift as time allows, finalizing a typed list of weekend shift responsibilities, determining hours of the shifts, and assigning a timeline to review how the shift is going and make adjustments. It took the group 2 hours to complete this task. She then reviewed the information to make sure that activities were aligned with the department processes and asked the work group to communicate the plan to the rest of the staff. The group needed a reminder when the time came (Jane kept it circled on her calendar) to revisit the changes that were made and gather input from others. At this point, a couple of minor modifications were made in the shift responsibilities, and those were communicated to the staff.

Establishing the Reporting Structure

Each project team should have clear direction on who to report to and how often. Set up electronic calendar alerts for this reporting process. You may also have the group present to your

Table 10-5. A Chair's How-to-Guide[a,b]

I. A Call to Order	The chair person announces the beginning of the meeting. It is requested that members turn off their electronic devices and silence their phones to presently attend to council business matters.
II. Roll Call	Check attendance utilizing the approved roster template. Accurate attendance verification is crucial at every meeting. Attendees initial on the date space of attendance for each meeting. Attendees not present will receive an X on their space.
III. Approval of the Minutes from the Last Meeting	The appointed scribe or chair person asks about previous minutes to learn of any additions or corrections. Members are expected to review minutes prior to meeting start to identify any action items for current meeting and to ensure accuracy. The chair person or designated scribe sends minutes to members and the department manager within 3 weeks after meeting adjournment. The chair person requests a motion to approve the minutes as they stand. A member makes a motion to approve the previous minutes. A member second's that motion to approve the previous minutes. All members vote on the motion.
IV. Review of the Current Meeting's Agenda	Agendas are created prior to the beginning of any council meeting using the approved agenda/minutes template. The agenda is sent out to members no later than 1 week prior to meeting. The chair person reviews the agenda topics with the council.
V. Old Business	First agenda item should consist of old business, which includes a question that was pending at the last session when it adjourned; any unfinished business that did not come up at the last session; or anything from last session that was not complete.
VI. New Business and Announcements	Additional agenda items will consist of new business and announcements. The chair person encourages that agenda items remain within their proposed timeframe. Follow the motion process for all decision-making business of the council.
VII. Adjournment	Adjournment ends not only the meeting but also the session. The next time the council convenes, it must start from the beginning of the agenda with old business. If additional time is necessary, an additional meeting is scheduled.

[a]Running an effective meeting is crucial to the success of introducing new processes and practices that improve nursing care delivery and promote desirable outcomes.

[b]Based on Robert's Rules of Order (http://www.robertsrules.org/).

Table 10-6. Project Team Roles and Responsibilities

Title	Role(s)
Project manager	The person designated to lead a project and work within defined parameters set by supervisor/manager/director

Responsibilities	

- Managing and leading the project team
- Recruiting project staff and content experts
- Developing and maintaining the project plan
- Managing project scope and change control
- Monitoring project progress and performance
- Coordinating and facilitating project meetings
- Providing status reports to pharmacy supervisor/manager/director
- Determining educational/training components needed
- Assigning a scribe to take meeting minutes

Title	Role(s)
Project team members	The staff who actively work on the project

Responsibilities	

- Providing functional expertise in a process
- Working with other staff as needed for input
- Documenting and analyzing current and future processes/systems
- Identifying information needs
- Training other staff

pharmacy leadership meeting on a scheduled timeline. Also, you need to determine what should be listed in your progress report. Do you want recorded minutes, a verbal report, an email summary of activities, or an updated progress report such as a Gantt chart? This simple bar chart graphically shows the progress of a project or work effort against a project schedule or timeline. The method of feedback you establish will depend on the urgency and scope of the project. If you are not actually a member of this project team, you need to watch for progress and offer support or guidance if the project is not moving forward as expected.

Case Example 2

Employee engagement is a key component in achieving a positive work environment. To facilitate this type of culture, it is important to bring decision-making abilities and ownership to front-line staff. Jim was looking for a way to bring more decision-making responsibilities to his staff members, which would in turn create

some accountability for their decisions. He realized that there were so many changes that the staff members wanted to address that he could not meet all of their expected timelines. Jim also realized that the best people to make the decisions are the ones doing the daily work. The nursing staff had instituted a shared governance process a few years earlier, so Jim decided to meet with this program's leader to discuss how they could adapt that model for his pharmacy department.

First, he created a document describing his pharmacy department's mission and scope of practice. The pharmacy leadership team decided to create four councils for the pharmacy department. They created the Culture Council (workplace attitudes), Clinical Practice Council, Operations Practice Council, and the Professional Growth and Development Council. A purpose statement and objectives were developed for each of these councils. Next, they created a formalized process for the councils including meeting schedules, agenda/minute/roster tools, reporting process, and quorum requirements for decision voting. Once they outlined these issues, they held an all-staff meeting and presented their council proposal to the staff. They decided to ask every pharmacy department employee to choose which council he or she wanted to join. Jim compiled council rosters and asked staff members to vote for the person in each council they felt was most suited to lead as chair and vice chair for the year. Once Jim had tallied the results, he approached the chair and vice chair nominees to see if they would be willing to serve. There was an overwhelming acceptance rate of 100% for those nominated for this leadership role. The councils were set up with authority to make and implement decisions on process and system changes that were approved by their councils. The pharmacy leadership team had decided that issues requiring resources had to be submitted to management for formal approval before implementation. This was clearly spelled out in our guidance documents. The councils started meeting on a monthly basis for an hour per month, with management allocating additional time as needed based on project requests. Any pharmacy member could generate agenda items to a specific council, or the management team could hand them to the group. This process was an overwhelming success, with employees who are actively engaged with the change process. This new structure also has led to employees holding each other accountable for the changes the council had generated.

Meeting Facilitation Methods

Facilitating meetings is a skill of its own. As a clinical coordinator, you may be charged with facilitating a group or helping others to develop facilitation skills. The main priorities of a facilitator are keeping within the **project scope**, getting everyone involved, and handling conflict management. A strong facilitator also ensures the work completed by the group is summarized, and there are clear assignments and timelines outlined. Facilitation skills can be utilized formally for large projects or informally to help keep smaller project discussions on task.

The *Facilitator Tool Kit* states that "As a facilitator, your job is to make the meeting easier for the participants. Your main task is to help the team or group increase its effective-

ness by improving its processes. A facilitator manages the method of the meeting rather than the content. Facilitators are concerned with how decisions are made instead of what decisions are reached."[6]

Facilitator Responsibilities

- Intervene if the discussion starts to fragment
- Identify and intervene in dysfunctional behavior
- Prevent dominance and include everyone
- Summarize discussions and conversations
- Bring closure to the meeting with an end result or action

Facilitation Challenges

- Continually focusing on and attending to the group
- Being comfortable with ambiguity and information overload
- Processing misperceptions and emotional reactions
- Focusing exclusively on process rather than content
- Helping the group develop so they can ultimately work without facilitation[6]

Project Scope

A facilitator keeps the team focused on the scope of the project. Teams can get off-task by identifying a new issue that may be more exciting than the issue they have been tasked to address. The facilitator must redirect them to the original issue by asking targeted questions on the original project or using the group's predetermined phrase when getting off-topic. Having a targeted objective to complete by the end of each meeting will keep the meeting on track. In addition, you can send out readings before the meeting to focus the team or have a **charter** for the project. A charter can help focus the team on the scope, so starting each meeting reviewing the charter will reset the team's focus and reduce the chance for scope creep (see **Figure 10-2**).

FIGURE 10-2. Sample Charter

Charter

Chair/team lead _____ Date initiated _____

Problem/mission statement

Scope

Deliverables

Measurements

Team members

Reporting structure

Meeting frequency

Target date for conclusion

Get Everyone Involved

There are several ways that a facilitator can get active involvement from all group members. You can use post-it notes asking team members to jot down their ideas on the notes and post them on a bulletin board. Other options include round-robin discussions or allowing people to speak up as they desire. As a facilitator, if you realize that someone is not contributing, you should take the initiative and ask for that person's ideas or thoughts. You may also utilize fun methods such as throwing a ball to someone, ask for an idea, and then pass it to another team member. It is important to avoid *groupthink*—a phenomenon that occurs when the desire for group consensus overrides people's common-sense desire to present alternatives, critique a position, or express an unpopular opinion. Here, the desire for group cohesion effectively drives out good decision making and problem solving. Utilizing effective facilitation methods to promote brainstorming and ideas is critical in preventing this problem.

You may also utilize strategies to get team members to all think as a different person. Assign someone to be a pharmacist, one a nurse, one a physician, and one a patient, and look at the project recommendations from different angles to determine if any important factors may not have been considered for certain solutions. The goal here is for ideas to be brought forward and potential challenges to be identified early in the decision-making process to avoid rework later.

Conflict Resolution

There will be times when project team members disagree in approaches to a project plan and cannot come to a resolution by themselves. As a clinical coordinator, you may be asked to step in and provide guidance. Some coordinators may feel that they should just take the project and complete it themselves. It serves the department best to help the team members through a conflict resolution process so they can finish the project and develop the skills necessary to work effectively in teams. The following are strategies for conflict resolution that may help to work through the issues:

- Discussion
- Written communication
- Mediation
- Compromise
- Voting

Many times, conflict may simply be a result of lack of communication. The first strategy for conflict resolution is to have the employees talk with each other so they can understand their thoughts and rationale. If this doesn't work, use a written communication process, mediation, compromise, or voting. One technique for voting is the *fist of five*. If the team is in complete support of the idea or topic, they can open their hand and vote five. If they are completely opposed to the idea, they can close their hand and vote zero as a fist. They can vote one finger to four fingers if they have a varying approval of the idea. This allows you to physically see the support or lack of support for an idea. Voting with your hands helps to get the discussion going and bring out the different perspectives so they can be discussed and addressed. It can also help to set a baseline of what will be approved, such as all ideas must be voted three or higher to be part of the final project. When simple measures of conflict management are not effective, you should bring another person (i.e., a witness) into the process and document your attempts for resolution.

Feedback

Before getting ready to go live with a new process or change, it is important to get feedback from other employees in the change process. How many times have you implemented a new process only to have forgotten how this change may affect others? Or you have been on the receiving end where it appears that there was not enough thought put into the solution. As a coordinator, you know that although often extensive effort is put into developing a solution, the decision makers are not the ones at the bedside or front line. It is important to hear from those that might be impacted by the solution. Changes that are made in pharmacy processes may affect not only pharmacists and pharmacy technicians but also nurses, physicians, the budget, and patients. Validating your change processes with various departments will ensure that other issues including safety and regulatory issues will be identified and addressed before implementing the change.

A method to obtain feedback from key stakeholders is to conduct an initiative review system (IRS). This technique is a structured way of formally asking for feedback and incorporating it into the project before it is implemented. This is similar to doing a failure mode and effects analysis, event tree analysis, or hazard identification. All these are formal process improvement techniques that can take a very long time to conduct, and often we do not have the opportunity for a long formal review. However, we need to have a method to provide feedback in a timely manner. The goal is to be proactive rather than reactive when implementing changes.

The IRS process logistics are as follows (**Figure 10-3**):

- Schedule sessions for the staff to attend in a location that is close and at times that are convenient.
- Either schedule staff members to attend or allow for walk-ins based on their schedule.
- Walk through each step of the proposed implementation.
- Have handouts if pertinent.
- Share policies if applicable.
- Role play if needed.
- Run through scenarios.
- Schedule each session for a brief amount of time (30 to 60 minutes).
- Conclude during the session; follow up if needed.

The IRS technique results in numerous successful change processes that can be implemented within the organization. Because staff could provide feedback and identify gaps in the process before implementation, a solid change was created that was widely entwined with staff ownership.

FIGURE 10-3. Initiative Review Session Form

Initiative: _____   _____

Date: _____ Facilitator: _____

Attendees: _____

_____

_____

Opportunities for improvement identified by the attendees:

1. _____

_____

2. _____

_____

3. _____

_____

4. _____

_____

Proposed solutions for each opportunity for improvement:

1. _____

_____

2. _____

_____

3. _____

_____

4. _____

_____

Additional ideas and suggestions from the staff:

1. _____

_____

2. _____

_____

3. _____

_____

Does the staff in attendance support the proposed solutions?

1. YES _____ NO _____

2. YES _____ NO _____

3. YES _____ NO _____

4. YES _____ NO _____

Communication

It is important to communicate ideas to your entire staff on what types of projects are taking place, the personnel on the project teams, and the progress that the teams are making in reaching goals. This can be communicated in staff meetings, emails, or even by having an active project board so that projects are clearly visible.

A project board is a visible way to keep project communication open. You can put colored paper up on your department's bulletin boards. The first section on the left is colored red, the middle section yellow, and the right section green. When an issue is identified that needs attention, anyone can post it on the bulletin board's red section. When that issue is picked up by someone to work on it, it gets moved to the yellow section posted with someone's name and a targeted resolution date. Once the issue is completed, it moves to the green section of the board. This concept is great for staff members to identify and share issues, pick an issue to work on that they are interested in, and watch the progress as items move from the red section to the green section. It is important that pharmacy management keeps this board active and discusses progress during staff meetings.

Projects also should be communicated to the executive who oversees the pharmacy department so he or she is familiar with the department's ongoing activities. You also should ensure that the quality department and appropriate nursing and physician committees are aware of pharmacy activities.

Measurement

Determining measurable goals can be difficult and cause projects to stall. Keep these simple, and measure something that is valuable to the department. Tracking progress on your projects is important to keep initiatives moving forward. The more visible you make project progression, the more effectively projects advance. For larger projects, you can use a performance improvement project planning form (**Figure 10-4**) to track movement toward our goals. For those initiatives that have the greatest value to the department or organization, you must track the measurement of success and celebrate them with staff when goals are reached. You can order lunch for the staff, give out coffee gift cards, congratulate the team publicly, or send personalized congratulations cards.

Summary

Strategic planning and project management are important operations of a pharmacy department to prioritize and organize resources. There are always plenty of projects for a clinical coordinator to manage. The most efficient way to move these projects toward your goals is to develop project teams. It is your responsibility to ensure that these teams are organized, have the correct team members, and have clearly defined goals to be able to succeed. The more effectively you set your system up, the more successful you will be in your role of project management.

PRACTICE TIPS

1. Align your department goals with those of the organization.

2. Delegate projects to teams, choosing the right project leader.

3. Define clear roles and responsibilities of project team members.

4. Monitor progress toward project goals and celebrate success as a team!

FIGURE 10-4. Performance Improvement Project Planning Form

Project Title:	
Name of Project Leader:	
Name of Department:	
Date:	

Model for Improvement:

What are we trying to accomplish?

How will we know that a change is an improvement?

What changes can we make that will result in improvement?

Act | Plan
Study | Do

What does your team want to accomplish?

Step 1. Problem versus process identification

Problem: _____
Process: _____

Step 2. Form team

Team members: _____

Step 3. Determine Aim statement: How Good? By When?

We will achieve the following results:
(Circle one) Increase/decrease/improve/reduce _____ by _____% within _____ timeframe.

Step 4. Flowchart the current process (See How to Flowchart on SharePoint PI Toolkit; attach completed flowchart)

Step 5. Develop opportunity statement

An opportunity exists to improve the process of _____ beginning with _____ and ending with _____. This effort should improve _____ for the _____ (customer). The process is important to work on now because _____.

How will we know that a change is an improvement?

Step 6. Establish outcome measures

Description of outcome measure(s): _____
Current baseline/total N-size/week or month: _____
Data collection method/display/frequency: _____
National benchmark/source: _____
Target score (based on Aim statement): _____

What changes can we make that will result in improvement?

Step 7. Selecting changes

After searching the literature for evidence-based practices, also take into consideration your clinical expertise and patient preferences to determine your tests of change (see Step 9).

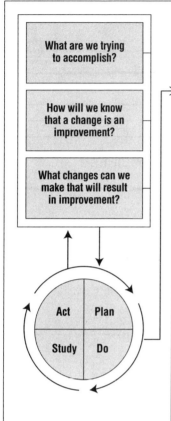

Step 8. Testing changes with Plan-Do-Study-Act (PDSA) cycles

For each test of change, complete the PDSA worksheet (found in SharePoint PI Toolkit). Use the PDSA worksheet to help your team document each test of change.

Note: Complete one PDSA worksheet for each test you conduct. Your team will test several different changes and each change will go through several PDSA cycles. Keep files (electronic and hard copy) of all PDSA worksheets for all changes your team tests.

Step 9. List all tests of change in table below:

Cycle #	Test of Change	Person Responsible	Completion Date

PI = performance improvement.

Source: Adapted from the Institute for Healthcare Improvement (2011). Project Planning Form and Science of Improvement: How to Improve. www.IHI.org. The Model for Improvement was developed by Associates in Process Improvement. Langley GL, Moen R, Nolan KM, et al. *The Improvement Guide: A Practical Approach to Enhancing Organizational Performance.* 2nd ed. San Francisco, CA: Jossey-Bass Publishers; 2009.

References

5. Zellmer WA, Walling RS. Pharmacy forecast 2013–2017: strategic planning advice for pharmacy departments in hospitals and health-systems. *Am J Health-Syst Pharm.* 2012;69(23):2083-2087.

6. The consensus of the Pharmacy Practice Model Summit. *Am J Health-Syst Pharm.* 2011; 68(12):1148-1152.

7. ASHP/ASHP Foundation Ambulatory Conference and Summit Consensus Recommendations, March 4, 2014. http://www.ashp.org/DocLibrary/PPMI/ AmCare-Summit-Preliminary-Recommendations.pdf. Accessed June 23, 2015.

8. ASHP. Practice advancement initiative. http://www. ashpmedia.org/ppmi/. Accessed June 23, 2015.

9. Schumock GT, Li EC, Suda KJ, et al. National trends in prescription drug expenditures and projections for 2015. *Am J Health-Syst Pharm.* 2015;72(9):717-736.

10. Facilitator tool kit: a guide for helping groups get results. http://oqi.wisc.edu/resourcelibrary/uploads/ resources/Facilitator%20Tool%20Kit.pdf. Accessed June 23, 2015.

Suggested Reading

Crane TG. *The Heart of Coaching: Using Transformational Coaching to Create a High-Performance Coaching Culture.* 2nd ed. San Diego, CA: FTA Press; 2012.

Dinkin S, Filner B, Maxwell L. *The Exchange Strategy for Managing Conflict in Healthcare: How to Defuse Emotions and Create Solutions When the Stakes Are High.* New York, NY: McGraw-Hill; 2012.

Kotter JP. *Leading Change.* Cambridge, MA; Harvard Review Press; 2012.

ASHP. Leadership development tools. http://www.ashp. org/menu/PracticePolicy/ResourceCenters/Pharmacy-Practice-Managers/LeadershipTools.aspx.

Patterson K, Grenny J, McMillan R, et al. *Crucial Conversations: Tools for Talking When Stakes Are High.* 2nd ed. New York, NY; McGraw-Hill; 2002.

Van Gorder C. *The Front-Line Leader: Building a High-Performance Organization from the Ground Up.* San Francisco, CA: Jossey-Bass; 2014.

CHAPTER 11

Implementing New Clinical Pharmacy Programs—Step by Step

Jenna M. Huggins and Laurimay L. Laroco

KEY TERMS

Business Plan—A detailed document outlining a new proposal for a service/business including benefits, costs, monitoring, and marketing.

Clinical Pharmacy Service—New process or workflow identified and implemented to enhance and/or support optimal patient care in an acute care, ambulatory, or community setting.

SWOT (<u>s</u>trengths, <u>w</u>eaknesses, <u>o</u>pportunities, <u>t</u>hreats) Analysis—A structured planning method that evaluates the pharmacy's strengths and weaknesses in the context of the opportunities and threats in the external environment.

Introduction

Clinical coordinators are often seen as the visionaries in the pharmacy department. A key job responsibility is researching and proposing how **clinical pharmacy services** may enhance patient care and outcomes in the hospital. Pharmacists are uniquely situated with opportunities to drive quality in the organization because of their access to patients, patient data, as well as their knowledge base of patients' quality outcome indicators. Clinical coordinators must effectively navigate the complexities of a health system to ensure that pharmacy services are presented as options in any situation but without overcommitting pharmacy services. Developing new clinical programs should be a process involving assessment, planning, and implementation phases with the coordinator making key contacts throughout the phases to ensure a new program's success (see **Figure 11-1**).

New Service Assessment

Environment Analysis

Before entertaining any ideas for new services, the first step is an environment scan: will the new service have added benefit or value? When you do an environment scan, you need to involve several different key parties. You must think about the end user as well as the different people that will impact end users over the course of being involved in the new service.

To present a well-rounded environment analysis, it is important to benchmark with similar institutions that may or may not have implemented your service. This analysis should include data, anecdotal lessons learned, etc. (see **Figure 11-2**). Ensure that the institutions chosen to benchmark are truly representative of a similar patient population and are of interest to hospital administrators (e.g., competitors and geographic location).

The environment analysis will also help prioritize your system's needs. For example, if the system is performing at an acceptable level on all readmission rates, but the core measure compliance for discharge medications is very low, this is where you should focus the attention of your pharmacy services. **Table 11-1** has examples of common organizational priorities/urgencies that pharmacists may get involved in. Once the organizational needs are prioritized, it is important for you as a clinical coordinator to take the ideas back to your core staff members for their ideas on how they might most effi-

FIGURE 11-1. Overall Flow Diagram in the Creation of a New Pharmacy Service

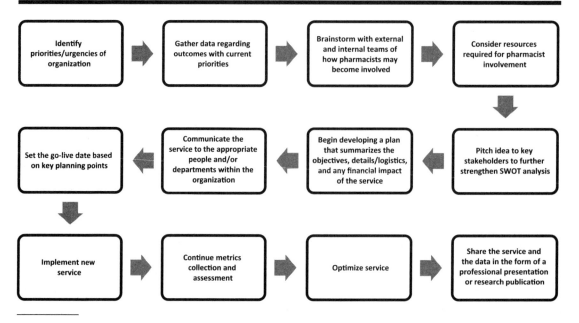

SWOT = **s**trengths, **w**eaknesses, **o**pportunities, **t**hreats.

FIGURE 11-2. Sample Benchmarking Checklist

	Institution #1	Institution #2	Institution #3
Name/location			
Contact/position title			
Service offered?			
Similar target population?			
Required staff resources			
Day/time service is offered			
Metric evaluation of the service			
Strengths			
Weaknesses			
Lessons learned			

Table 11-1. Example SWOT Analysis for Code Blue Response[a]

Strengths	Weaknesses
■ Pharmacist knowledge of pharmacotherapy at codes ■ Pharmacist knowledge of medication concentrations and mixing/final check ■ Nurses are free to take care of other patient care issues ■ Pharmacist direct link to main pharmacy for medications out of the crash cart	■ Different pharmacists with different skill levels ■ Additional person in small room for a code ■ Unable to provide 24/7 coverage due to night shift staffing
Opportunities	**Threats**
■ Development of simulation lab pharmacist-specific ACLS training to bring staff up to speed ■ Updating to code blue policy regarding team members ■ Expansion to other code response (trauma, stroke) ■ Providing dosing card on side of cart in case a pharmacist is not present	■ Nurses typically run medications out of cart ■ Physician trust if one incompetent pharmacist participates

ACLS = advanced cardiovascular life support; SWOT = strengths, weaknesses, opportunities, threats.

[a]Examples of potential pharmacy services identified by a SWOT analysis: code stroke response for ED; HF/AMI readmissions programs for hospital CMS reimbursement; transitions of care services; HCAHPS scores; ASP program; and ancillary services (i.e., code trauma or code blue response).

ciently and effectively impact those priorities. These discussions and brainstorming sessions will help them feel like they are a key part of the development process and improve employee retention. This usually translates to the program having a higher likelihood of success down the road when the roll-out of the service actually occurs. The worst thing is to force a new process on your core staff team without their buy-in, as these often quickly fail.

SWOT Analysis and Data Gathering

One useful tool to ensure a complete environment scan is done for the targeted health system or service line is a **SWOT** (**s**trengths, **w**eaknesses, **o**pportunities, **t**hreats) **analysis** (see Table 11-1). The SWOT analysis will help analyze the strengths of your new service, the weaknesses that you have and have not considered (with the help of others), external opportunities that the new program will present, and external threats that the program may face while trying to be successful.

The most important aspect of a SWOT analysis is gathering accurate data. Hospital data are very important in supporting any new service. Specific examples include up-to-date readmissions data (if your service involves care to reduce readmissions) or door-to-needle times for tissue plasminogen activator (tPA) if the new program will involve pharmacists with tPA admixture and administration (refer to Table 11-1). These data will help define the clinical program's strengths and opportunities as part of the larger SWOT analysis. Data may be generated from the idea itself, or the data—such as that from an organization's strategic plan or balanced scorecard—may generate the idea. Either way, it is vital that the data reinforce the current strategic plan or develop a future strategic plan. It is important to know what value the pharmacy services can provide and how to align them with the organization's strategic direction and goals. Data also may not be available if this is a new service mandated by a new federal regulation. In these situations, the idea must be generated to meet regulation requirements rather than to improve data for your health system.

If data from the health system are required to implement an idea, the clinical coordinator must establish contacts early in the process. An example of generating contacts is being proactive on committees that meet monthly regarding stroke, heart failure, acute myocardial infarction, critical care services, etc. You can then stay up-to-date on service line deficiencies and simultaneously establish key relationships. Being involved with the key groups is also a great way to involve pharmacy. For example, when a conversation involves improving patient care and pharmacists could lend assistance, volunteer your potential services.

SWOT Analysis and Resources

The weaknesses must also be addressed for the SWOT analysis and overall environment scan. Although employees are our greatest strength, their cost is often viewed as a weakness of any new clinical program. Therefore, necessary resources such as pharmacists or pharmacy technician full-time equivalents (FTEs) should be considered in the assessment phase. You must know how many hours you can cover a specific service. In the case of code stroke pharmacist coverage, can you provide this service 24/7? If a service is not full-time, you must have a clear plan to provide a similar level of service on the off-hours, especially if the service is related to a new inpatient clinical program. If a plan for coverage is not addressed, hospital and pharmacy leadership will focus on this as a threat to the program's success. Included in resource requirements will be training requirements. Will the training be extensive and require additional staff to fill current roles? Or is the training done as part of the pharmacists' or pharmacy technicians' normal daily schedule? Administration will have a more difficult time accepting a program that is not resource neutral (augmentation of your current staff members' duties) and/or requires backfilling positions for training purposes.

Feedback on New Service Idea

Finally, to round out the assessment phase, you need to ensure all key stakeholders have been involved. It is important to delay this until after the initial meetings during the environment analysis, and once your idea is slightly more solidified. However, before planning the new service, you want to briefly pitch your idea to the key individuals and teams so that all parties give meaningful input. Ensure that key stakeholders include both those who support your idea as well as those who disagree or question its validity. This will help you identify more opportunities and threats for your SWOT analysis as well as strategies to either capitalize on the strengths or ward off the threats that could cause your clinical program to fail. For example, if pharmacist involvement in code blue response is your new clinical program, and nursing leadership wants pharmacist coverage 24/7 even though the pharmacy department cannot support this, you at least now know to include a clear solution in your planning phase. An example of how to mitigate this and work with the nursing staff would be to provide crash-cart mixing reference on all of the crash carts when pharmacy staff is not able to attend. You should not let the entire initiative stop because of one feedback, but use this to determine how to identify a solution that is acceptable to all and still provides a high level of patient care. This helps prevent an idea from failing in the end because of one downfall. The meetings with these key stakeholders should be a brief elevator pitch that includes a quick overview of your idea, what data support the need for the new service, the potential benefits/outcomes, resources required, and tentative timeline you have explored for the need of this service.

New Service Planning

Business Plan Development

After a thorough assessment, identification, and preliminary acceptance of a new service by your department and other appropriate stakeholders, creating a plan to successfully establish the service is essential. This process should begin with creating a plan that contains many elements similar to a **business plan**. The business plan is beneficial in outlining the main objective of this service and summarizing the benefits to patient care and the organization. The plan should also demonstrate how your core team members directly contribute to the process and how the process fits into their daily workflow and goals. Consider coordinating time to meet with senior executives once you are close to finalizing your business plan so that you can make the proposal to them if the service would need their buy-in. As pharmacists, we need to take more accountability for our actions and outcomes; with a new service, this is the best time to demonstrate to senior leaders how pharmacy can take responsibility and lead in exceptional patient outcomes. Remember, when communicating with the senior executives (C-Suite), start with the final recommendation and then review the background if they want to hear more. Executives prefer a different style of communication rather than how pharmacists have been taught to provide the evidence first and then the final recommendation last. Inclusion of any financial requirements of the department and organization should be disclosed in this plan as well (see **Table 11-2** for a sample business/new service plan). In preparing the business

plan, consider a mission statement for this service. Some may find it useful to describe your new service in one statement prior to creating the actual business plan. It also may be a very simple exercise to test the clarity of the service's concept. If you cannot concisely and confidently describe the concept in one statement, then it may indicate some potential challenges that may not have been considered. Usual elements of a mission statement include the target population, the professional values that will guide this positive impact on patient care, the type of service, the specific goal of the service, and the community or hospital team's view of this service.[1,2]

Executive Summary

Typical business plans begin with an executive summary of the service. This should be a high-level overview including a proposal of the program, benefits to the organization, the impact on your employee's workload, and any financial impact. In general, the summary should be succinct with a sufficient amount of detail to gain the reader's interest and buy-in. Although the executive summary is the first section of the business plan, it is often the last piece created, so the author has a chance to review the entire plan and maybe even rethink some aspects of the plan.

Background

The business plan's background is generally a description of the new service and an opportunity to provide specific details on the service's positive impact on the organization, your employees, other staff, and ultimately the patients and their family members. Consider beginning the background stating the problem you are trying to fix. Behind every new service is an issue. Utilization of any specific data or examples that resulted from the issue may further allow the reader to relate. After establishing the problem, switch gears and lay out the specific healthcare statistics, epidemiology, and impact on healthcare costs that could directly correlate to this service. Furthermore, providing literature on outcomes, both clinical and financial, of similar services in other institutions could also provide more evidence on the likely success of this service.

Table 11-2. Elements of the Layout of a Business/New Pharmacy Service Plan

Element	Key Components to Include
Executive summary	■ Purpose of the plan ■ New service and its advantages ■ Target patient population ■ Management team ■ Financial projections ■ Funding requirements
Background (new service description)	■ Key stakeholders ■ Advisors ■ Acute objective of the service ■ Long-term objective of the service ■ SWOT analysis
Patient population analysis	■ Target patient population ■ Trends and/or benchmarking in other healthcare institutions ■ Competitive advantages ■ Benefits to targeted patient population
Promotion/marketing strategy	■ Communication to key stakeholders ■ Income sources, if applicable ■ Advertising strategy to other departments impacted by service and entire institution
Management team	■ Management team and department structure ■ Outline of the management team's qualifications and experience ■ The educational background and specialized training or skills of staff members directly involved in executing the new service
Staffing and operations	■ Outline of resources/staffing requirements ■ Training plan ■ Operations plan ■ Methodology/logistics of new service's process ■ Estimation of time needed to complete the new service per patient
Financial projections	■ Costs versus revenues ■ Hard versus soft savings
New service pipeline	■ Assessment of acute target of service ■ Assessment of potential for growth of service to other patient populations and/or additional areas of the institution

SWOT = **s**trengths, **w**eaknesses, **o**pportunities, **t**hreats.

Source: See references 1 and 2 for more information.

Patient Population Analysis

After describing the background, you should redirect the reader to focus on why it was initially supported and what aspect of the organization it will positively impact the most. If the assessment phase established that the organization is focused on improving a specific aspect of patient care, then emphasize this to ensure the reader knows you are in line with the organization's goals to improve that specific aspect of the patient's care. If the assessment phase identified improvements in being more Joint Commission compliant, then ensure that the new service impacts this compliance in some positive manner, whether directly or indirectly. This would be described in the element of the business plan labeled "Patient Population Analysis" (see Table 11-2).

Marketing Strategies

Marketing strategies should include initial discussions with the affected core pharmacy staff. Obtaining support from your staff and using information gained from the assessment and planning phases are the first key steps in making the service a success. Without gaining support from the core staff who will be executing the service, the plan can never be implemented. Promotion to key stakeholders in the project is also important to gain support from your management team and/or higher administration, if needed. This will support and assist in buy-in of the service that may be needed when a department or others present pushback on the service's development. This step will also include discussion with income sources, if applicable, and promotion of the service with other departments affected by the new service.

Management Structure Overseeing the Service

Providing the projected structure of your management/leadership team to oversee this new service is also vital. This will allow an organization to understand who will be responsible for implementing and maintaining the service, as well as the general background and expertise required of the pharmacist staff who will execute this high level of service on a daily basis. The organization may gain further trust by reviewing the existing required certifications, background, and education needed to execute the new service.

Staffing and Operations

The staffing and operations section should outline the required resources needed to implement the service and fulfill the service on a daily basis. Resources include staff requirements, days/times for the service to be provided, any additional staff needed, and any equipment or products that will be utilized. Of course, this section should also review the proposed training plan for the staff and an outline of the daily activities that will occur to achieve completion of the service. Furthermore, an estimate of the time required to provide the service per patient should be included so the reader is aware other required tasks of the day are not affected. This may also be important in expanding the service to other areas of the organization.

Financial Projections

Financial considerations must be included in your plan. This section should list predicted costs, revenues, and any cost savings, including both hard and soft savings (see **Table 11-3**). If additional staffing requirements are needed, this may need to be re-emphasized in this section so that it is included in any financial estimation. Any additional required funding may be included here, such as any funds needed for equipment or products.

New Service Pipeline

Lastly, you should highlight the impact that the new service will have on the future of the organization. Ending your proposal with excitement and optimism of the growth of the service will hopefully develop excitement in your reader as well. This section should include the organization's areas that this service could potentially cover. This may include more resources and funding, but it is a chance to highlight the growth of its impact on enhancing patient care and satisfaction.

Table 11-3. Hard Versus Soft Savings (Cost Avoidance)

Soft Savings (put numbers to your metrics of improving hospital measures)

- Core measures, readmissions, Joint Commission, etc.
- Length of stay
- Prevention of medication errors, using benchmarking and help of quality reporting/finance
- Patient satisfaction
- Provider satisfaction
- Operational efficiency (who does your service free up to do other things: nursing, physician, etc.?)

Hard Savings

- Prevention of drug waste
- Prevention of drug usage, etc.

Other Considerations During the Creation of a Business Plan

While creating the business plan, two considerations should be discussed. A proposal of a pilot of the new service prior to the actual go-live date could be entertained. This is an opportunity for the coordinator and the reader of the plan to still be able to implement a service if the required resources are not fully in place or might take an undetermined amount of time to fully obtain. Therefore, beginning a service could still be implemented but with possible restrictions depending on the resources currently available. The second consideration is to develop a timeline and/or pilot timeline to ensure the proposal meets any strict deadlines established by your department or institution. The timeline should include each step of the process/plan and the expected time each step would take. Figuring out a go-live date for the process gives the coordinator a chance to reprioritize other goals and projects and remanage time and resources if needed.

Financial Plan Development

For any initiation of a clinical program, both costs and potential revenues/cost savings will be a key focus for any leadership team and must be a part of your business plan. Emphasis on this portion of the business plan will give your clinical program credibility with both your upper management as well as senior leadership outside of the department. With financial indicators, you can demonstrate that you understand the big picture of how your new program will impact the overall organization. Typically, you can choose one or two financial indicators to provide a general basis of the program's costs/revenues (see **Figure 11-3**). Revenue and expenses are typically projected for the first 3 to 5 years of the project. Return on investment (ROI) is one of the most common financial indicators and is simple to calculate and understand when presented to various audiences. The ROI divides the net benefit by the total net of expenses or costs of the new clinical service. Because pharmacy often creates soft savings such as length-of-stay decreases, safety catches, and quality improvement for core measures, it is important to review literature for published soft savings that can be used for your new clinical service if it is not a

direct revenue-generating service. For example, a new service to provide discharge counseling and follow-up by phone may not have direct revenue by billing, but with each decreased readmission, one may estimate cost savings of $1,000/patient not readmitted for the hospital as a soft savings based on published literature. Therefore, if the service helps prevent eight patients from being readmitted per month, the estimated soft savings would be $8,000. If you allocated a 0.5 FTE (estimated $50,000/year or $6,000/month cost) pharmacist to provide this service, your ROI would be $8,000 to $6,000/6,000 = 33% ROI.

Financial indicators are only as useful as the data put into the calculations for revenues and cost. For the cost of a new clinical service, you will need to include both supply and labor costs. These can further be divided into start-up, fixed, and variable costs if necessary. Start-up costs typically include supply costs (e.g., desks, computers, and testing materials, etc.), which can also include items such as tubing and pumps if it involves new medications or processes to run new medications. Start-up costs also include labor costs, particularly those spent on training staff. Once training is completed, labor costs may remain fixed if the FTE is dedicated to the service in perpetuity, or they may be variable costs based on how often the service is utilized (e.g., consult dosing service).

The largest cost factor is typically your key resource of pharmacists or pharmacy technicians. Labor costs should be minimized if at all possible, and often you may be asked to start a new service without any additional FTEs. See Figure 11-3 for a summary of examples of financial considerations for a new service. One novel way to start a new service without additional FTEs is to create a pharmacy student-driven service. With pharmacy schools needing increased rotation sites for their students, this is a prime opportunity to put talent to use and create a strong rotation that students will enjoy. Consider requesting a student each month, including nontraditional months such as December, so that your service labor costs will be minimal. In addition to creating a low-cost option to implement this, it will provide a strong clinical service where pharmacy students can apply their knowledge (once you ensure they have the competency to run the service). In

FIGURE 11-3. Financial Planning

Costs	Revenue

▪ Space/desk requirement cost_____
 ▪ Technology cost_____
 ▪ Medication cost_____
 ▪ Supply cost (pumps, tubing, etc.)_____
 ▪ Labor costs
    ▪ Hours/week × staff payment/hour_____
 ▪ Training costs
    ▪ Hours of training × staff payment for backfill/
      hour_____
	▪ Billing for service revenue per patient_____/pt
	
	 Hard savings:
	
	 ▪ Medication cost savings_____/(year/month/etc.)
	 ▪ Waste prevention:cost of waste____ × units saved
	
	 Soft savings:
	
	 ▪ Decreased LOS _____/day × days saved
	 ▪ Decreased readmissions _____/readmission × patient
	   readmission prevented/(year/month/etc.)
	 ▪ Medication error prevention: cost saved per error
	 ▪ Operational savings: time freed up for physician ×
	   revenue generated by time
	 ▪ Core measure compliance
	 ▪ Patient/provider satisfaction (HCAHPS scores improved
	   and value)

HCAHPS = Hospital Consumer Assessment of Healthcare Providers and Systems; LOS = length of stay; pt = patient.

either case of extending your current pharmacy staff's workload or using pharmacy students, ensure that your pharmacists or pharmacy staff members record time spent on their activities because this information will help justify FTE funding if needed in the future. You should also consider any training time that may pull staff out of other staffing models and whether or not these times need to be backfilled or just incorporated into the pharmacists' normal day. Staff members will face an adjustment with the new services and worry about working new activities into their day, so assure them that you will help prioritize their workflow during training. You should continuously stress the importance of the service—especially with administration on board and monitoring outcomes.

Other variable costs relate to volume of the service or drug usage (e.g., Does your new service increase or decrease utilization of drugs, especially high-cost medications?). However, if your new service is noted to decrease the cost of medications, this would actually go under revenue as *hard savings*.

Revenue is ideal but may not be generated with pharmacy services. Some of the methods where pharmacists have generated

revenue include discharge concierge services and billing for services in ambulatory care clinics. The revenue with these is more direct. Soft and hard savings are typically the major components of financial calculations in the place of revenue for clinical programs for health systems. Hard savings are calculated savings from drug savings, drug waste, or the use of a less expensive agent, while soft savings are calculated based on what the service is projected to save. See Table 11-3 for an example of hard versus soft savings that may be used as revenue in a financial calculation. Finally, consider other sources of revenue such as student-precepting revenue from schools of pharmacy.

Training for Success

One of the largest time commitments to any new service is educating your staff charged with providing or in some way supporting the new service. As previously stated, buy-in of the service not only comes from your organization's leadership but also from your actual employees. The education plan is extremely important and should emphasize the positive impact it will have on patient care and, ultimately, the success of the organization. When planning an education strategy, decisions to consider include the time this service should take place; which part of the staff will be directly impacted by this service; does each pharmacist require the same type of educational strategies to appropriately train the particular service; and who will provide the education. Furthermore, an evaluation of the need for an initial and annual competency on this service should be determined, depending on departmental, institutional, and regulatory requirements. Also, remember if students are providing this service, they will need the same level of education and competency.

Scheduling of Service

Determination of when this service will take place on a daily basis is critical and directly impacts the scale of the education plan. Depending on the service, the needs of the institution, and the resources available, some services may be 24/7, while others may need to be limited to certain days or hours of the week. Even further, there may be some services that start off by finding volunteers willing to be trained for the service, which can obviously affect when the service will be available. For example, if the service consistently requires a pharmacist to accurately and quickly prepare a thrombolytic for an acute ischemic stroke patient in the emergency department (ED), then this service would likely need to be provided all day/every day as determined by the appropriate key stakeholders, department goals, team goals, institution goals, and regulatory goals seen in the assessment phase. As you would suspect, services that are provided for a longer duration will require a higher number of pharmacists on staff, throughout the different shifts each day, to be trained on the service.

Selecting Staff to Train

Once you determine when this service will be provided, it will help you decide who needs training. Whether you decide to educate part or all of the pharmacist staff, it is wise to consider future needs for backup assistance when considering partial staff education. As we all know, every day brings new challenges, and urgencies/emergencies within one's usual workflow will occur or callouts will happen in the schedule. Therefore, to provide this service

consistently with the least barriers as possible, it would be prudent to train others in addition to the core staff to assist in unforeseen occasions. Be careful in choosing these backups to ensure that they are generally available in the schedule, such as a combination of FTEs and part-time and supplemental employees (always considering your weekend staffing mix). Of course, include yourself as a consistent backup to this service, so that you also stay in tune to the process, identify ways to continue to improve the process, and continue to show support for the service and your team.

Creation of Training Elements

When creating the actual educational documents, make sure you consider any differences in the service that will be provided. Also, consider any other healthcare staff this service will impact. In the example of the code stroke service, you have determined that this is a 24/7 service that pharmacy will provide to ED code strokes. You determine you only have a decentralized pharmacist model in the ED from 7 a.m. to 11 p.m. Therefore, you need to educate all pharmacists on the day, evening, and night shift. Because of this assessment, you realize that the educational documents required will be different for the day and evening shift pharmacists as they are decentralized in the ED and will have a different process in obtaining, preparing, and dispensing the thrombolytic drug. In contrast, the night shift staff who are not decentralized will have another process for obtaining, preparing, and dispensing the thrombolytic drug from the main pharmacy. This difference in process needs to be accurately reflected in the educational documents and communicated clearly to the key stakeholders supporting the service and the ED nursing staff, because the medication will be dispensed in slightly different ways depending on the shift. In addition, you may need to create educational documents for the other services if they are going to participate. You also need to keep these materials updated to orient new employees and provide regular updates to your staff and other departments to ensure everyone knows the details of the service and remains competent in providing services.

Your education strategy is particularly important to ensure your staff members are prepared to execute the service successfully and recognize that their roles in this service and the daily progress will provide long-term impacts in patient care, the success of the organization, and their professional growth. The education program will depend on the service and staff baseline knowledge as well as inclusion of all necessary resources to ensure staff success. The educational program may not always address all of the unforeseen future questions, but it should be a detailed guide for the majority of the situations your staff will encounter. You can create an FAQ (frequently asked questions) document and post this on your department's intranet or other electronic resource prior to the go-live date and after the service is live for questions that might arise. You should emphasize this is a new service and communication of any unforeseen situations or unanswered questions will be addressed, either during the training sessions or after it goes live.

Educational programs may include several types of learning to both inspire and engage the trainees to be successful. Didactic lectures, audio-based/webinar-type lectures, hands-on education, utilization of simulation labs if available, case-based training, or a combination of these may be implemented. You may want to consider providing a pre-educational assessment to assist you in gauging the group's exact needs so that you can use your training time wisely. Refer to Chapter 9: Development and Assessment of Competency regarding techniques for education and competency assessment. Obviously, the go-live date, the number of staff members to educate, and the preparation of these educational tools need to be considered when planning the educational sessions. For example, the pharmacy service for pharmacists to assist during trauma responses—depending on the baseline knowledge of the group—may include a combination of pretest, didactic, and audio lectures; hands-on training; and post-test to assess if the group is adequately prepared for trauma response. Again, keep in mind (1) the need for a regularly scheduled competency assessment to ensure the staff remains competent in the service, and (2) a time where new information can be communicated and implemented in the service. It may also be a service you may want to consider adding to the training of new hires.

Selecting Content Experts

Because physically conducting the educational program will take a potentially large amount of time and dedication to complete, you need to consider if you will lead all or part of the education or if the "train-the-trainer" strategy should be considered in some or all parts of the education. This strategy moves several individuals who know the material and service to a higher level where they can educate others. These individuals also can be referred to as *superusers* because they are experts in the service and the materials. This will depend on the actual timeline until the go-live date, the number of staff members to be educated initially, and the actual components of the educational program.

Develop Tools for Measuring Outcomes

The only way you can demonstrate the benefits of this service is to ensure you have some type of plan in measuring the outcomes of the service. The outcome of the service directly correlates to the main objective of the service. In the code stroke example, the main objective of the service was to ultimately decrease the door-to-needle time of the administration of a thrombolytic drug for acute ischemic stroke patients in the ED. If this is the main objective, then measurements of the door-to-needle times for every thrombolytic drug for an ED code stroke during all hours will need to be measured and collected. Choosing specific metrics of the service should be discussed among the initial key stakeholders of this service and your department to ensure it includes all the important aspects of the service. If you are implementing discharge processes to reduce readmissions for myocardial infarction or heart failure, quarterly readmissions data will be the key outcome to review. Remember to consider specific department or institutional goals, as well as any specific regulatory goals or standards. Metrics of a service are imperative to demonstrate its impact on patient care; display how each pharmacist's efforts on a daily basis contribute to the overall progress of patient care and the service; and manifest the results of a service to the initial key stakeholders. You should only appreciate the metrics that may potentially show little to no impact as was initially hypothesized. This would be your opportunity to determine what barriers will prevent the goal from being reached. Therefore, you must know how to collect metrics, when to collect metrics, and who will evaluate them in a reasonable time after the go-live date to measure success, barriers to the service, and future actions. If this service starts out as a pilot program, ensure that metrics are collected in at least 6 months to a year so that results can be evaluated and shared with the key stakeholders in a timely fashion. Refer to Chapter 13: Evaluation and Monitoring of Clinical Interventions for additional information regarding measurement.

Because metrics are another component that needs dedication and time to record, you should strongly consider partnering with one or more of the key stakeholders who support this service to assist and/or provide resources to help gather data. You should have already built a strong relationship with your quality department as they will easily have access to the most data for any public reporting. After talking with the quality department and other stakeholders, you may find out that reports with metrics you are interested in already exist. It would not be surprising to find that the need for this service was generated from a report. Furthermore, using the institution's existing technology to generate key reports that directly measure what is needed will potentially save a tremendous amount of time.

Action taken may include a few avenues. If metrics demonstrate achievement and success in the program, then you should consider reviewing the need for more resources to provide this service to more areas of the institution, during more hours of the day, or for more days of the week. If metrics demonstrate no significant changes to the baseline metrics prior to the service, then an analysis—very similar to what was reviewed in the assessment phase—should be performed to identify ways to improve, potential training on changes to the process, and a re-evaluation of the service post changes.

Communication of the New Service

Another element of planning is communication of this new service to the appropriate people and/or departments within the organization. After thoroughly developing your business plan on the successful implementation and assessment of this new service, you are ready to communicate it to your own department. Much like adding a new drug to formulary, a new service requires all areas within pharmacy to review and assess how it will affect their own areas including pharmacy operations, technology, clinical services, and finance. For example, if the new code stroke service will require operations to assist in assembling and/or stocking a code stroke kit, then this process will need to be detailed. For a code blue response, clearly operations will be involved to supply the resources for training as well as ensuring the carts are appropriately stocked with medications and resource cards if needed. If the technology team needs to add in a code stroke entry into the pharmacy order-verification system, then this will need to be identified and planned accordingly to what the pharmacist will need on a daily basis. If the clinical team identifies the need for volunteers to assist in the stroke education and/or thrombolytic lecture in the training program, or even volunteer their time to actually be a part of the service, then this would need to be delineated in the plan. Lastly, if there are any financial needs in the implementation of this service, it will definitely need to be discussed prior to implementation. Determining whether the impact is a one-time cost impact or if there could be any continuous or future impacts to the success of the service should be reviewed. Keep in mind that the latter information may cause a small delay on the go-live date of the service or a longer-than-anticpated delay. Either way, it is best for these types of "bumps in the road" to be smoothed out as much as possible versus dealing with them after the go-live date. Communicating regular updates on the service's progress after the go-live date to your pharmacy management group is key to ensuring they stay informed of their staff's daily progress and are prepared to speak on its progress during management meetings.

Prior to implementation, you will want to reidentify your key stakeholders in the process and ensure they are on top of the plan that will hopefully implement the service successfully. They will feel more comfortable and optimistic on the process if they are able to actually review a plan in writing prior to implementation. To reiterate what was mentioned in the planning phase, it is important to loop in the stakeholders who demonstrated hesitancy in the start of this new service. Seeing the plan will increase their confidence in the service and may ease their minds about the specific items they expressed hesitancy on initially.

Furthermore, there may be other departments at your institution directly affected by this new service. Take the time to examine every detail of the new service and assess how each one might potentially affect the daily workflow of not only your pharmacist staff, but also the other healthcare professionals: nursing, physicians, respiratory therapists, laboratory technicians, etc. Once these departments are identified, take the time to create a brief summary of this service's objective, outline the various activities of the pharmacist, and emphasize the areas that may change or affect their workflow. You should identify each department's key leadership and set up a meeting to discuss your summary. Key leadership should include, at a minimum, the director, a manager, and a supervisor/educator. You should empower and rely heavily on this group to educate their staff on this new service, the potential changes of their staff's workflow, and the implementation of a go-live date. You should be willing and prepared to assist in reviewing the education to their staff to ensure it accurately reflects and supports your new service plan. See **Figure 11-4** for an example of an intradepartmental communication checklist to ensure all elements within the pharmacy management team and with other departments are addressed.

Implementation and Monitoring

Now, the moment we all have been waiting for—the setting of the go-live date! At this point, you may have been smooth-sailing with your planning or you may have experienced a little turbulence. Either way, you made it through the assessment and the planning. You should have adequate information to assist in making a reasonable go-live date. Keep in mind the major aspects that may directly impact your go-live date: planning, implementing, and the completion of the training program; communication, assessment, and completion of responsibilities identified within

your pharmacy management team; ensuring that the key stakeholders and other affected departments and their staff members are informed; and ensuring any needed means of collecting data are ready. Also, if there are any changes that should be reflected on the actual daily work schedule of your pharmacist staff, this will need to be done prior to the go-live date as well to avoid confusion. Once all the latter has been taken into account and you have determined the amount of time needed for each aspect to be completed through adequate means of communication, then a go-live date can be proposed and communicated to your department leadership and staff, the key stakeholders, and other departments affected by this service. Of utmost importance, schedule times to meet with the core pharmacist staff during staff meetings, core group meetings, department meetings, and/or one-on-one meetings to ensure everyone has gone through appropriate training and is prepared and confident to execute the new service. If you have staff members who are not 100% competent, you need to work with them one-on-one and provide extra assistance and guidance. Set clear goals and if they do not show improvement, you should contact and work with your human resources department. Make sure you document your meetings with the individuals as well as your plan to ensure forward progress. For more information on human resources management, refer to Chapter 7: Human Resources and People Management.

Another point to consider prior to the go-live date would be implementing a smaller version of a pilot or a test run to work out any last-minute kinks or potential barriers not addressed in the planning phase.

As the primary coordinator of this service, it is essential that you are available to your staff not only on the first day of the go-live, but also for the first 1 to 2 weeks after the go-live. This, of course, will depend on how smoothly the process has gone during both the first week and the first weekend after the go-live date. You need to physically visit the areas of the organization where the service has begun and discuss with the pharmacy staff members and other healthcare professionals how the new service has impacted their workflows and patient care/satisfaction. This is referred to as *walking rounds*. This rounding time may include

FIGURE 11-4. Communication Checklist of New Pharmacy Service

Area Involved	Activities Assigned	Deadline for Any Assigned Activities	Assigned to	Complete (√ and date)
Pharmacy operations				
Pharmacy clinical				
Pharmacy technology				
Financial				
Systemwide pharmacy management				
Other organization departments affected by new service				
Hospital administration and/or other key stakeholders				

Source: Original version used with permission from WakeMed Health & Hospitals Pharmacy Department, November 2014.

actually performing the service if the staff requires extra support on the new process or helping with their other daily responsibilities so they can focus on the new service. This is your opportunity to take notes on items to follow up on, such as positive notes of achievement and notes of both constructive and negative feedback from your staff and other department's staff. Adding the status of this new service to the scheduled pharmacy management meeting's agenda for an indefinite amount of time, depending on how well it is progressing, may

be a good idea to ensure your leadership group stays informed.

After the go-live date or maybe even after a pilot of the service begins, remember that the success of this service lies with your employees and their actions to improve patient care. As a coordinator, it is your responsibility to ensure that your staff members are recognizing the impact of their actions on this new service and ultimately the care of their patients. The only way to allow them to recognize this is to make sure they have very clear goals each day that may be directly related to this new service. Then, make sure you are available and checking in on your staff members to ensure they have enough resources to meet these goals. If employees are also responsible for the data collection of this service, make sure they understand and have the time to input this information on a daily basis. At the end of their shift, ask for their feedback and see what goals they were able to achieve. Their feedback should be clues to you on ways to improve the process. Therefore, the data collected are not only for the key stakeholders, higher administration, or for your pharmacy management team, but they are also for your core team to use in implementing tasks. Once you gather this information, it is important to share your findings and resolutions with the staff. By sharing this information with them, they can take pride in their achievements and see how it contributes to the bigger picture of why they chose this profession and why they provide this new service to positively impact the patient care on a daily basis. In turn, this will hopefully fuel their motivation to keep the service going for a long time. It is okay if everything does not go perfectly, but it is important to quickly identify what is not working, obtain feedback, develop a solution, implement it, and then re-evaluate to make sure that what you changed generated improvement.

For the future, data collection may play an important role in sharing the information with other institutions interested in a similar service or even the process of implementing a new service. The power of sharing this information in a publication may be vital for other institutions seeking to implement these services. See **Appendix 11-A** for an example go-live checklist.

Summary

Implementing new clinical pharmacy programs is one of the many responsibilities of a pharmacy clinical coordinator. It is likely also one of the main inspirations of the clinical coordinator to be in this role. These clinical pharmacy programs are meant to not only inspire the coordinator and their staff, but also to inspire key stakeholders and leaders in an organization to support innovative ways that continue to challenge healthcare systems in improving patient care. Therefore, proper steps should be taken when considering the creation and implementation of new pharmacy programs (see Figure 11-1 for an overall flow diagram in the creation of a new pharmacy service). The steps include a high-level assessment of the needs of the organization, planning a robust proposal of all aspects of this new service, and careful implementation of the program. All these phases equally contribute to the successful creation of a service and its longevity. If you have been successful (or even if you have not been successful), consider sharing your work in a poster or publication. It is equally important to share even if something did not work so that others can learn from your experience. Sharing what you do helps the overall healthcare profession to further our impact on positive patient care.

PRACTICE TIPS

1. Invest time in fostering relationships with other department leaders when planning new initiatives.

2. Communicate regularly with your management team and the core staff performing the new service throughout the planning and implementation process to ensure successful go-lives.

3. Obtain and address meaningful feedback before and after go-live dates on the new service process to provide new perspectives that may not have been considered and could be essential in optimizing the process.

4. Don't give up! Some projects may not be successful in the initial stages of the implementation. Adjustments to the process after the go-live date is natural and should be made if necessary.

References

1. *The Dynamics of Pharmaceutical Care: Enriching Patients' Health. Monograph 23: Writing a Business Plan for a New Pharmacy Service.* Washington, DC: American Pharmacists Association; 2007.

2. Harris IM, Baker E, Berry TM, et al. Developing a business-practice model for pharmacy services in ambulatory settings. *Pharmacotherapy.* 2008;28(2):7e-34e.

Suggested Reading

DeCoske M, Tryon J, White SJ. *The Pharmacy Leadership Field Guide: Cases and Advice for Everyday Situations.* Bethesda, MD: ASHP; 2011.

Liedtka J. *Designing for Growth: A Design Thinking Tool Kit for Managers.* New York, NY: Columbia University Press; 2011.

Ries E. *The Lean Startup: How Today's Entrepreneurs Use Continuous Innovation to Create Radically Successful Businesses.* New York, NY: Crown Publishing Group; 2011.

Appendix 11-A

Example of a Go-Live Checklist

Time to Begin Prior to Go-Live	Activity
4 weeks prior to go-live	■ Ensure all elements of the communication checklist have been addressed/assigned to the appropriate pharmacy teams and/or other department teams ■ Ensure the data collection tool has been completed with all preliminary elements in place as decided in the planning phase ■ Ensure all elements of data collection are collectable either in the technology system or manually
3 weeks prior to go-live	■ Ensure all education of the staff outlined in the business plan is complete ■ Ensure all elements of the communication checklist are in process ■ Test the new service process at each step outlined in the training to double-check the logistics of the process and/or identify any unforeseen issues ■ Begin to address any unforeseen issues identified in the previous step ■ Utilize the data collection tool to assess if all elements can either be collected in the current technology system or manually collected (depending on what was decided in the planning phase)
2 weeks prior to go-live	■ Ensure all elements of the communication checklist are in process ■ Address any unforeseen issues from the checklist ■ Re-address any unforeseen issues in the new service process identified last week ■ Schedule staff meeting, core group meeting, and/or one-on-one meetings with pharmacy staff to ensure comfort in the upcoming new service
1 week prior to go-live	■ Ensure all elements of the communication checklist are complete ■ Ensure any unforeseen issues in the new process have been addressed ■ Continue to assess pharmacy staff comfort in the process
Week of go-live	■ Recommunicate with pharmacy department and other affected departments to ensure all assigned tasks are complete
Go-live day!	■ Be available and be prepared to do physical rounds on go-live day and daily thereafter for a variable amount of time after go-live day ■ Talk with pharmacy staff and other healthcare professionals involved during rounds
After go-live	■ Provide ongoing rounding ■ Provide ongoing metric evaluation ■ Provide ongoing education and competency assessment ■ Provide ongoing process improvement assessments within pharmacy department and other departments ■ Provide regular updates to pharmacy management team and other key stakeholders/departments ■ Continue to assess service expansion opportunities ■ Look forward to research opportunities, poster presentations, publications, etc.

CHAPTER 12

Programs That Work: Clinical Pharmacy Services 101

Carrie A. Berge and Steven S. Carlisle

KEY TERMS

Antimicrobial Stewardship—Program(s) designed to improve the appropriate use of anti-infective agents while decreasing microbial resistance and improving patient outcomes.

High-Risk Medications—Medications that have an increased risk of producing patient harm if used incorrectly.

Pharmacokinetics—Interaction of a drug and the body involving the properties of absorption, distribution, metabolism, and excretion.

Therapeutic Drug Monitoring (TDM)—Measuring and evaluating blood levels of selected medications to ensure safe and effective therapy.

Transitions of Care (TOC)—The movement of a patient between settings within a healthcare system.

Introduction

The value of clinical pharmacy services has been repeatedly demonstrated in the medical literature and regulatory and accrediting agencies such as the Centers for Medicare & Medicaid Services (CMS) and The Joint Commission (TJC) require many of them.[1-3] Justifying the implementation of these services can be a challenging endeavor for pharmacist leadership and the pharmacy department (see Chapter 11: Implementing New Clinical Pharmacy Programs—Step-by-Step for discussion of this process). The goal of this chapter is to provide practical, ground-level advice on the implementation of selected clinical services as well as strategies for building and initiating these programs.

The selection of clinical programs to offer at your institution should be based not only on the program's known value or the requirement(s), but also on the unique aspects inherent to your facility including your patient population; characteristics (education, experience) and quantity of your pharmacist and technician staff; and availability of resources. The value of clinical pharmacy programs is clear; however, every program cannot be implemented by every institution. Ideally, this chapter will provide you with a ready-to-use guide for a framework of clinical programs within your institution.

Antimicrobial Stewardship

Antimicrobial stewardship is a "coordinated program that promotes the appropriate use of antimicrobials (including antibiotics), improves patient outcomes, reduces microbial resistance, and decreases the spread of infections caused by multidrug-resistant organisms."[4]

How to Get Started: Antimicrobial Stewardship

Pharmacists guiding and monitoring all use of antimicrobials is a key clinical service need in all health systems. There are a wealth of organization resources and literature to guide a clinical coordinator in establishing or refining a stewardship program. ASHP has helpfully created a resource center at www.leadstewardship.org/resources.php for implementing antimicrobial stewardship programs in health systems.[5] Links will direct you to resources from the Centers

for Disease Control and Prevention (CDC) who publishes the Core Elements of Hospital Antibiotic Stewardship programs and the most current guidelines, policy statements, compendiums, and regulations from relevant organizations such as ASHP, Infectious Diseases Society of America, the Society for Healthcare Epidemiology of America, and TJC.[6,7]

Stewardship Program Checklist

To establish a baseline assessment of your institution's status against best stewardship practices, the CDC published a checklist for core elements of hospital stewardship programs (available at http://www.cdc.gov/getsmart/healthcare/implementation/checklist.html).[8] Use this tool as your baseline assessment. The identified gaps will lead you to the opportunities for short-term and long-term performance improvement plans (PIPs).

Resources for Stewardship

One of the key issues any clinical coordinator will face with a clinical service enhancement or implementation is resources. Antimicrobial stewardship specifically asks for a pharmacist leader as part of the core program components. For some large health systems, this will be a full-time PGY2 (postgraduate year 2), infectious disease, residency-trained pharmacist who might report to a clinical coordinator as well as to an inpatient operational manager depending on your organizational structure. There are alternative models that will also provide successful stewardship. In some models, the clinical coordinator leads and monitors the stewardship initiatives but trains the entire staff to have an active role carrying it out 24/7. In some systems without a dedicated specialist, it is a shared responsibility between critical care and internal medicine lead pharmacists.

Stewardship Tips

- Turn your baseline assessment tool into an ongoing stewardship team status report.
  - Green—What is in place and measureable
  - Yellow—Elements requiring further refinement
  - Red—Items not yet implemented

- Insert your PIP/action plans into the status report for all yellow and red elements.

- Designate who is leading each PIP/action plan and the expected timelines for implementation or next update.

- Many larger health systems form dedicated stewardship committees to organize their team activities, review outcomes, and plan new initiatives. Others may focus on stewardship on a regular schedule at their Pharmacy and Therapeutics (P&T) committee or other clinical performance improvement committees in the health system.

- Order sets (either electronic or preprinted) become essential in guiding antimicrobial therapy. Be sure you or your stewardship pharmacist leader is part of facilitating the development, implementation, and monitoring of all antimicrobial orders for all service lines in your health system.

- Network on association list servers or with your mentors and colleagues for sample order sets, procedures, or other stewardship project examples to gather starting points that inspire you and your stewardship team.

There are additional clinical surveillance tools that can interface with your electronic medical record (EMR) and pathology/microbiology information systems. These tools can enhance efficiencies for stewardship daily interventions as well as ongoing measurable outcomes. Some current vendors in this area are Premier's Theradoc product and BD's MedMined program.

Pharmacokinetics and Therapeutic Drug Monitoring

No topic has more thoroughly integrated itself in the fabric of clinical pharmacy than pharmacokinetic drug monitoring. This concept has become such a key component to many facilities' clinical pharmacy services that it is hard to imagine a facility providing clinical pharmacy services without including **pharmacokinetics** and medication monitoring. The value of these services has been thoroughly described in the medical literature and definitively supports provision of these services.[9-11] The overreaching goal of a **therapeutic drug monitoring** (TDM) program is to ensure the safe and effective use of potentially dangerous medications. This section will provide practical guidance on how to build a TDM monitoring program that works and is sustainable.

No term in pharmacy produces more trepidation and anxiety than *pharmacokinetics*. This began in our pharmacy school days and, for many, continues through our careers, probably stemming from the obvious connection between pharmacokinetics and advanced mathematics. It is important to realize many critical aspects of a TDM program can be provided with little or no use of advanced mathematics. All pharmacists can and should perform these services.

Designing the TDM Program

As stated previously, facility-specific and staff-specific characteristics must be considered when implementing any clinical program. A benefit in the area of TDM, which is true for many services discussed in this chapter, is the longevity of these programs has resulted in extensive information available on facility-specific implementation. A prudent first step in implementation is to network with similar institutions about how they implemented these programs. Most facilities are eager to share experiences and will often provide copies of policies and procedures, guidance on overcoming obstacles, and first-hand insight into what works and what did not. This information will prove invaluable and go far in simplifying the creation of a new service. With this as a guide, you can search for available guidance on the topic from a variety of sources: other facilities, professional societies, regulatory and accrediting agencies, and medical literature. This information will be the frame on which you build your program. Potential steps in the TDM program creation can be found in **Table 12-1**. The steps represented in this table can be easily adjusted to meet the implementation requirements for many clinical programs discussed in this chapter.

Selection of Medications for Monitoring

You should select which medications to monitor in a TDM program based on the general

Table 12-1. Checklist for Creation of a TDM Program

Task	Potential Information Sources
Search for TDM program examples	Medical literature, similar facilities, professional societies
Select medications for inclusion	Medical literature, facility high-risk/high-alert list, facility medication safety reports
Select program design/scope: monitor/report, pharmacy to dose, combination	Staffing data, pharmacy practice model, staff background/experience
Identify pharmacist roles and responsibilities	Professional societies, medical literature, similar facilities
Evaluate/obtain needed resources	Staffing possibilities, technology options
Educate staff	In-house experts, local experts, online resources
Educate providers/nurses	Facility medical/nursing leadership

TDM = therapeutic drug monitoring.

medical literature on this topic as well as facility-specific factors. Clearly, the vast majority of TDM programs include aminoglycosides and vancomycin. It is hard to imagine an acute care facility not having some use of these medications. Even small use of these medications would warrant serious consideration for inclusion in your TDM program. Other medications that are commonly included in TDM programs include phenytoin, lithium, heparin, digoxin, and warfarin.[12-14]

The selection of medications to include should be data driven. These data should come from the medical literature as well from your own institution. Institution-specific data to aid in selection include medication usage patterns, a facility high-risk medication list, and medical specialty/patient demographics. The addition of a facility-specific list of selected high-risk/high-alert medications to your TDM program is a useful way to meet the requirements to identify and monitor these types of medications. CMS and the Institute for Safe Medication Practices have created lists of high-risk/high-alert medications that can be used as a template for selection of institutionally relevant high-risk/high-alert medications for monitoring.[15,16]

Basic TDM Program Design

An early decision is to identify the method your institution will use to provide TDM services. There are two overreaching concepts utilized in

TDM programs: (1) monitor-and-report and (2) pharmacy-to-dose. Each of these designs offers benefits and drawbacks and both may be used within the same facility.

Monitor-and-report design. Pharmacists monitor patients who are receiving TDM medications and report significant findings to the medical team caring for the patient. This list of patients on these medications can either be generated by a traditional list report or through a surveillance system that has clinical decision support logic, which provides more than just a list of the patients and medications. Using clinical decision support allows you to add rules that will only display the patients when certain criteria are met and also provide guidance on dosing recommendations. It is much easier to provide a traditional list and more time-consuming to build rules, alerts, and clinical decision support, but these can often be more valuable for the most efficient workflow. These reportable findings are based on medication toxicity/efficacy characteristics of the TDM medications and can include initial and ongoing laboratory tests such as blood urea nitrogen (BUN), serum creatinine (SCr), creatinine clearance (CrCl), white blood cell (WBC) count, and ordered drug levels. In this design, the pharmacist's responsibility is to ensure the medical team orders the appropriate monitoring, and the team is made aware of any changes in the monitoring parameters. The pharmacist can suggest changes in TDM medication doses to the medical team, but the final responsibility for dose modification rests with the medical team alone.

The monitor-and-report design offers many benefits to a pharmacy. This methodology can be implemented with a predominantly generalist pharmacist staff and often can be performed adequately in a 24/7 manner in conjunction with the pharmacy's normal operations. Drawbacks include being a passive system where the medical team has the majority of decision-making responsibility. All changes come from the medical team, and the potential exists for important dose change recommendations to be overlooked. This could result in a patient experiencing toxicity or inadequate dosing.

Pharmacy-to-dose concept. In this system, pharmacy is allowed to order appropriate laboratory monitoring and adjust the patient's medication doses accordingly. Your facilities' appropriate medication oversight body (often the P&T committee) should approve and your state's regulations should allow all program activities.

Benefits include greater assurance that patient doses will be adjusted appropriately based on relevant patient monitoring and, possibly, greater job satisfaction among the pharmacy staff. There are many potential drawbacks because there is a greater impact on pharmacy workflow, and it may require additional staff to implement and maintain this style of TDM. Additionally, the generalist pharmacy staff may require additional training to perform these tasks. Specialized training may be needed to prepare your pharmacy staff to appropriately document interventions and notes in the legal medical record. These two styles can exist in concert, and having both within one facility may be a way to provide comprehensive TDM services utilizing many pharmacy models: decentralized services, clinical pharmacy specialists, and/or high-risk areas (e.g., neonatal intensive care units).

Scope of TDM Services

Each facility must determine how and where they will implement TDM services. Options include implementation throughout the entire facility or only within select areas. This decision can be based on facility-specific risk strati-

fication and staffing. A word of caution with regard to partial implementation—excluding certain areas of your facility from this safety-focused initiative may be challenging to defend. An alternative path may be to implement a monitor/report-based system in low-risk areas and a pharmacist-to-dose system in high-risk areas. This approach may be the way to address the days/times for provision of TDM services. Clearly, the gold standard is to provide comprehensive services in a 24/7 manner. If this is not feasible, a mix of monitor-and-report and pharmacy-to-dose may be appropriate.

Identify Pharmacist Roles and Responsibilities

A key component to implementing a TDM program is the creation of appropriate roles and responsibilities for your pharmacist staff. To start this process, talk with similar institutions and learn from their experiences. Colleagues who have experienced the process will provide valuable guidance on what each pharmacist will do and how they will accomplish the TDM program's requirements. Professional societies often create policy statements or guidelines on many topics within the provision of pharmacy services. These policies and guidelines are great tools for the creation and justification of clinical pharmacy services. ASHP's Statement on the Pharmacist's Role in Clinical Pharmacokinetic Monitoring provides recommended responsibilities and roles for generalist and specialist pharmacists in the area of TDM.[17]

Evaluate/Obtain Needed Resources

The resources needed for implementing a TDM program will vary depending on the scope and method you choose. The types of resources needed involve personnel, information sources (books, subscriptions), and technology for calculation and decision support. A pivotal question to answer involves defining adequate staffing levels for the desired services. Can you provide the TDM services you desire with the staff you have, or will you need to add personnel? Clearly, adding personnel to any pharmacy will be a challenge. Requesting additional staff may be necessary, but it will probably not occur quickly. Consider implementing a manageable TDM program with available staff while you wait for approval/hiring of additional staff.

Information and decision support resources include books, journal subscriptions, and computer-based TDM programs. Satisfactory pharmacokinetics resources are readily available and in many cases free of charge (for examples, see **Table 12-2**). Obtaining the best and most current resources in this arena is key to providing stellar TDM services. The most competent pharmacists may find themselves handcuffed if the available resources are inadequate to support their efforts.

Staff Education/Competency

The crucial component to the successful provision of TDM services involves staff education and competency. It is critical to train your staff to be fully competent in providing these services. If your current staff includes specialist pharmacists who are fluent in these activities, they may serve as your primary educators. Another method for educating your staff would be you (as the clinical coordinator) designing and providing the education. Educating from within offers numerous advantages in terms of cost savings, speed of education completion, and flexibility. Alternatively, external resources can be utilized. A wonderful resource is the Nebraska Medical Center Department of Pharmacy's *Pharmacokinetic Training Packet for Pharmacists* (available at http://www.nebraskamed.com/app_files/pdf/careers/education-programs/asp/pk_trainingpacket_2012.pdf).[18]

Initial and annual competency verification for all pharmacists participating in TDM activities must be performed and documented. This will ensure that all involved staff are up-to-date in providing these critical services as well as ensuring that you are fully prepared for competency assessment questions that can occur during a CMS and/or TJC inspection.

In conclusion, TDM services are an integral component of clinical pharmacy services. It is possible for any institution to implement a comprehensive, effective, and sustainable TDM program. Appropriate planning and preparation will allow your facility to build this program in an efficient manner with limited impact on pharmacy operations.

Renal Dose Monitoring and Adjustment

A very common component of an institution's clinical pharmacy program is the monitoring and adjustment of medication doses based on a patient's renal function. This program is a frequent cornerstone of clinical programs due to the obvious links to patient safety, **high-risk medications**, and a clear correlation between the dosing of many medications and renal function. A well-designed and thoughtfully implemented renal dosing program can be an integral component to an institution's medication safety program. This section will discuss potential implementation strategies and issues involved in the creation of a facility-specific renal monitoring and dosing program.

Table 12-2. Examples of TDM Information and Decision Support Resources

Sources	Website	Description
The Merck Manual	http://www.merckmanuals.com/professional	Resource for basic information
Pharmacokinetic and Pharmacodynamic Resources	http://www.pharmpk.com/	Diverse collection of routinely updated information
Resource Clinical	http://www.resourceclinical.com/clinical-pharmacokinetics-and-pharmacodynamics.html	Diverse collection of pharmacokinetic training and support
RxKinetics	http://www.rxkinetics.com/	Kinetics software
University of Utah Health Care	http://pharmacyservices.utah.edu/rxweblinks/	Kinetics software and calculators

TDM = therapeutic drug monitoring.

Designing the Renal Dosing Program

Before implementing any clinical program you must consider all relevant facility- and staff-specific characteristics. Pharmacy renal dosing programs are a staple in the pantry of clinical services offered by many institutions. Due to this frequent occurrence in the pharmacy community, you will probably have a wealth of similar institutions available to contact for first-hand information on issues involving the design, implementation, and maintenance of a renal dosing program. Your search for examples and details of pharmacy renal dosing programs should not be limited to other institutions. Investigating information available from professional societies, regulatory and accrediting agencies, and the medical literature is critical in the creation of any clinical program. The following sections describe the potential steps in the creation of a renal dosing program.

Selection of Medications for Dose Adjustment and Monitoring

No topic in the pharmacy and medical literature has been better researched than the interplay between medications and renal function. There are numerous sources detailing the need to adjust the dose of medications based on renal function. Any list of medications requiring renal dosage adjustment will be quite large. A readily accessible source regarding renal dosing is the *Drug Information Handbook*, which contains dosing information for countless medications as well as renal function assessment information.[19] The process for selecting medications should include reviewing data obtained from your specific institution, such as previous medication incidents and safety reports related to medication dosing and renal function. Data from these sources will provide clear evidence of drugs that are of known risk in your facility. Additional data that will prove useful include medication usage patterns, facility high-risk medication lists, and medical specialty/patient demographics.

Basic Renal Dosing and Monitoring Program Design

As with many clinical programs, there are multiple ways to implement a renal dosing and monitoring program. Within the arena of renal dosing and monitoring, the two major options are *prospec-*

tive review and *renal dosing and monitoring protocols.* Each of these designs brings unique advantages and challenges. These two designs may also both be used within a facility.

Prospective review for renal monitoring and dosing involves an institution's pharmacists monitoring all patients (i.e., or select patient groups, CrCl <50 mL/min) for medication use impacted by renal function. Pharmacists will review and document relevant patient laboratory values (SCr, BUN, CrCl) and current doses of selected medications. These details are then communicated to the medical team caring for the patient. The pharmacist's role in this model is to communicate the monitored data to the medical team. The responsibility to change medication doses will remain the responsibility of the medical team. The pharmacist may be asked to provide dosing recommendations.

Prospective monitoring offers significant advantages. This program is easily implemented with a generalist pharmacist staff and can be relatively easily accomplished each day with limited disruption to the normal pharmacy operations. A limitation to this system is whether medications are dosed appropriately because the possibility exists for a critical medication dose change request to be missed or delayed.

Renal dosing and monitoring protocols offer an alternative method for ensuring safe and effective medication dosing based on renal function or risk of renal damage. In this protocol-driven system, the pharmacist staff is granted authority to monitor and dose selected medications based on potential impact by and on the renal status of the patient. This type of program must be approved by the institution's P&T committee (or your appropriate medication oversight body).

Protocol-based renal dosing and monitoring programs provide greater, direct involvement in the provision of safe dosing with respect to renal function. A protocol-based renal dosing program will have a much greater impact on established pharmacy workflow and may require additional staff to ensure the protocol requirements can be effectively met while still completing all other required pharmacy functions. Also, additional training will be required to ensure the pharmacist staff has the required knowledge to appropriately manage the protocol activities and correctly document interventions and notes in the medical record.

Both of these methods can coexist within a facility. Often, the medical staff has the opportunity to select one or the other method for each patient. Keep in mind, the ability to select protocol-based renal dosing services will require your pharmacy to provide the services whenever they are requested.

Scope of Renal Dosing and Monitoring Services

Because you need to provide this service to all patients, you must take that into consideration when deciding how to implement a renal dosing and monitoring program. Offering different levels of care to different groups of patients or during different times/days (nights/weekends excluded) will be an extremely challenging position to justify. Great care must be utilized to ensure the system you chose to implement is sustainable with your current available staff.

Identify Pharmacist Roles and Responsibilities

When implementing a renal dosing and monitoring program, you must clearly delineate the roles and responsibilities for your pharmacist staff. Talking with similar institutions can provide a wealth of information useful in creating these roles and responsibilities. The appropriate roles and responsibilities of pharmacists in the provision of a renal dosing and monitoring service can include reviewing patient medical records, ordering appropriate laboratory monitoring, and documenting in the medical records. Potential pharmacist activities in a renal dosing and monitoring program should be specified and detailed in a departmental policy. An exceptional example of a comprehensive, yet easy-to-follow, renal dosing policy can be found at the University of Kentucky Medical Center Department of Pharmacy (http://www.hosp.uky.edu/pharmacy/departpolicy/PH02-07.pdf.).[20]

Evaluate/Obtain Needed Resources

As with the implementation of any new program, available resources must be considered when you are designing a renal dosing and monitoring program. A crucial step is to ensure you have the staff to do the job. Implementing a new program stresses the current staff's ability

to perform all required pharmacy duties and can potentially yield unfavorable results in other areas of pharmacy services. Using your current staff's unique attributes will ensure creating a more sustainable renal dosing program. A pharmacy must have appropriate knowledge and decision support resources (commonly maintained by all hospital pharmacies) including books, journal subscriptions, and information providing the pharmacist staff online sites to find up-to-date renal dosing information.

Staff Education/Competency

To effectively provide a renal dosing and monitoring service, the pharmacist must be appropriately trained. Many skills and competencies required to provide these services are general pharmacist abilities that everyone should possess. Prior to any pharmacist providing these services, you must ensure he or she is competent in providing these services. You may have in-house experts who can provide staff education, including clinical pharmacy specialists or others with additional training/experience. External educational resources can be utilized, such as locating local experts from a neighboring hospital or college of pharmacy and inviting them to provide an educational program. Initial and annual competency verification for all pharmacists participating in renal dosing activities should be performed and documented. Creating and maintaining appropriate documentation of staff competencies and education is a must for the accreditation and inspection visits your pharmacy will face (see Chapter 6: Accreditation, Medication Management, and the Clinical Coordinator).

In conclusion, a renal dosing and monitoring program is commonly considered to be a critical piece of any pharmacy clinical program. It is possible to design a program to provide heightened patient safety while considering pharmacy resources and sustainability. Renal dosing programs that consider P&T protocols allowing pharmacists to automatically dose and order laboratory tests as needed are a foundation pharmacy service that all pharmacists can provide.

Anticoagulation Services

The use of anticoagulants is a key clinical service needed in all health systems. There is a plethora of organizational resources and literature to guide a clinical coordinator in establishing or refining anticoagulation programs (see **Table 12-3**). Examples exist in the literature for inpatient, transitional, and clinic service models. ASHP has helpfully created a resource center (at www.ashp.org/anticoagulation) that host's scientific articles, guidelines, and sources for education and training.[21] Links will direct you to the key guidelines from the American College of Chest Physicians and other resource links to other policy statements, compendiums, and regulations from relevant organizations such as TJC.[22]

TJC has specific regulations for hospitals that must reduce the likelihood of patient harm associated with the use of anticoagulant therapy and published a sentinel event alert in 2008 regarding preventing errors related to commonly used anticoagulants.[23] One of TJC's recommended key risk-reduction strategies is implementing a pharmacist-managed anticoagulant service to help discharged patients receiving warfarin therapy and to assist staff caring for patients on anticoagulants.[23] Dager and Gulseth summarized two institution's approaches to implementing inpatient pharmacist-based anticoagulation programs and recommended key steps to consider in developing or enhancing your currently offered services.[24]

Anticoagulation Services Tips

- Customize your service needs to the populations served. Do you offer both inpatient and outpatient services or are your patients going to transition to a different outpatient setting?

- Determine the level of pharmacist involvement in preventing venous thromboembolism in hospitalized patients. ASHP has a recent therapeutic position statement that provides a summary and key recommendations.[25]

- Build strong relationships with your pathology colleagues regarding all testing capabilities within your health system from phlebotomy or point-of-care testing.

- Use an interdisciplinary performance improvement team for all anticoagulation activities. Some institutions use the P&T committee or unique anticoagulation subcommittees.

- Build tools within your EMR or written chart to facilitate standardized anticoagulation ordering and monitoring.

- Determine the scope of pharmacist activities. It could range from consult service to full pharmacist dosing and monitoring of specific anticoagulants and all communication and documentation with the medical team.

- Have specific quality measures and reports in place prior to starting any new service change.

- Ensure adequate staff training and continual competency evaluations.

Table 12-3. Recommended External Sites for Anticoagulation Service Resources[a]

Source	Website
American College of Chest Physicians[26]	http://chestjournal.chestpubs.org (search for most current supplement)
Anticoagulation Forum[27]	http://www.acforum.org
Clotcare[28]	http://www.clotcare.com
University of Washington Department of Pharmacy Services[29]	http://depts.washington.edu/anticoag/home

[a]See Suggested Reading for additional ASHP publications.

Emergency Response

One of the more recent innovations in clinical pharmacy involves the active participation of the pharmacist on an emergency response team. The medical literature has shown significant pharmacy-response rates to code blue situations for over 20 years.[30] Pharmacist emergency response has now become commonplace in stroke-response and rapid-response teams. Additionally, including pharmacists as a member of an interdisciplinary emergency team assists in meeting the ASHP minimum standard for pharmacies in hospitals with respect to pharmacy response to medical emergencies.[31]

Designing a Pharmacist Emergency Response Program

Even though pharmacist emergency response is a newer addition to the choir of clinical pharmacy services, it is well represented in the clinical pharmacy community. You, therefore, have the benefit of querying similar institutions and utilizing these readily available sources to provide an easy way to begin your program's design. Additional sources on designing a pharmacist emergency response program are professional societies, regulatory and accrediting agencies, and the medical literature.

Selection of Types of Pharmacist Emergency Response

A major decision in creating your institution's specific pharmacist emergency response program involves selecting the type of emergencies your pharmacists will respond to. There is no perfect, cookie-cutter response to this question. Each facility, regardless of similarities to other facilities, is 100% unique. Any pharmacist emergency response program is destined for failure if you do not adequately address your facility's special concerns and needs.

The types of emergency scenarios you chose to require a pharmacist response should be based on your facility's type of services. You must decide if rare occurrences, like malignant hyperthermia, should be included in the pharmacist emergency response program. These decisions can be facilitated by looking at the types of patients and your institution's medical specialties. Additionally, you should base the decision regarding emergency-type inclusion on data from your facility's medication safety program (to identify high-risk medications and situations). Guidance can also be found by looking at your institution's types of emergency response programs. Basically, strong consideration should be paid to adding a pharmacist to all emergency response teams within your facility. The current healthcare environment strives to maximize interdisciplinary care in a variety of emergency scenarios. Pharmacists participate in far more than just the traditional code blue programs to include stroke, trauma, ST segment elevation myocardial infarction, sepsis, and general rapid-response team programs.

Basic Emergency Pharmacist Response Program Design

After you have selected the types of emergency situations requiring pharmacist response, the next step is designing the methodology. Key components to consider include selection of pharmacists who will respond to emergency situations; identification of where/when the services will be offered; creating appropriate policies and guidance for the service's initiation and maintenance; and developing competency and evaluating it on a regular basis to ensure the pharmacists are providing the response to positively impact patient outcomes.

Each facility will have varying levels of pharmacist staff approval on the requirement to respond to emergency situations. Some will feel thrilled with the opportunity while others may react somewhere along the range of apathy to hostility; and many will feel this is an obvious opportunity to utilize a pharmacist's unique skills while others may see this as an area where pharmacists do not belong. Many misgivings can be effectively managed by appropriate education and training. You may find it necessary to aggressively market these new programs to gain acceptance. In the end, it is necessary to decide who should respond and what their consistent role is. Any pharmacist emergency response program will function more efficiently if all pharmacists share the responsibility of providing this critical service.

By its definition, it is obvious that emergency response can be required any day at any time. Most pharmacies operate with limited staff overnight, weekends, and holidays. It is tempting to consider creating a pharmacy emergency response program that also is more limited during those times. But implementing an emergency pharmacy response program less than 24/7 in nature will be challenging to defend. An alternative approach is to create a program narrow enough in scope (with regard to areas of coverage and expectations of response) so it can be fully activated at any time of every day of the week. Additionally, the system you choose to implement should be 100% sustainable with the current staff available to you.

Identify Pharmacist Roles and Responsibilities

The roles and responsibilities for all pharmacists participating in the emergency pharmacist response program must be clearly identified. As mentioned previously, you may face widely differing views on this program. Many who are not fully supportive may be swayed with a well-designed policy spelling out what is expected of them. The appropriate roles and responsibilities can include providing backup emergency medications, assisting with medication selection, and administration of medications. Pharmacy activities and expectations in a pharmacist emergency response program should be specified and detailed in a departmental policy. Suggested components of a pharmacy policy for pharmacist emergency response should include the following:

- Response locations and pharmacist assignments
- Notification methods
- Pharmacist responsibilities
- Orientation and training
- Emergency medication stocking procedures

Staff Education/Competency

Providing effective pharmacist emergency response requires pharmacists to be appropriately trained for their required duties. Advanced cardiac life support (ACLS), a wonderful cornerstone for this training, effectively adds to the knowledge base of those who complete the course and should be a minimum requirement for pharmacists participating in the program.

ACLS is often provided free of charge in many hospitals and offered throughout the year. This adds to the ease with which staff members can be educated. Critical care and/or emergency experts on your staff can provide additional pharmacy-specific education. You should ensure the training program includes appropriate operational information as well. The pharmacist responder needs to be comfortable with medication preparation, ordering, and storage requirements as well as more clinical skills. Some organizations have recognized that ACLS focuses more on the diagnosis of the rhythms and less on the physical preparation of medications. To ensure pharmacists are prepared to respond, they need to know more than just the ACLS course, so consider creating your own educational program and work with your emergency response oversight committee to obtain approval for an alternative educational program.

A critical component to include in your training program is the requirement for the newly trained pharmacist to first function as an observer only. Watching a more established pharmacist responder (prior to functioning as the sole responder) will provide opportunities for questions and will also boost confidence. Some health systems have also incorporated simulation laboratory scenarios into their code response program. Components of your pharmacist emergency response education should provide the training to adequately perform the required tasks in your pharmacist emergency response policy. The education needs to also focus on the pharmacist's role in the preparation and dosing of the medications. You can have your pharmacists either attend ACLS and augment with your own sessions focused on the key aspects for pharmacists, or you can create your own education session and have the code response leadership approve it. Initial and annual competency verification for all pharmacists participating in emergency pharmacist response should be performed and documented.

In conclusion, appropriate pharmacist emergency response programs can be designed for all pharmacy institutions. Special care should be paid to ensure all staff receives the training required to make them comfortable and knowledgeable in providing these services.

Transitions of Care

Transitions of care (TOC) describes various care actions dealing with the movement of a patient between settings within a healthcare system. Each transition creates an opportunity for clinical pharmacy involvement with a patient's medication management needs and avoiding adverse outcomes.

Getting Started with TOC

There have been recent changes to how health systems are reimbursed for patient outcomes and care. Due to penalties for hospital re-admission rates above expected levels, health systems, payors, and quality organizations are testing new models of interdisciplinary care to prevent adverse events after discharge. These changes have created new roles and opportunities for pharmacists to assist with TOC. The Agency for Healthcare Research and Quality set four goals for patients and caregivers to decrease preventable readmissions:

1. "Know what medications to take and be able to take it
2. Know the signs of danger and know whom to call if they occur
3. Have a prompt follow-up appointment and be able to keep it
4. Understand and be able to follow a self-care program"[32]

In reviewing the available resource centers and toolkits available for TOC (see **Table 12-4**), you can clearly link many of the pharmacist-provided activities to meet these four patient goals.

Transitions-of-Care Tips

- Invest time in predicting adequate resource calculations. Discharge assessments, counseling, and follow-up phone calls can require extensive pharmacist time commitments especially with high-risk patients.
- Have predetermined data collection measures and agreed-on reporting metrics and data sources.
- Partner with your information technology department to automate/integrate into your EMR as many steps of your TOC program as possible.

- Make the pharmacist a strong team member of providers, nurses, case managers, and social workers involved in all medication-related elements of safe TOC.
- Consider the following examples to use pharmacy students and technicians in your TOC services to gather patient information and support the pharmacist's activities:
  - Technicians can gather medication reconciliation data from patients and family members, call retail pharmacies for past medication histories, etc.
  - Students can assist with discharge counseling and discharge calls once trained and evaluated in performing the service.
  - Pharmacists and pharmacy students can focus on the heart failure, acute myocardial infarction, and stroke patients to prepare their discharge medication lists and prescriptions, provide discharge instructions and counseling, and coordinate with the retail pharmacies to avoid medication errors between the acute care setting and the transition to home.
  - For heart failure patients (or any other focused patient population), you can ensure they are scheduled to see a pharmacist in the ambulatory setting within 1 week after discharge. If you are not able to see them in clinic or do not have pharmacists in the clinic, consider developing a business plan to demonstrate the reduction of readmissions and improvements that a pharmacist can provide to these patient populations. Another option is to call the patients in your focused patient population to review their medications, answer questions, ensure all prescriptions were picked up, and check that medications are taken as intended and

Table 12-4. Resource Centers and Toolkits for Transitions of Care

Resource Title[a]	What You Will Find
ASHP Transitions of Care Resource Center[33]	Case studies, posters, and presentations, publications
ASHP website: Best Practices from the ASHP-APhA Medication Management in Care Transitions Initiative[34]	56-page report on eight institutional TOC program descriptions including common barriers and elements of success
Re-Engineered Discharge (RED) Toolkit[35]	Seven tools to assist a health-system team in focusing on RED-suggested, 12 mutually-reinforcing actions regarding discharge processes **Components of Project RED** ▪ Ascertain need for and obtain language assistance ▪ Make appointments for follow-up care (e.g., medical appointments, post discharge tests/labs) ▪ Plan for the follow-up of results from tests or labs that are pending at discharge ▪ Organize postdischarge outpatient services and medical equipment ▪ Identify the correct medicines and a plan for the patient to obtain them ▪ Reconcile the discharge plan with national guidelines ▪ Create a written discharge plan that the patient can understand ▪ Educate the patient about the diagnosis and medicines ▪ Review with the patient what to do if a problem arises ▪ Assess the degree of the patient's understanding of the discharge plan ▪ Expedite transmission of the discharge summary to clinicians accepting care of the patient ▪ Provide telephone reinforcement of the discharge plan
ACCP White Paper: Improving Care Transitions: Current Practice and Future Opportunities for Pharmacists[32]	▪ Challenges in care transitions ▪ Potential at risk populations ▪ TOC models ▪ Potential pharmacist roles in inpatient settings, long-term care, ambulatory care, community pharmacies, and home healthcare ▪ Recommendations for system changes to improve TOC ▪ Potential reimbursement ▪ Information technology
CMS Transitional Care Management Services[36]	Document describing new billing codes and qualifying encounters for patients discharged from inpatient hospital settings
TJC Transitions of Care Portal[37]	Links to publications on TOC, examples of TJC programs with TOC

ACCP = American College of Clinical Pharmacology; APhA = American Pharmacists Association; ASHP = American Society of Health-System Pharmacists; CMS = Centers for Medicare & Medicaid Services; RED = re-engineered discharge; TJC = The Joint Commission; TOC = transitions of care.

[a]Website addresses are available in the References at the end of the chapter.

other medications were stopped as necessary.

- In the emergency department (ED), the focus is on the acute problem, not chronic issues. However, if there is no process to address the chronic issues, then the patient will readmit to the ED and cost the healthcare system a lot more. A pharmacist or pharmacy student can review all the patients in the ED and communicate with the patient's primary care physicians (if they do not have a primary care physician, they can have case management assign one). The pharmacist or pharmacy student can fax the primary care physician his or her review recommendations and then follow up to make sure they were received and if there were any changes. This process can work for primary care physician offices that are owned by the health system or private physicians as long as you communicate with them about your TOC process and how it will benefit the patient care.

HCAHPS and Pain Management

Pain and how well it is managed is increasingly a regulatory, media, and safety focus for health systems. In 2006, CMS implemented the HCAHPS (Hospital Consumer Assessment of Healthcare Providers and Systems) Survey.[38,39] "*HCAHPS* (pronounced H-caps) is a 32-item survey instrument and data collection methodology for measuring patients' perceptions of their hospital experience."[40] How well hospital staff help patients manage their pain as measured by the comparative HCAHPS scores is a key dimension in the survey. TJC has also focused on pain management with requirements in its standards sections as well as issuing a Sentinel Event alert in 2012 regarding hospitals' safe use of opioids.[40] Each measurement area is an opportunity for pharmacists and the development of clinical services around successful pain management.

Determine your health system's HCAHPS scores to see if you are doing well or whether pain management is an area for improvement in your health system. If scores are low for the question, How often was pain well controlled?, services or measures to consider include medication-use evaluations to determine agents used, effectiveness, adverse events, and opportunities for improvements such as order sets, consultative pharmacist services, knowledge gaps, etc. If scores are low for the question, Did the staff do everything they could to help with a patient's pain?, you should consider a review of pain assessment and escalation procedures, acute or chronic pain clinical guidelines development, and adjuvant or alternative therapies available to the care team. You should review safety event trends, such as moderate sedation adverse events, opioid-related prescribing, administration, monitoring events, and use of reversal agents. Additional areas to review include current number of readmissions related to pain management and internal regulatory survey readiness tracer or rounding activities for pain management measures. These reviewed areas should provide opportunities where clinical pharmacist expertise could be best utilized to improve patient outcomes.

Service or process changes for improving HCAHPS scores and pain management include the following:

- Placing a pharmacist with an anesthesiologist in a postoperative acute pain service.[41]
- Intravenous (IV) to oral (PO) conversion assistance
- Interdisciplinary pain consult service with a pharmacist for all types of pain needs
- Palliative care services both in the inpatient setting as well as transitioning to clinic or hospice care to prevent costly readmissions
- Order-set standardization for patient-controlled analgesia, epidurals, IV, and PO opioid orders
- Clinical guideline development for different types of pain (e.g., muscle skeletal, neuropathic, non-narcotic options, multimodal adjuvant therapies)

- Diversion monitoring programs
- Educational programs on pain management topics for all interdisciplinary team members
- The institution's use of sedation assessment scales and technology
- Technology options to enhance safe use of opioids within your EMR
- Patient education materials during hospitalization and for discharge

In conclusion, most health systems will have opportunities in pain management. By using your health-system internal data, you can strategically plan where to get started and quickly show value in patient outcomes and enhanced safe medication use.

IV to PO Conversion

One commonly included piece of an institution's clinical pharmacy programs is IV to PO conversion program. This program can provide benefits in patient satisfaction, ease of administration, and cost of therapy. This strategy utilizes the fact many medications are equally effective in PO formulations. Additionally, significant cost savings may be realized using an appropriately designed IV to PO program. For each patient switched, literature has shown up to $3,300 in decreased total hospital costs.[42]

Designing the IV to PO Program

The significant possible cost savings make these programs very popular within the pharmacy community. Designing a very effective IV to PO program can be a fairly simple endeavor to implement.[43] The efforts of similar institutions are readily available sources of information on creating and implementing your program. Nearby institutions usually are eager to share their success stories. Searching the medical literature and professional societies also can yield good information to use in designing your program.

Selection of Medications for an IV to PO Program

The literature is replete with examples of medications commonly included in IV to PO programs. These medications are commonly represented by antibiotics, histamine blockers, and proton pump inhibitors. The process for selecting medications to include in an IV to PO program should be based on data specific to your institution. These data can include cost, length of stay, and medication usage rates. Involving facility-specific data will ensure you select medications with the most impact on your facility.

Basic IV to PO Program Design

Common mechanisms for designing an IV to PO program are sequential therapy (switch from an IV medication to the same PO medication), switch therapy (switch from an IV medication to an equivalent PO medication of a different class), and step-down therapy (switching from an IV medication to a similar medication of the same or a different class). Your IV to PO program can include each of these types or you can pick the most suitable type for your institution. Physician acceptance is an important component to the program you design.

A key component of any IV to PO program involves ensuring appropriate patients are selected for inclusion and exclusion. Specific inclusion and exclusion criteria must ensure those chosen for IV to PO conversion maximize the opportunity for safe and effective therapy with PO agents and minimize the potential for treatment failures or adverse events. A critical inclusion criterion is the ability to take PO medications. Other inclusion criteria include improving clinical status and the expectation that the patient will be able to comply with the PO regimen. Exclusion criteria include critically ill patients, certain disease states requiring higher than normal medication concentrations (endocarditis, central nervous system infections, osteomyelitis), and active gastrointestinal bleeding.

Another key concept to consider in the IV to PO program design is the level of autonomy given to pharmacists implementing the program. An IV to PO program may be designed to allow the pharmacist automatic conversion of selected agents in appropriate patients without communication with the medical team. This type of program requires considerable pharmacist effort but also allows for the greatest results. Pharmacy will control the program's implementation. If this program is implemented, it is crucial to include a clear method for members of the medical team to choose to opt out for individual patients.

Alternative program design options include varying levels of pharmacist autonomy and preconversion requirements for medical team authority. A drawback for these programs will be potentially decreased numbers of appropriate conversions.

IV to PO conversion programs can be implemented in a computer provided order-entry (CPOE) model or in a paper-based system. Clearly, a CPOE-based system affords greater ease of program implementation and documentation along with greater decision support (automatic notification of patient inclusion/exclusion criteria, automatic notification of appropriate medication for conversion). In a non-CPOE system, there will be increased complexity due to the data collection aspect of program initiation for each patient. Appropriate IV to PO program paper orders will smooth this process.

Scope of IV to PO Program

The relatively short list of medications to include in an IV to PO conversion program, along with the relative ease of determining patient inclusion/exclusion status, should make this a program to implement facilitywide in a 24/7 manner. This will allow your facility to avoid the many potential pitfalls accompanying an attempt to limit potentially beneficial services to only selected patients or during certain days/times.

Identify Pharmacist Roles and Responsibilities

As with any program, chance for overall success will be optimized if pharmacists are provided with a clear list of their required roles and responsibilities. Identifying common program roles and responsibilities at similar facilities is a great way to begin creating your facilities list. These pharmacist roles and responsibilities may include reviewing patient medical records, ordering the IV to PO conversion, communicating with the medical team regarding the conversion, and notifying the nursing staff of all IV to PO conversions.

Potential pharmacist activities should be appropriately detailed in a departmental policy

covering the IV to PO program. Policy topics include the following:

- Pharmacist responsibilities
  - Follow P &T committee policy covering IV to PO conversion program.
  - Review daily list of identified patients for potential inclusion.
  - Write (or enter) order for conversion in appropriate patients.
  - Inform medical/nursing team of the conversion.
  - Ensure automatic conversion order appears in the medical record.
- Inclusion/exclusion criteria
- Medications for automatic conversion

Staff Education/Competency

Appropriate and detailed staff education is necessary for any IV to PO program to function effectively. The fairly concrete nature of inclusion/exclusion criteria and a relatively small list of medications to consider will simplify required education. A key component to any staff education program for IV to PO conversions is ensuring that pharmacy leadership will support all participating pharmacists in their execution of autonomous actions within the program. This will alleviate staff members' concerns over potential repercussions for their appropriate actions.

The skills and competencies required are general pharmacist abilities all should possess. Prior to any pharmacist providing these services, you must ensure they are competent in these services. In-house experts will probably provide all required education and training for implementation of an IV to PO program. Those with infectious disease experiences are often well-suited to provide this training. Initial and annual competency verification for all pharmacists participating in IV to PO program activities should be performed and documented.

In conclusion, providing a comprehensive IV to PO conversion program offers significant institutional advantages in the areas of cost savings, decreased length of stay, ease of medication administration, and patient satisfaction. These benefits, and the need for few additional resources to implement the program, make this program an attractive option for inclusion in clinical pharmacy programs.

Participation in Team Rounding

Inclusion of pharmacists on medical teams for daily patient rounds has produced positive outcomes in the areas of decreased adverse drug events and cost savings. These programs have become increasingly common due to significant acceptance within the medical community and support from both medical and pharmacy groups.[44-46] These positive characteristics must be balanced against the significant amount of time and effort required to maintain a comprehensive pharmacist-rounding program. Undoubtedly, a pharmacist-rounding program can be a very important component to your pharmacy's educational services. Your staff's rounding activities will provide wonderful mentoring and teaching situations with the pharmacy students at your institution.

Designing the Pharmacist-Rounding Program

More than with any other clinical program, facility-specific staff characteristics must be considered before implementing a pharmacist-rounding program. Staff numbers, experience and educational background, your institution's pharmacy practice model, and staff desire for participation must be addressed. Investigating similar institutions' pharmacist-rounding programs is a great way to get some key insight into possibilities for designing your own program.

Basic Pharmacist-Rounding Program Design

Before implementing a pharmacist-rounding program, investigate how rounding is currently accomplished at your medial facility. The following, facility-specific, medical team-rounding information should be obtained prior to designing your pharmacy-rounding program:

- Number/services represented of each team
- Names/contact information for leaders of rounding services
- Style of rounding utilized by each team (walking, sit-down)

- How often teams round and times of day for rounding
- Location of rounding activities
- Usual duration of rounding activities
- Willingness to accept pharmacist addition to team

After you have compiled all the required data regarding the current state of team rounding in your facility, you can begin to create a program to include members of your pharmacist staff in these rounds. Many facilities have begun including daily interdisciplinary team rounds in their patient care activities. This is an attractive location for insertion of a pharmacist. Benefits of placing a pharmacist in this setting with a defined time/place/duration (very useful in limiting effect on pharmacy operations) offers the opportunity for pharmacist input to be immediately shared with all members of the medical team.

Additionally, the growth of hospitalist services has significantly changed the dynamic of the team-rounding services. The impact of your facility's hospitalist services should be considered as you design and implement a pharmacist-rounding program. A strong relationship exists between pharmacy and hospitalist communities. This is evidenced by the ASHP–Society of Hospital Medicine (SHM) joint statement on pharmacist collaboration.[47] Some facilities perform rounding activities in multiple locations at various times of the day. Integrating a pharmacist into these activities will prove challenging. Significant numbers of staff and large time commitments may be required. Each facility must determine how, and to what degree, to implement a pharmacist team-rounding program in multiple areas.

Invaluable clinical input should be provided even in places and situations where face-to-face rounding programs do not exist. Each pharmacist has a wealth of daily opportunities to identify, evaluate, and act on critical patient-specific pharmaceutical care opportunities by proactively reviewing all patients (or select patient types) during a shift and identifying key intervention opportunities such as antimicrobial therapy, anticoagulation, TDM, IV to PO, renal dosing, and others. Potential interventions can then be communicated to the medical team via telephone or other institutionally supported method.

Scope of a Pharmacist-Rounding Program

Creation of a pharmacist-rounding program can take many forms. Individual facilities must ensure they can continue to provide all traditionally required pharmacy services in the face of the increased requirements of the pharmacist-rounding program. An initial critical step in program design/implementation involves deciding on the scope of pharmacist-rounding services. Overriding facility-specific details (staffing numbers, practice model) may make it impossible to implement this program in all areas. Facility-specific data can assist in determining the best locations for implementing these services. These data include location of medical teaching services, patient safety data such as incident reports, and location of high-risk patient types.

Identify Pharmacist Roles and Responsibilities

It is critical to create a thorough and comprehensive list of pharmacist roles and responsibilities in rounding program including times and locations for rounding, data required for rounding activities, expected contributions, and anticipated duration of rounds. Meeting with the medical leaders of the involved rounding services is a great way to ensure you know what your customers (the rounding teams gaining pharmacist participation) are looking for in the collaboration. As with other programs, talking with similar institutions will yield much information regarding the creation of appropriate roles and responsibilities. The previously mentioned *ASHP–SHM Statement on Hospitalist-Pharmacist Collaboration* provides some examples of desired pharmacist responsibilities in a medical team collaboration[47]:

- Providing consultative services that foster appropriate, evidence-based medication selection
- Providing drug information consultation to physicians, nurses, and other clinicians
- Managing medication protocols under collaborative practice agreements.
- Assisting in the development of treatment protocols
- Monitoring therapeutic responses

- Continuously assessing and managing adverse drug reactions
- Gathering medication histories
- Reconciling medications as patients move across the continuum of hospital care
- Providing patient and caretaker education, including discharge counseling and follow-up

Evaluate/Obtain Needed Resources

Additional technology resources may be helpful in the successful implementation of a pharmacist-rounding program. Portable devices (laptops, tablets) will prove invaluable to your pharmacists who are participating in these rounds. These devices will allow immediate access to requested drug information and medical literature and (if they can access the pharmacy computer system and EMR) real-time ordering/changing of medication therapy and documentation. Provision for the performance of these operational activities while rounding will greatly limit disruptions to pharmacy workflow.

Staff Education/Competency

All pharmacists have the skills needed to effectively provide beneficial pharmacotherapy information in a team-rounding activity. Obviously, every pharmacist is not identical and each will bring a unique level of knowledge and interest to the rounding activities. Appropriate education and training will provide each pharmacist the required framework to effectively and efficiently function in this environment. This training should include refresher training on obtaining drug information and patient demographic information for the unit(s) they will be rounding. Additionally, it may be valuable to provide some training on effective communication strategy. Information of this type will assist in ensuring your staff members present their recommendations in the best possible manner. This will not only increase the acceptance rate for recommendations, but also increase the medical team members' respect of your pharmacy staff.

In conclusion, providing pharmacist-rounding services is an attractive way to include pharmacist knowledge and expertise on the front-lines of patient care. Significant cost savings and cost avoidance, along with decreased adverse drug events and increased staff job satisfaction, can be realized through these efforts. Designing and implementing a successful and comprehensive pharmacist-rounding program must involve the consideration of individual staff characteristics and pharmacy practice model.

Nutrition Support

Pharmacist leadership with interdisciplinary nutrition support services (NSS) has been a key clinical service in many health systems for years. As a new clinical coordinator, you may be asked only to assess what is in place and review any opportunities for improvement or your organization could decide to insource parenteral nutrition (PN) (nutrition provided intravenously) production as a cost savings initiative and suddenly you have to assist in linking a clinical service to an operational change.

The key guidelines to review in any NSS setup, review, or refinement are from the American Society of Parenteral and Enteral Nutrition.[48] The society's publications and updates can guide you on specific patient-population needs, how to respond to shortages, or how to order and label PN. Another resource is the Department of Pharmacy for University of Kentucky Healthcare, which shares its Adult Nutrition Support Services manual online (available at http://www.hosp.uky.edu/pharmacy/departpolicy/PH02-07.pdf.)[49,50]

Nutrition Support Tips

- Have clinical pharmacist participation on the NSS team in your institution.

- Ensure P&T committee oversight of all order sets or protocols, safety events, and clinical outcomes involved with PN support.

- Determine if your NSS will be provided via a consult with providers still entering the daily orders or via a consult/protocol service with pharmacists and/or dietitians delegated to assessment, ordering, and monitoring actions.

- Have a daily cutoff time for all PN orders to ensure enough time for internal review and production or for outsourced production and delivery back to your institution.

- Have a standardized first day PN option(s) for all populations served by your health system for orders arriving beyond the cutoff time.

- Team up with the sterile IV compounding leader(s) in your institution to ensure all NSS patient care communication and insourced/outsourced production is continually monitored for patient safety.

Summary

Implementation of new clinical programs and services within a pharmacy system is always a challenging and somewhat stressful endeavor. Benefits from the successful implementation of these programs are many and diverse. They include improved patient outcomes, increased cost savings, and heightened job satisfaction among the pharmacy staff. With appropriate preparation and planning, all hospital pharmacies can implement a selection of these programs while meeting the unique and varied requirements of their facilities.

References

1. Perez A, Doloresco F, Hoffman JM, et al. ACCP: economic evaluations of clinical pharmacy services: 2001–2005. *Pharmacotherapy.* 2009;29(1):128.

2. Bond CA, Raehl CL, Franke T. Clinical pharmacy services and hospital mortality rates. *Pharmacotherapy.* 1999;19(5):556-564.

3. Bond CA, Raehl CL. Clinical pharmacy services, pharmacy staffing, and hospital mortality rates. *Pharmacotherapy.* 2007;27(4):481-493.

4. Association for Professionals in Infection Control & Epidemiology. Antimicrobial stewardship. www.apic. org. Accessed March 30, 2015.

5. Antimicrobial stewardship. ASHP Resource Center website. http://www.leadstewardship.org/resources. php. Accessed November 30, 2014.

6. Core elements of hospital antibiotic stewardship programs. CDC website. http://www.cdc.gov/getsmart/healthcare/implementation/core-elements.html. March 4, 2014 update. Accessed November 30, 2014.

7. Society for Healthcare Epidemiology of America; Infectious Diseases Society of America; and Pediatric Infectious Diseases Society. Policy statement on antimicrobial stewardship. *Infec Control Hosp Epidemiol.* 2012;33(4):322-327.

8. Checklist for core elements of hospital antibiotic stewardship programs. CDC website. http://www.cdc.

gov/getsmart/healthcare/implementation/checklist. html. March 3, 2014 update. Accessed November 30, 2014.

9. Rybak M, Lomaestro B, Rotschafer JC, et al. Therapeutic monitoring of vancomycin in adult patients: a consensus review of the American Society of Health-System Pharmacists, The Infectious Diseases Society of America, and the Society of Infectious Diseases Pharmacists. *Am J Health-Syst Pharm.* 2009;66(1):82-98.

10. Nicolau DP, Freeman CD, Belliveau PP, et al. Experience with a once-daily aminoglycoside program administered to 2,184 adult patients. *Antimicrob Agents Chemother.* 1995;39(3):650-655.

11. Wong G, Sime FB, Lipman J, et al. How do we use therapeutic drug monitoring to improve outcomes from severe infections in critically ill patients? *BMC Infect Dis.* 2014;14:288.

12. Gross AS. Best practice in therapeutic drug monitoring. *Br J Clin Pharmacol.* 1998;46(2):95-99.

13. Kang JS, Lee MH. Overview of therapeutic drug monitoring. *Korean J Intern Med.* 2009;24(1):1-10.

14. Ghiculescu RA. Therapeutic drug monitoring: which drugs, why and how to do it. *Aust Prescr.* 2008;31:42-44.

15. Centers for Medicare & Medicaid Services. Use of high-risk medication in the elderly (DAE). http://www.cms.gov/Medicare/Medicare-Fee-for-Service-Payment/PhysicianFeedbackProgram/Downloads/Elderly-High-Risk-Medications-DAE.pdf. Accessed November 27, 2014.

16. Institute for Safe Medication Practices. List of high-alert medications in acute care settings. http://www.ismp.org/tools/highalertmedications.pdf. Accessed November 27, 2014.

17. American Society of Health-System Pharmacists. ASHP statement on the pharmacist's role in clinical pharmacokinetic monitoring. *Am J Health-Syst Pharm.* 1998;55(16):1726-1727.

18. Hermsen ED, Gross A. Pharmacokinetic training packet for pharmacists. http://www.nebraskamed.com/app_files/pdf/careers/education-programs/asp/pk_trainingpacket_2012.pdf.

19. Corbett AH, Dana WJ, Fuller MA, et al (eds). *Drug Information Handbook: A Clinically Relevant Resource for All Healthcare Professionals.* 23rd ed. Hudson, OH: Lexi-Comp; 2014.

20. Winstead K. Procedure PH-02-15 renal dosing program. University of Kentucky Pharmacy Department website. https://www.hosp.uky.edu/pharmacy/departpolicy/PH02-15.pdf. Accessed November 30, 2014.

21. ASHP Resource Center Anticoagulation website. http://www.ashp.org/menu/PracticePolicy/Resource-Centers/Anticoagulation. Accessed November 30, 2014.

22. The Joint Commission. Hospital 2014 national patient safety goals. www.tjc.org. Accessed November 30, 2014.

23. The Joint Commission. Preventing errors related to commonly used anticoagulants. www.tjc.org. Sentinel Event Alert (Sept 24, 2008;41). Accessed November 30, 2014.

24. Dager WE, Gulseth MP. Implementing anticoagulation management by pharmacists in the inpatient setting. *Am J Health-Syst Pharm.* 2007;64(10):1071-1079.

25. Mahan CE, Spyropoulos AC. ASHP therapeutic position statement on the role of pharmacotherapy in preventing venous thromboembolism in hospitalized patients. *Am J Health-Syst Pharm.* 2012;69(24):2174-2190.

26. Antithrombotic therapy and prevention of thrombosis. American College of Chest Physicians website. http://journal.publications.chestnet.org/issue.aspx?journalid=99&issueid. February 2012; 9th ed:141(2_suppl). Accessed November 30, 2014.

27. Anticoagulation Forum website. http://www.acforum.org. Accessed November 30, 2014.

28. Clotcare website. http://www.clotcare.com. Accessed November 30, 2014.

29. UW medicine pharmacy services. Anticoagulation Services website. http://depts.washington.edu/anti-coag/home/. Accessed November 30, 2014.

30. Raehl CL, Bond CA, Pitterele ME. National clinical pharmacy services study. *Pharmacotherapy.* 1998;18(2):302-326.

31. American Society of Health-System Pharmacists. ASHP guidelines: minimum standard for pharmacies in hospitals. *Am J Health-Syst Pharm.* 2013;70(18):1619-1630.

32. Hume AL, Kirwin J, Bieber HL, et al. Improving care transitions: current practice and future opportunities for pharmacists. *Pharmacotherapy.* 2012;32(11):e326-337.

33. ASHP. Transitions of care resource center. http://www.ashp.org/menu/PracticePolicy/ResourceCenters/Transitions-of-Care. Accessed November 30, 2014.

34. Best practices from the ASHP-APhA medication management in care transitions initiative. February 2013. ASHP website. http://www.ashp.org/DocLibrary/Policy/Transitions-of-Care/ASHP-APhA-Report.pdf. Accessed November 30, 2014.

35. Re-engineered discharge (RED) toolkit. May 2014. Agency for Healthcare Research and Quality website. http://www.ahrq.gov/professionals/systems/hospital/red/toolkit/index.html. Accessed November 30, 2014.

36. Transitional care management services. June 2013. ICN 908628. Centers for Medicare & Medicaid Services website. http://www.nacns.org/docs/TransCareMgmtFAQ.pdf. Accessed November 30, 2014.

37. The Joint Commission Transitions of Care Portal website. http://www.jointcommission.org/toc.aspx. Accessed November 30, 2014.

38. Centers for Medicare & Medicaid Services. HCAHPS fact sheet. August 2013. www.hcahpsonline.org. Accessed November 30, 2014.

39. Hospital Consumer Assessment of Healthcare Providers and Systems (HCAHPS). Mailed Survey. www.hcahpsonline.org. Updated March 2014. Accessed November 30, 2014.

40. The Joint Commission. Safe use of opioids: sentinel event alert. August 8, 2012, issue 49. www.joint-commission.org. Accessed November 30, 2014.

41. Fan T, Elgourt T. Pain management pharmacy service in a community hospital. *Am J Health-Syst Pharm.* 2008;65(16):1560-1565.

42. Kuti JL, Lee TN, Nightingale C, et al. Pharmaco-economics of a pharmacist managed program for automatically converting levofloxacin route from IV to oral. *Am J Health-Syst Pharm.* 2002;59(22):2209-2215.

43. Kuper K. Initiating IV to PO switches. *Pharmacy Purchasing Products.* 2011;8:2-4.

44. Kucukarsian SN, Peters M, Mlynarek M, et al. Pharmacists on rounding teams reduce preventable adverse drug events in hospital general medicine units. *Arch Intern Med.* 2003;163(17):2014-2018.

45. Patel R, Butler K, Garrett D, et al. The impact of a pharmacist's participation on hospitalists' rounds. *Hosp Pharm.* 2010;45:129-134.

46. Society of Critical Care Medicine and the American College of Clinical Pharmacy. Position paper on critical care pharmacy services. *Pharmacotherapy.* 2000;20(11):400-406.

47. Cobaugh DJ, Amin A, Bookwalter T, et al. ASHP-SHM joint statement on hospitalist-pharmacist collaboration. *Am J Health-Syst Pharm.* 2008;65(3):260-263.

48. Mirtallo J, Canada T, Johnson D, et al; Task Force for the Revision of Safe Practices for Parenteral Nutrition. Safe practices for parenteral nutrition. *JPEN J Parenter Enteral Nutr.* 2004;28(6):S39-S70.

49. Magnuson B, Flomenhoft DR, De Villiers W, et al. University of Kentucky pharmacy services adult nutrition handbook. University of Kentucky Healthcare website. http://www.hosp.uky.edu/pharmacy/nss/default.html. Accessed November 30, 2014.

50. Magnuson B, Armistead J. Procedure PH-02-07 nutrition support. University of Kentucky Pharmacy Department website. http://www.hosp.uky.edu/pharmacy/departpolicy/PH02-07.pdf. Accessed November 30, 2014.

Suggested Reading

Dager WE, Gulseth MP, Nutescu EA. *Anticoagulation Therapy: A Point-of-Care Guide.* Bethesda, MD: ASHP; 2011.

Gulseth MP. *Managing Anticoagulation Patients in the Hospital.* Bethesda, MD: ASHP; 2007.

CHAPTER 13

Evaluation and Monitoring of Clinical Interventions

Kate M. Schaafsma

KEY TERMS

Benchmarking—The practice to evaluate or check by comparison with a standard.

Clinical Intervention—An action related to the observation and treatment of patients to improve the patient's situation and to avoid an adverse drug event or prevent a medication error.

Control Plan—A written summary that describes what is needed to keep an improved process at its current level.

Cycle Time—The total time from the beginning to the end of your process, as defined by you and your customer. Cycle time includes process time, during which a unit is acted on to bring it closer to an output, and delay time, during which a unit of work is spent waiting to take the next action.

Medication-Use Process—A complex process that comprises the subprocesses of medication prescribing, order processing, dispensing, administration, and effects monitoring.

Process Owner—A person who has ultimate responsibility for the performance of a process in realizing its objectives.

Scorecard—A statistical record used to measure achievement or progress toward a particular goal. Dashboard is a graphical summary of various pieces of important information, typically used to give an overview of a business.

Stakeholder—A person with an interest or concern in something.

Takt Time—The rate at which a finished product needs to be completed to meet customer demand.

Introduction to Clinical Pharmacy Services

Clinical pharmacy services optimize medication therapy use and promote health, wellness, and disease prevention.[1] The services we provide as pharmacists are comprised of both distributional and clinical work. Our vision for pharmacists in the health-system setting is to be accountable for the **medication-use process**, ranging from distributive to clinical services and beyond. The pharmacists' expertise in managing the medication-use process provides high-quality, safe, and effective patient care. The clinical services offered across and between hospital and health-system settings vary in what is offered and in the extent of the services offered. Bond and Raehl suggest pharmacists must provide clinical pharmacy services associated with reductions in patient mortality, drug and total cost of care, and in length of stay and medication errors.[2] The services they reviewed included drug information, adverse drug reaction management, drug protocol management, participating in medical rounds, and admission drug histories. Over the past decade, a number of other clinical services have demonstrated the value of pharmacists within the healthcare setting, including pharmacist discharge medication counseling, pharmacokinetics, anticoagulation management, immunization services, and managing drug-related problems.

At your hospital or health system, pharmacists may be participating in numerous clinical pharmacy services. To achieve and sustain these services, you must identify how to maintain the pharmacists' roles to allow for agile and responsive meeting of customer or patient needs. To provide the best clinical services in your practice setting, you must provide key **clinical interventions** that improve your patients' outcomes and guide your peers to perform best practices, improve processes, and demonstrate value.

Defining a Clinical Intervention

The transition from distributional to clinical pharmacy services has manifested over several decades. Clinical pharmacy services are comprised of a variety of clinical interventions. *Clinical* is defined as relating to the observation and treatment of actual patients rather than theoretical or laboratory studies, and *intervention* is defined as actions taken to improve a situation.[2-4] Combined, *clinical intervention* is an action related to the observation and treatment of patients to improve the patients' situation. It also includes actions taken to prevent a medication error. Your primary role as a clinical coordinator is to ensure that you are optimizing the pharmacist expertise and utilizing resources to achieve the best clinical, financial, and humanistic outcome for your patients. To identify, implement, and sustain these outcomes, you must continuously monitor and evaluate performance as well as processes.

Benefits of Monitoring and Evaluating Clinical Interventions

As a clinical coordinator, you may find yourself asking why you spend so much time gathering, collating, analyzing, and stressing over clinical intervention data and results. The benefits of monitoring and evaluating clinical interventions enable you to provide high-quality and consistent services to your patients. The benefits include the following:

- Validate outcome or output based on use of resources dedicated to a service productivity and utilization of allocated resources.
- Be prepared for consultant visits and difficult economic times in which resource allocation is questioned.
- Inform key decision makers on the value proposition that pharmacy clinical interventions contribute to the patient, organization, and community.
- Involve and engage staff to the purpose and value to patients via the work performed to improve the patients' experience and avoid an adverse drug event or prevent a medication error.
- Build pharmacists' awareness of skills, knowledge, and impact in improving patients' outcomes and optimizing patient care.
- Exhibit responsibility and accountability for the medication-use processes.
- Participate in continuous process improvement activities.

- Demonstrate responsiveness, agility, and flexibility during times of growth or decline in service to meet patient demand.
- Be prepared to make educated financial and outcome-driven decisions.
- Provide visionary leadership through forecasting based on understanding the service, intervention, and impact on patient outcomes.
- Support innovative service development to optimize healthcare delivery to patients.

Your continuous efforts to monitor and evaluate clinical interventions will not only vastly improve the service you provide to patients, but it will also equip you with the data to advocate for those services across the organization—both internally within your department and externally to **stakeholders**. Efforts will also help to advance the profession and allow for excellence in practice.

Evaluation of Clinical Interventions

The evaluation of clinical interventions begins with thorough planning. The amount of preparation done to understand and evaluate the clinical intervention(s) will produce a more effective and efficient evaluation and monitoring practice. The planning process will allow you to openly discuss and uncover barriers while developing a feasible plan for gathering and compiling relevant data. Once you have the data, combining it with the experience you can offer patients allows you to not only justify the means to provide the clinical intervention, but also to build awareness of the pharmacist's value.

Define the Clinical Intervention

Begin by defining the purpose of what you want your clinical intervention to achieve. If you are having trouble clearly defining the purpose, it may help to further explore the problem that the pharmacy service or outcome would help you to achieve. By developing a full understanding of the challenge or defining the output, you will be better able to concisely define the purpose in addition to identifying a more efficient way to resolve the problem.

A useful tool to define the clinical intervention is the 5 Ws and 2Hs (5W2H) or who, what, when, where, why, how, and how much, a tool utilized in Lean methodology.[5] The 5W2H tool is a problem definition tool utilized to ensure full understanding of the problem you are attempting to resolve and the clinical intervention. To utilize the tool, you will develop questions that begin with who, what, where, when, why, how, and how much. Then, finish the questions with phrases that describe the problem your clinical intervention is attempting to resolve. Be specific and clear as you answer each situation question within the tool. Upon completion of the 5W2H tool, you will have concisely defined the purpose you strive to achieve. This tool also will help to identify potential barriers and the logistics of completing the clinical intervention. (See **Table 13-1**.)

Describe the Clinical Intervention Process

After using the 5W2H tool to clarify and define your clinical intervention, you will want to map out the process steps necessary to complete it. To best evaluate the clinical intervention, you will need to develop a thorough understanding of the process steps. Map out the clinical intervention process from beginning to end, preferably on paper with a pencil and eraser or by using sticky notes that can easily be adjusted (see **Figure 13-1**). At times, you may find that it is easier to start from the end of your process and work backward. The process steps will include actions taken both by the pharmacy team in addition to other team members. Depending on the process you are mapping out, the span of time of the processes may range anywhere from minutes, to hours, to weeks.

Based on your knowledge and the complexity of the process, and how many roles are involved, you may find that it is beneficial to develop the process map with a small group of stakeholders who know the process intimately. Developing the process map as a group confirms that all steps are accounted for. Group discussion also helps to build awareness of the various functions of different roles in the process. For example, if a prescriber and pharmacist discuss the process a pharmacist

Table 13-1. 5W2H Problem Definition Tool—Example: Completing Medication Reconciliation

Question	Clinical Intervention–Specific Question
Who?	Who does complete medication reconciliation? Who will do medication reconciliation? Who has to approve medication reconciliation?
What?	What is done to complete medication reconciliation? What is essential to complete medication reconciliation?
When?	When does medication reconciliation start? When does medication reconciliation end? When is medication reconciliation repeated?
Where?	Where does medication reconciliation get done? Where is medication reconciliation documented?
Why?	Why do we do medication reconciliation?
How?	How is medication reconciliation done?
How much?	How many medication reconciliations are completed? How much does it cost?

Source: For more information, see http://healthit.ahrq.gov/health-it-tools-and-resources/workflow-assessment-health-it-toolkit/all-workflow-tools/5w2h.

FIGURE 13-1. Process Map Development

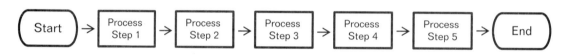

Source: See references 6 and 7 for more information.

uses to dose warfarin, the prescriber may better understand why certain documentation is necessary, or the pharmacist may identify a more efficient method for collecting the necessary information to complete the medication order assessment (see **Figure 13-2**).

Once you have the clinical intervention process map, the next step is to create a SIPOC (**s**uppliers, **i**nputs, **p**rocesses, **o**utputs, and **c**ustomers) diagram.[6,7] The SIPOC diagram aids in identifying who and what is needed to complete each process step of your clinical intervention (see **Figure 13-3**). To complete a SIPOC diagram, identify each process step in the middle column, clearly noting start and stop. Next, indicate the inputs required to complete each process step and the outputs received at the completion of each process step. The inputs and outputs of the process steps include knowledge, skills, equipment, materials, services, and information. Finally, indicate who is supplying the resources or inputs to complete each process step as well as who is the customer of the output of each process step. During the identification of suppliers and customers, confirm that your pharmacists have access to the resources needed to complete the process steps. This may be a good time to ensure that what is generated at each step as an output meets the customers' needs to allow for process continuation. In addition to visually communicating the process, you should identify inputs needed but not received as well as outputs received but not needed. Both may indicate a sign of waste that is critical in developing an efficient clinical intervention. An example of a SIPOC diagram for the medication-order process is presented in **Table 13-2**. Each process step should flow in sequential order. Customers will transition to suppliers throughout the sequence. At this point, if you have not included your team in the

FIGURE 13-2. Process Map Development—Example: Pharmacist Warfarin Dosing

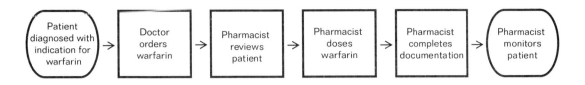

FIGURE 13-3. SIPOC Diagram

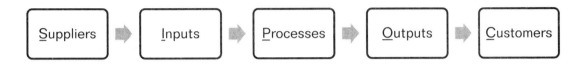

Table 13-2. SIPOC Diagram—Example: Process a Medication Order

Suppliers	Inputs	Processes	Outputs	Customers
Definition: Supplier provides inputs into a process step	*Definition:* Inputs include key materials, information, and services to functionally complete a process	*Definition:* Process steps describe the key high-level actions taken to achieve a target (each process should be a combination of a verb and a noun)	*Definition:* Outputs include key product, materials, information, or services produced from each process step	*Definition:* Customer receives outputs from each process step
Prescriber, patient	Patient assessment	Patient condition diagnosed	Patient vitals, symptoms, and signs	Patient, prescriber
Patient, prescriber	Clinical knowledge, patient presentation	Treatment decision	Treatment options	Pharmacist, nurse
Pharmacist, nurse, prescriber	Treatment options	Medication ordered	Electronic order, medication name, dose, route, frequency	Pharmacist
Pharmacist, patient	Patient chart, electronic medication order, laboratory results, clinical knowledge, evidence-based guidelines	Pharmacist review	Medication order assessment	Pharmacist
Pharmacist	Documentation of pharmacist review and verification with electronic signature	Pharmacist verification	Safe and effective medication order	Patient, nurse

Source: See references 6 and 7 for more information.

preparation of the diagram, it is a good time to have the team validate that you have correctly accounted for the information compiled.

With a process map and SIPOC diagram in hand, you have the opportunity to understand how the process steps are interrelated. Evaluate if the process can be made more effective. Verify that resources are allocated to pharmacy team members to complete the process step or clinical intervention. It is important to evaluate whether each step in the process is contributing to the end result as *value-added*, or if the step can be eliminated as *nonvalue-added* or *waste*. This allows you to make the process more efficient by eliminating steps that do not create value. The process map and SIPOC diagram are tools that will aid in the development of your data management plan as described later in this chapter. Before we start to measure, we need to define the *why* and the *value* of our clinical intervention.

Define the Value of the Clinical Intervention

In healthcare, *value* has been defined as quality provided to the patient through clinical, financial, or humanistic outcomes divided by the cost to all purchasers of care.

$$\text{Value} = \frac{\text{Quality (Clinical, Financial, Humanistic Outcomes)}}{\text{Payment (cost to all purchasers of healthcare)}}$$

Value is what you, your organization, and your decision makers deem as important.[8] To determine if your clinical intervention is going to add value, you must understand the leadership vision and your organization's strategic goals. As defined above, value is made up of quality, including the clinical, financial, and humanistic outcomes. Clinical outcomes include physiological measures, mortality, clinical events, and readmissions. For example, pharmacist participation in the patient-centered medical home managing diabetes may improve adherence to diabetes medications and decrease patient HgA1C results. Financial outcomes include direct costs, such as medication and labor costs, and indirect costs, such as attrition and administrative costs. The pharmacist's completion of a therapeutic interchange from a nonformulary to a formulary medication order may improve adherence to the drug budget and decrease medication costs. Humanistic outcomes describe the

experience, patient or provider satisfaction, patient functional status, and quality of life. A pharmacist postdischarge, comprehensive medication review with a complex patient may improve patient satisfaction with discharge information (see **Figure 13-4**).

After defining the clinical intervention and laying out the process, you will begin work to translate how your clinical intervention will add value to your patients. Create SMART (**s**pecific, **m**easurable, **a**ssignable, **r**ealistic, and **t**imely) goals or targets to define the clinical intervention's value in addition to evaluating progress.[9] A goal could be to improve patient satisfaction by 0.5% within 1 year. Although the value of completing the clinical intervention for your patients may be clear to you and pharmacists on your team, it will be necessary to justify why pharmacy resources should be dedicated to the clinical task. It is critical to continuously build awareness and develop others' understanding of the value that you have dedicated to key pharmacy resources. The more stakeholders are aware of and understand the value of the pharmacists' work, the more prepared the stakeholders will be to use pharmacists' resources to embrace accountability for the medication-use process.

Stakeholder Analysis

The completion of a stakeholder analysis is often overlooked. It may seem intuitive or duplicative in nature; however, it is a simple, yet critical, activity to evaluating each clinical intervention that defines your department's clinical services and who is invested in the process (see **Table 13-3**). A *stakeholder* is anyone with an interest or concern in something.[8] A *stakeholder analysis* is a method to identify not only the suppliers and customers of your process and/or outcome but also to identify those who may hold the key to your clinical intervention's success. Once stakeholders are identified, you will then want to understand the power, influence, or interest each stakeholder or group of stakeholders has. Finally, you will want to work to understand how to communicate and engage with your stakeholders.

Benefits of a stakeholder analysis include developing a shared purpose and understanding of the intervention's significance and its communication and the ability to predict and

FIGURE 13-4. Examples of Pharmacist-Driven Clinical Interventions to Create Value

Clinical Outcomes

- Pharmacist medication management for patients with HIV and high virologic load can improve patients' medication adherence rates and decrease the virologic load
- Pharmacist medication management for solid organ transplant patients' graft life of the transplanted organ

Financial Outcomes

- Specialty pharmacist medication management program increases specialty medication prescritpion capture to improve prescription-generated revenue
- Acute care pharmacists perform therapeutic interchanges, intravenous to oral conversions, and antimicrobial stop dates to achieve cost avoidance.

Humanistic Outcomes

- Patient medication discharge counseling improves patients' satisfaction
- Medication reconciliation completed prior to the initial patient visit improves provider satisfaction
- AIDET, LAST, and Managing Up improves patient satisfaction

AIDET = Acknowledge, Introduce, Duration, Explanation, and Thank You; HIV = human immunodeficiency virus; LAST = Listen, Apologize, Solve, Thank You.

comprehend the response when completing the intervention. The analysis demonstrates an understanding of who is directly or indirectly involved in your practicing setting. It also provides a detailed description as to who may be in support or against the clinical intervention. As you evaluate how to measure and communicate your results, it is important to understand how the key stakeholders define success. The stakeholder analysis gives you a different perspective on who the clinical intervention will impact and how to best measure and report the evaluation.

Measuring Clinical Interventions

How will you select what you will use to assess your clinical intervention? The process measures will tell you if the intervention is being completed the way you expected, and the outcome measures will tell you if the intervention is achieving your targeted goal. To identify your clinical intervention measures, use the process map and your SIPOC diagram. You may want to start at the beginning or end of the process. It is important to identify measurements that will shed light on the process, its experience, and its outcome. Once you identify potential measures, you should determine the measures' feasibility and relevance to narrow down your list. You may also want to review

the list from the stakeholder's perspective to identify a communication plan.

The outcome of your process should fix a problem or create value from the clinical, financial, or humanistic perspective. Value is determined by the organization's culture and strategic focus. You will want to determine the outcomes necessary to describe the value. Based on the type, complexity, and number of process steps to complete the intervention, you may have one or multiple outcome measures. When defining the outcome measures, you want measurements that you can assess in an accurate, complete, feasible, and relevant manner. Based on the type of outcome data evaluated, you may want to target safety, quality, efficiency, or metrics that capture each of these characteristics.

It is critical to measure the clinical intervention's outcome by determining its impact or effect on the healthcare system in terms of the patient(s), healthcare team, organization, or a population. It is also critical to assess the outcome from the clinical, financial, and humanistic perspective. Outcome measures can be determined by considering who or what the initial problem impacted that the clinical intervention was put in place to resolve. Consider the impact and value of the result to the patient in addition to other healthcare team

Table 13-3. Stakeholder Analysis Template—Example: Pharmacist Discharge Reconciliation

Stakeholder	Role	Expectations	Interest	Benefits/ Positive Influence	Concerns/ Negative Influence	Communication Plan/Manage Expectations
Jake Green, PharmD	Pharmacists	Accurate medication list and easy, feasible process	Participant, supplier of information to patient	Adds value to the patient	Documentation is time-consuming	Clinical pharmacist dashboard
Stacy Blue, MD	Provider	Discharge decision maker	Participant, supplier of information to other team members	Add value to patient, minimize postdischarge questions	Delay in discharge, added volume of clarifications	Workgroup dissemination of information, meetings, Intranet
Buck Yellow, RN	Nurses	Timely communication of discharge decision and medication orders	Participant	Provide medication education support	Delay in patient care, multiple suppliers of information	Scorecard, workgroup dissemination of information
Jim Purple	Case manager	Patient access to discharge needs	Support discharge medication patient assistance	Correct medication list	Delay in patient care, variety of practices based on patient setting	Workgroup dissemination of information
Melissa Orange	Social worker	Patient placement at time of discharge	Support discharge medication patient assistance	Correct medication list	Delay in patient care, variety of practices based on patient setting	Workgroup dissemination of information
Sean Grey	Transport	Patient transport plans before discharge decision	Patient ready status	None	Delay in patient discharge process	Intranet, general messaging
Kathy Black, RN	COO, executive suite	Efficient bed turnover and accurate medication management	Accurate, timely discharge process	Accurate medication list, TJC status	Manage labor costs	Project status report out, scorecard

MD = doctor of medicine; PharmD = doctor of pharmacy; RN = registered nurse; TJC = The Joint Commission.

members. If possible, align patient outcomes to those the prescribers use to measure value or success. The use of surrogate measures may be necessary based on the ease, efficiency, or qualitative ability to measure a specific outcome. You and your stakeholders need to clearly state and understand the description of the relation between the surrogate and the outcome. For example, for a pharmacist providing oral chemotherapy patient education and adherence, phone calls could measure patient adherence. Patient adherence would be a surrogate measure of the patient's cancer diagnosis management.

In addition to evaluating the clinical intervention's outcome, it is just as important to measure and evaluate the process itself. For each process step, you could count the times it occurs, the times it occurs successfully, and how well it is done, among many other outcomes. Each process can be evaluated in many ways; it is important to measure the process in a way that is relevant and meaningful to you and your stakeholders. If the clinical intervention achieves a regulatory or compliance standard, you must evaluate the process's completion through documentation. In the instance where measurement will indicate a process step completion, you will want to measure the quantity and quality of documentation. For example, when measuring a pharmacist's impact on the ability to de-escalate antibiotic therapy based on the use of a new laboratory technology, a process measure would be to evaluate the times pharmacists on different shifts received notification that a laboratory result was significant. In addition to measuring the process steps, each item on the SIPOC diagram and the process steps should be evaluated for measurement. The metrics describing the inputs and outputs should be intuitive and meaningful for the stakeholders to make decisions (e.g., the time it takes a pharmacist to complete medication reconciliation). Evaluate how you measure what resources go into completing the clinical intervention. Examples of common healthcare inputs include time, people, medications, and supplies. The time and volume of patients with completed medication reconciliation within one day is much more meaningful than simply the number of pharmacists who completed medication reconciliations. Often, you can use inputs and outputs as a way to measure the process steps. For example, when a pharmacist completes medication reconciliation, you may count the number of times a record is accessed to determine the volume of inputs to complete a medication history or the number of medication reconciliation notes as the number of times the activity was completed.

As the clinical coordinator, along with others supporting the clinical intervention, you must understand how and how many resources are dedicated to complete the service. You will also need to accurately speak about the quantity and quality of the work being completed. Productivity is a process measure that will be important for decision making. Specifically, productivity should relate the amount of work and time needed to complete a clinical intervention to the staff's time to do work.

To develop productivity metrics, you must consider the amount of work to be completed in addition to the resources and time needed to complete the work. Within an 8-hour day, consider how much time is available for the staff to complete the intervention in addition to the other components of the role. For example, if a pharmacist is scheduled for an 8-hour shift, 30 minutes allocated to lunch, 30 minutes allocated to breaks, the pharmacist will effectively have 7 hours of time to allocate to the intervention. This is referred to as **takt time**, which is available time for production by required units of production.[2] The organization rate of discharges is approximately 70 patients per day, and each discharge requires approximately 20 minutes of pharmacist time. This is referred to as **cycle time**. Based on the takt and cycle time, approximately 3.3 pharmacists would be required each day to complete the discharge work. The metric for completing discharge reconciliation in this example would be the number of discharges completed per day.

Productivity, if measured over time, can demonstrate improved processes, performance, and justify resource allocation. When combining the quality of the intervention with the quantity of interventions completed, the measurements can describe how the pharmacist's clinical intervention adds value to patient care. Identifying measurements that your stakeholders find valuable will also be important to obtain support of your clinical intervention. To do so, you must understand the value proposition for each stakeholder (see **Figure 13-5**).

As you get started identifying potential metrics, do not re-create the wheel if you do not have to. Seek out how others measure your clinical intervention. Not only will using similar methods to measure the intervention allow you the ease of something known and tried, but you also have access to lessons learned and the end result benefit to compare performance. Others that are completing the clinical intervention may have different processes and systems, but the benefits of learning from others successes and failures will save you time and energy. The diversity of systems and processes may result in a clinical intervention that is not measured in a way that allows

FIGURE 13-5. Value Proposition Example—Medication Reconciliation

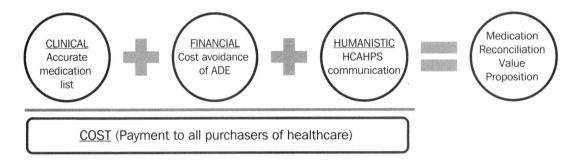

ADE = adverse drug event; HCAHPS = Hospital Consumer Assessment of Healthcare Providers and Systems; med = medication.

you to apply what other pharmacists have concluded. It is helpful to also investigate how other healthcare providers measure work or how other industries measure performance. By exploring other measurements, you may find insight into defining a metric that can be well understood and feasible to measure.

For some clinical interventions, you may want to consider relating how to measure your intervention to a similar process or outcome to one in another role or setting. When we conduct clinical trials, we often use similar laboratory values or design methods. Our literature has advanced as we share results and relate the studies by using similar metrics and methods. Similar valuations can also help when you communicate progress or results to stakeholders. If you translate your metrics into language your stakeholders understand, your message will be better understood. For example, when completing medication reconciliation across healthcare settings, a variety of healthcare roles are involved, and how each role interacts with the patients may differ. When expanding pharmacy-driven medication reconciliation to ambulatory areas, you may want to identify first how medication reconciliation was measured on the inpatient setting, then use the metrics to define a methodology for evaluating medication reconciliation in the ambulatory care setting. Another helpful comparison may be the comparison of acute care order verification processes and measurements to outpatient prescription order verification processes.

Check that you have accounted for everything to complete the necessary process steps.

It may be easy to overlook time, supplies, and equipment required to prepare for the clinical intervention. As we continue to offer more robust clinical pharmacy services, we must adjust efficiency, quality, accuracy, or all three to meet patient needs. Evaluating the resources are required to complete the clinical intervention; you will likely find that there are best practices in how to achieve the highest quality with the most efficiency. Using the results of the evaluation of inputs will help you drive service development and growth based on decisions to most effectively use resources.

Instances when new knowledge in a field is presented or new technical advances improve workflow are key times to re-evaluate inputs and productivity. A good example of the need to re-evaluate inputs and productivity is the introduction of prescriber order-entry, which replaced pharmacy staff transcribing medication orders and required adjusting evaluation of productivity for medication review and verification. The structure and framework to evaluate and track our clinical interventions must remain agile to change over time. As our equipment and resources change, our tools to measure and evaluate also must change to provide an accurate assessment.

A list of process and outcome metrics is listed in **Table 13-4**. Once you develop a complete list of process and outcome metrics, it will be critical to evaluate which metrics will be essential to report to stakeholders. Each metric should be specific, measurable, and relevant to the stakeholders of the clinical intervention. An example of a list of work measurements for

Table 13-4. Work Measurement Table

Metrics			
Input	**Process**	**Output**	**Outcome**
Volume	Cycle time	Productivity	Efficiency
Resource	Resource utilization	Volume	Effectiveness
Time	Volume	Timeliness	Readiness
Supplies	Orders/Prescriptions	Usefulness	Capacity
Equipment			Satisfaction
Cost			Cost
			Safety

Table 13-5. Clinical Intervention Measurements—Example: Code Response

Metrics			
Input	**Process**	**Output**	**Outcome**
Code medications	Median time to code response	Number of patients resuscitated	% of codes followed ACLS guidelines
Code supplies	Number of pharmacists present at each code	Completed code documentation forms	% of patient survival without admission to ICU
Pharmacist time	Median duration of code response	Used code trays and carts	Provider and nursing satisfaction
Pharmacy technician time	Number of codes	Number of medications prepared	
Code tray and cart		Number of medication questions answered	

ACLS = advanced cardiovascular life support; ICU = intensive care unit.

pharmacist participation in code response is presented in **Table 13-5**. Although you might identify 10 measures under each heading, it is important to identify the key measurements significant to the stakeholders.

Clinical Intervention Data Collection Plan

Now that you have defined the measurements to describe the success of the clinical intervention, develop a data collection plan (see **Table 13-6**). Describe each measure with a concise statement, determine the units for each measure, and indicate the measure based on what it is assessing. For each measure,

determine how the data will be collected. By defining your process and measurements, you should have a clear understanding how to obtain the data you hope to measure. Become aware and optimize the use of your system as much as possible. When possible, utilize data fields, orders, or other discrete information that can be pulled into reports to automate your data and make it easier to analyze. Most systems used in pharmacy areas now have a variety of data elements and reporting capabilities. Some systems also have the ability to track clinical interventions, documentation, and actions taken while other systems take

Table 13-6. Data Collection Plan—Medication Reconciliation

Metric	Description	Type of Metric	Where It Comes From	Who Is Responsible	How Measured	Frequency	Assumptions
Patient satisfaction	Patients' satisfaction with medication information	Outcome	Patient satisfaction survey vendor	Clinical coordinator	Percentage of top box score	Monthly	Confounders
Medication reconciliation	Patients with completed medication reconciliation	Process	Electronic health record generated report counting number of medication review button or medication list notes filed	Clinical coordinator	Number of patients with completed medication reconciliation	Monthly	Review note file type; first note indicates medication reconciliation; second note indicates patient education
Adverse drug events (ADEs)	Identified ADEs	Output	Online event reports reviewed and extracted based on type	Clinical coordinator	Number of ADEs identified, further described by type, severity, etc.	Weekly	Depends on the ADE reports

the initial data pulled into a report and query against stated assumptions such as safety, time, and cost savings to produce a ready-to-analyze report. For example, certain electronic health records (EHR) allow pharmacists to document intervention tracking tools. Based on the programing of these tools within the EHR, time, weight, and other values can be assigned to particular types or subtypes of interventions.

If you do not have the tools or reports created to automate your data collection, you will still want to develop a data collection plan. With the data collection plan, you can work with resources around your organization to create reports and pull data to facilitate the measurement of your clinical interventions. At times, it may be necessary to complete manual data collection to define the metric or to clarify what you are attempting to measure for the report builders. To successfully continuously monitor clinical interventions, gaining

access to a resource with a skillset to build and adjust reports in a timely and effective manner is critical.

Who will be responsible for obtaining, cleaning, and managing the data? Often in healthcare settings, data must be filtered and organized to accurately portray the measurement. It is best to include information used to obtain the data, such as key words or a search path, in addition to assumptions made when sorting the data. Even if this information is maintained solely by the individual managing the data, it is useful to have this documented as factors within data and processes change over time.

An individual should be assigned the responsibility to understand how and where to obtain the data to describe the measures in addition to how frequently to obtain the data. This information should include which system(s) the data are retrieved from and in what format. Assumptions when interpreting the data should be documented within the data collection plan as well. It is also vital to know if information is derived from multiple systems. Efficient access and feasibility of data collection leads to a more complete and efficient data evaluation.

Identify a specific target or goal for each measure. Based on the complexity and stability of measures, consider making the target a stretch goal, including incremental milestones to be achieved. By identifying a tolerance around the target that you wish to achieve, you will be prepared to respond appropriately. The tolerance you define will describe the variance either at one end or both ends of your measurement. Both the target and tolerance are useful in evaluating when you need to respond or investigate to manage a change to the clinical intervention. A more mature process will likely have a wide or less stringent tolerance level.

For each measure you identify as critical, construct your performance tracking plan by compiling the following list of descriptors:

- Description of the measure (e.g., percent of antimicrobial agents pharmacist verified with a stop date)

- Units of the measure (e.g., number of agents pharmacist verified with a stop date per period of time)

- Collection frequency of the measure (i.e., daily, weekly, monthly)

- Source of data (e.g., EHR report generated describing total number of antimicrobial agents pharmacist verified, number entered with and without a stop day, and period of time)

- Target for measure (e.g., target is 75% of antimicrobial agents pharmacist verified)

- Tolerance for measure (e.g., tolerance is 65% of antimicrobial agents pharmacist verified)

- Process owner (e.g., clinical coordinator)

Depending on the size and structure of your department or organization, there are probably key individuals to help you gain access to data to describe your clinical interventions. At most sites, data analysis resides with the pharmacy, quality, or informatics department. Seek these individuals out and build a relationship with them. A data analyst is someone who

can help to identify which data points can be generated from the various systems used to complete clinical interventions in addition to automating reports based on a frequency that helps support your process.

Be prepared to adjust the data collection plan as necessary. As you become more knowledgeable about the process of providing the clinical intervention, the awareness and in-depth understanding of the data management plan will improve. This may ease your data collection plan. At times, you may also find that additional data are necessary to fully evaluate the clinical intervention. It is critical to ensure that your data management plan is agile and responsive, particularly when changes are being applied to the clinical intervention. Based on the involvement and interest of your stakeholders, you may want to share your data collection plan with them to gather feedback and input on additional information they would like or perhaps weed out information they are not interested in.

A clear understanding of the measurements and how each is retrieved is critical to a complete interpretation of your data. By documenting this process of retrieval, you must understand it completely to write it out and you can use this description to communicate the plan to others. It is important to decide if the data will pushed out to the **process owner** or if you must pull it out. The frequency of monitoring depends on the volume of occurrence and timing of occurrence. Identify one individual as the process owner. This could be you, as the clinical coordinator, or a designee. The selection of a process owner provides clarity and accountability to the process stakeholders. This person is the "go-to" and is relied on to provide updates as well as to escalate concerns or the need for help when data fall outside of defined tolerance. Develop a **control plan** that maintains this information while also containing a response plan for both positive and negative results (**Table 13-7**). A control plan is a written summary about what is needed to keep an improved process at its current performance so you are prepared to speak to positive and negative results. A control plan not only enables you as the clinical coordinator to monitor performance prepared, but it also prepares you for changes that your team or environment may encounter.

Table 13-7. Control Plan—Example: Medication Reconciliation

Process (or subprocess)	Control Item (input/ output)	Control Methods	Responsibility	Target	Specification Limits (tolerance)	Response
Patient discharge medication education	% patients educated on medications at discharge	Monthly scorecard	Clinical coordinator	85%	75%	Identify reasons for not completing; discuss with pharmacists completing discharge medication reconciliation
Patient medication reconciliation	% patients with complete discharge medication reconciliation	Monthly scorecard	Clinical coordinator	95%	90%	Identify reasons for not completing; discuss with pharmacists completing discharge medication reconciliation
Prescription capture	% discharge prescription capture	Monthly scorecard	Clinical coordinator	45%	40% to 5%	If <80% or >85%, discuss with pharmacists and evaluate change
Patient satisfaction	% patient top box satisfaction	Monthly scorecard	Clinical coordinator	82%	80% to 85%	If <80% or >85%, discuss with pharmacists and evaluate change

Attributes of Clinical Intervention Measures

A final step in defining measures is to validate your data. Your evaluation is only as good as the measures you choose to assess it. Not only should you consider the significance of what you are measuring from the clinical, financial, or humanistic perspective, but you should also want to ensure the measures are specific and sensitive to the impact you are trying to make. Reflect and consider the relevance and applicability of the measure. The measure should produce reliable, valid, comprehensible, and feasible data. Specifically, it is critical to have a clearly stated numerator and denominator to provide the measure's context. The validation process should include reviewing the results with participants within the process such as a supplier or customer. When validating data, make sure the data collection process is free of bias and confusion, which can skew the results.

Data Analysis

With the completed data-obtaining process and a final (or initial) data set in hand, you can begin to analyze your data. Data analysis should answer these five questions:

1. Is your clinical intervention being completed?
2. How well is it being completed?
3. Is your clinical intervention making the impact you expected to see?
4. What barriers exist?
5. What changes could improve its outcome?

The first step to complete data analysis is determining the tool to help you to best understand the story your data are telling. Select a tool to portray your results in an accurate, intuitive, and easily understood manner. As is the case when evaluating clinical literature, the appropriate tool or test is critical to ensure accurate data assessment. The tool must be appropriate to measure the difference or impact of the clinical intervention. The selected tool should provide an answer in terms your clinical intervention was intended to resolve. Evaluate your expected outcome within the context of the problem or issue you are attempting to resolve. Depending on whether the measure is a process or outcome oriented, you may need to evaluate the data over time or compare to a control group.

On initial evaluation of the clinical intervention, you may find incomplete data if certain steps of completing the clinical intervention are not done. If the actual observation does not match your expected observation, identify where the process is breaking down. After identifying the process step in question, involve the customers, suppliers, stakeholders, and team to better understand what is causing the process breakdown.

Once you have identified that your intervention is occurring, review the clinical intervention measures and, depending on their strength, determine how well the clinical intervention is being completed. As you begin to analyze the data collected, it is important to balance the various data points in context of the work being done. It is important to ensure that your data analysis completely describes the intervention's effect based on the context of your evaluation. Often scalability and sustainability of the clinical intervention determines how well the clinical intervention is being completed or its impact. To identify where improvement needs to occur, it is crucial to differentiate the five questions mentioned above and understand what could be improved to achieve the target outcome. If you have done your due diligence to establish and conduct a sound evaluation, use the results to make a decision. Do not become paralyzed in your analysis; instead review the data analysis, discuss with your team, and take action on your results.

Data Analysis Tools

Data analytics can be intimidating, and the tools can be scary if you are not using them consistently. The key to data analysis is to select the right tool to analyze your measures to describe the assessment and demonstrate the desired result. The following are several tools commonly used to assess and interpret data:

- **Descriptive data analysis**—Provides guidance on the performance of the metrics based on the target established. Once the process to complete the clinical intervention is stable, descriptive data can easily be placed into a **scorecard** or dashboard to describe performance of the clinical intervention over time.

- **Pareto analysis**—Also known as the *80/20 rule*. A prioritization data analysis tool to determine if a discrepancy exists between various causes. It is a simple and quick tool to use. Data analysis can be completed quickly from a spreadsheet (e.g., evaluation of the volume of incomplete intravenous to oral conversions (see **Figure 13-6**).[10]

- **Histogram**—A data analysis tool that graphically represents data distribution. It can evaluate the stability and performance of a process or evaluate if the intervention is making an impact on the output or outcome of the goal. In **Figure 13-7**, a histogram is used to describe the type of and severity of adverse drug events reported.[11]

- **Control chart**—A graph used to study how a process or performance of process changes over time. Once a clinical intervention is established, a control chart can determine if the process is performing consistently, improving, or getting worse over time. In **Figure 13-8**, a control chart is used to describe average discharge prescription capture per week over 2 years. As illustrated, by adjusting the upper control limit and lower control limit, you can establish tolerance based on process changes introduced to improve the metrics performance.[12]

Monitoring of Clinical Interventions

For this chapter's purposes, the sections of evaluation and monitoring have been differenti-

FIGURE 13-6. Pareto Analysis—Incomplete Intravenous to Oral Conversions

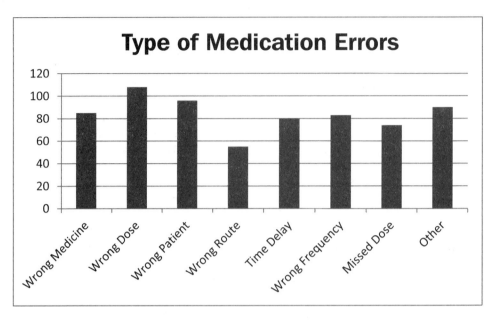

Source: See reference 10 for more information.

FIGURE 13-7. Histogram—Type of Medication Errors

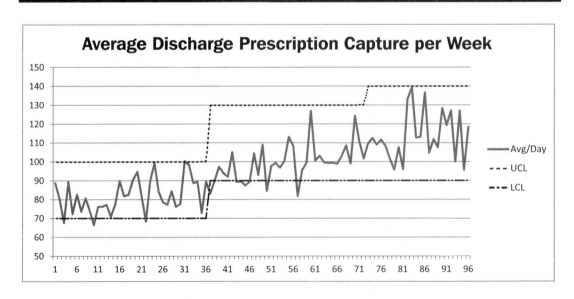

Source: See reference 11 for more information.

FIGURE 13-8. Control Chart—Average Discharge Prescription Capture per Week

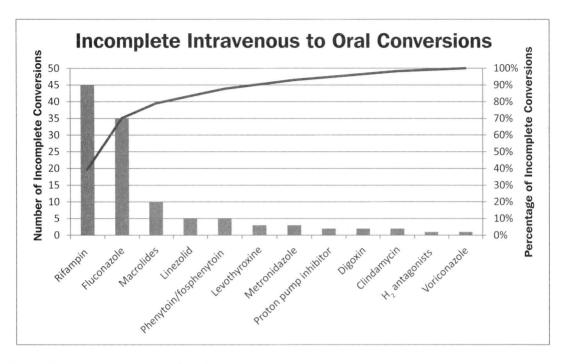

Source: See reference 12 for more information.

ated. Continuous monitoring or tracking of clinical interventions provides clarity as to what is accomplished over time. The reason to monitor performance is multipurpose ranging from justification of resource allocation to validating a process to achieve a regulatory standard. There should be a specific purpose and intent in monitoring performance of clinical interventions.

Pharmacists provide daily clinical interventions to improve patient outcomes, and as a leader, you must evaluate these interventions daily. Once you devise a plan to demonstrate the clinical intervention's value, you must continually monitor performance to ensure it is getting done and done well. Certain interventions or activities that we perform as pharmacists have immediate impact and action, such as review and verification of a medication order. For these activities, monitoring for completion may not be as important; however, for complex activities such as antimicrobial stewardship, anticoagulation management, and medication management, if performance is not monitored, performance may slowly change and you may not be aware until it is too late.

To develop a continuous monitoring plan, begin by identifying the metrics to help you maintain an understanding of the process performance and the outcome of the clinical intervention. Identify and monitor metrics that indicate a potential risk to patient safety, effectiveness, and cost. Metrics that indicate a change in performance that indicates a risk of patient safety, effectiveness, or cost, may be identified to monitor. Another important factor to consider is whether the completed clinical intervention is compliant with a regulatory standard. For example, if pharmacist review of postoperative anticoagulation management supports compliance with a value-based purchasing clinical process metric, this measurement should probably be included in the clinical intervention monitoring. If the number of monitored interventions becomes extensive and you decide to remove some, eliminate metrics that describe outdated processes or processes that perform well and consistently over time.

Each intervention that is critical to success should be included in your monitoring plan. The number of metrics for each clinical intervention should be based on the complexity and maturity of the process. The initial number of metrics may be high, so as understanding and maturity increases, strive to select two to three control measures for each clinical intervention.

When selecting control measures, you should reflect on the clinical intervention's purpose, SIPOC, baseline evaluation, and stakeholder's analysis. To determine alignment and whether a measure will be useful, ask for feedback from the pharmacists completing the intervention and the stakeholders. You may need to select different measures to report to different audiences. For example, when reporting to executive leadership on a discharge reconciliation program, you may report on total costs of readmissions avoided while for front-line staff you may want to report the number of interventions completed or medication errors caught. Consider the importance of selecting a measure that is easily understood, accurate, relevant, and easily communicated to your stakeholders, customers, and suppliers.

The completion of an evaluation and explanation of productivity with measures aligning the organization's mission and purpose help to gain executive and stakeholder support. This explanation will make it easier to tie use of valuable resources to mission and purpose. Ultimately, make sure you are measuring items that support the work you are asking pharmacists to perform, and share the data with them.

A critical reason to monitor performance of clinical interventions is to support the justification for current or additional resources for patient care. For each clinical intervention that requires a significant amount of time to complete, ensure that one metric clearly aligns with how the pharmacists' performance of completing the intervention adds value to the organization's mission. These interventions and roles should also be tied directly back to the pharmacy team member's job description and performance evaluation. By establishing alignment, monitoring performance and communicating the significance of the clinical intervention, you will support justification of current or future resources.

Process Owners

Each clinical intervention with significance for monitoring should be assigned to a process owner. A *process owner* is a person who has the responsibility for the performance of a process and has the authority to make necessary changes to achieve performance.[6] As the clinical coordinator, you may be the process owner of the pharmacist responsibilities, or you may choose to assign certain members of your team to be process owners of clinical interventions. For example, the clinical coordinator may be responsible for monitoring antibiotic stop dates, therapeutic interchanges, and discharge education while the operations coordinator may be responsible for first dose turnaround time and stock-outs. It is important that each clinical intervention or process deemed critical is assigned a process owner to monitor performance and indicate when change or adjustment is necessary to maintain or improve performance.

Scorecards or Dashboards

A scorecard or dashboard, like your car's dashboard, displays important and actionable information.[13] A scorecard or dashboard of clinical interventions can provide a quick and intuitive way to communicate performance. Its goal is to communicate strategic priorities and establish clear expectations for performance. Translating the monitoring plan into a dashboard can help to illustrate and communicate performance to a variety of audiences. The visual tool can also ensure a more complete and efficient performance assessment. The key to a user-friendly scorecard is that it can tell a story that you can post on one page or a poster. In other words, how can you link the results together to describe how the work and workload of pharmacists impact patient care? The utilization of colors to indicate positive versus negative outcomes or the extent of performance allows the viewer to interpret and respond quickly. The visual tools used to display the information on the dashboard should be easily prepared, updated, and interpreted. One benefit of using a dashboard is the ability to quickly communicate key information for stakeholders to assess and make decisions. If the dashboard becomes too complicated, too long, or too confusing, the dashboard will not be useful and should be updated.

Key components of a dashboard include a description of the measurements, guidance on expectations of performance or the target of the clinical intervention, and baseline and current performance of the clinical information. If possible, dashboards within your pharmacy system can provide immediate feedback on performance. The dashboards displayed on a daily basis often help to ensure that daily functions and tasks are completed. When this reporting functionality is not available within your system or needs to include data that cannot be generated from your pharmacy system, printing or writing out daily performance can be effective. For example, if your daily target is to complete six to eight comprehensive medication reviews, documenting on a calendar the volume completed each day can be a quick reference and way to monitor performance.

Other monitoring plans can also be found within the dashboard of a pharmacy system. Reports can be requested and built to display performance. To the extent that you are able, build dashboards that front-line workers can access as needed. Instructions for more timely change and time management can easily occur when a performance dashboard exists at the worker's finger tips.

More advanced or complex dashboards likely need to live outside of the computer system, particularly if including data from a variety of sources. The dashboards should be stored in a location that allows them to be easily retrievable and reviewed. The preparation of a dashboard should be designated to an individual or a small group of collaborating individuals. To provide for consistent, timely, and meaningful use of the dashboard, data should be updated on a consistent schedule with a particular time or frequency to be reviewed.

Various types of scorecards and dashboards, from line charts to tables to spreadsheets, can be used to illustrate performance. Key elements include clearly presenting (1) baseline measurements; (2) ongoing measurements; (3) target measurements; (4) direction of the target; and (5) information on how to interpret the measure. In **Figure 13-9**, the strategic priority scorecard indicates performance based on key strategic priorities. For example, indicating performance using green (for strong or good), yellow (for intermediate or okay), and red (for poor or bad), may help your audience to more quickly interpret results and focus on metrics that improvement is required. If you have multiple charts within a scorecard, it may be helpful to use specific colors or textures to indicate information consistently.

To Benchmark or Not to Benchmark

Benchmarking is the practice to evaluate or check by comparison with a standard.[14,15] Benchmarking allows you the opportunity to evaluate performance through comparison of internal or external data. Both help to validate and track performance as well as to establish targets. It enables the identification of best practices. The process of benchmarking can be utilized to identify gaps in care and provide insight to areas of strength and opportunities for improvement. Benchmarking combined with pharmacist clinical interventions can allow for significant improvement in caring for patients. For example, when performance data are compared with external data, differences in practices can identify opportunities to improve patient care. One example of utilizing benchmarking can be through drug utilization reviews. At a high level, comparing two similar organizations, differences in drug utilization can lead to the identification and support for the advancement in pharmacist intervention to improve patient outcomes. One example is comparing use of a high-cost agent such as thymoglobulin in transplant patients based on indication. Benchmarking can identify differences in practice that allow pharmacists to better utilize clinical evidence to review and make recommendations for medication therapy changes.

The Benefits of Internal Benchmarking

Know the variables or variations in practice, know how to use available measurements, and know how to measure change in performance over time. To complete internal benchmarking, a substantial amount of work is required to develop baseline and continuous performance monitoring. If you are using internal benchmarking to compare different areas of practice, this must also be incorporated into your data collection and analysis plan.

The Benefits of External Benchmarking

Track performance against similar practices in other settings, target opportunities for improvement, and identify best practices. To effec-

FIGURE 13-9. Clinical Intervention Monitoring Scorecard Examples

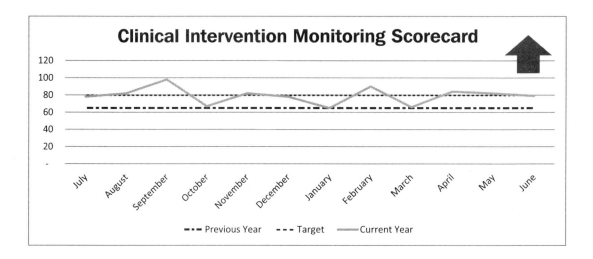

Strategic Priority Scorecard																
Strategic Priority	Goal	Baseline Performance	Target Performance	Actual Performance	JUL	AUG	SEPT	OCT	NOV	DEC	JAN	FEB	MAR	APR	MAY	JUN
Finance	Antimicrobial expense	119,098	125,000	129,083	134,000	122,000	119,000	131,000	122,000	131,000	127,000	126,000	118,000	132,000	154,000	133,000
Finance	Labor expense	650,000	660,000	654,583	651,000	651,000	652,000	655,000	665,000	649,000	653,000	655,000	655,000	654,000	655,000	660,000
Quality	Rate of C. difficile	15.0%	12.0%	12.2%	15.0%	14.2%	14.2%	13.4%	9.8%	11.1%	9.8%	11.2%	12.0%	14.5%	8.1%	13.1%
Patient satisfaction	Patient satisfaction	79.5%	81.8%	80.8%	82.0%	83.4%	78.1%	79.4%	82.1%	80.4%	79.5%	81.9%	82.4%	79.5%	81.5%	79.9%
Workplace excellence	Employee engagement	4.12	4.15	4.16	N/A	N/A	N/A	N/A	N/A	N/A	N/A	N/A	N/A	4.16	N/A	N/A

N/A = not applicable.

In Figure 13-9, the Strategic Priority Scorecard indicates performance based on key strategic priorities. Color may be applied to provide quick guidance to your audience on performance. For example, color may be applied to each box, similar to a green, yellow, and red stoplight.

tively apply external benchmarking, you must compare fundamentally similar data describing similar services. Often, the data produced or collected to make comparisons are generated from different sources, types, systems, and methodologies. For example, one organization may report comparative data from financial sources while another reports data from operational documentation. It is important to understand in detail how the data are related and compared to ensure accurate interpretation. When you compare your services and interventions to outside organizations or departments, ensure that you can identify any fundamental differences.

A key concept to apply for external benchmarking is best described by comparing "apples to apples." Data evaluation can be easier when described by both a numerator and denomi-

nator. As described above, it is important to ensure that data collection is described with similar measurements. For example, the performance can be very different if one nursing unit is compared to an entire hospital or if a surgical floor is compared to a palliative floor.

Evaluate the demographics between the two comparators; at times, you may want to consider the impact of multiple comparators that offer similar services. Variation found when completing external benchmarking should prompt questions to encourage more in-depth analysis. Although the use of an equivalent comparison group is helpful, you may still come across differentiated service or factors that account for the variation. The completion of external benchmarking is also an opportunity to collaborate with stakeholders to validate the data. The most beneficial uses of benchmarking are identifying opportunities for performance improvement, specifically around resource allocation. It can quickly create buy-in and a sense of urgency when framed with the correct data and messaging.

When benchmarking, keep in mind that numerous factors can influence large variation in processes and outcomes. Based on the practice setting, role, and intervention, benchmarking may have to consider creating options. This may lead to an inaccurate benchmarking process, if the comparison is incompletely presented. Focus on identifying value-added services. Align performance measurements with monitoring so that you do not silo yourself.

Continuous Process Improvement

A final step in establishing a process for monitoring performance is to determine how you will embed continuous process improvement. Not only is continuous process improvement one of the major reasons we track performance, but it is also required by many regulatory and accrediting bodies. Part of the rationale for establishing a target and tolerance level for each measurement, is the ability to respond with a more intensive review if the measure falls out of tolerance. In addition, by establishing the target for each clinical intervention and evaluating key indicators surrounding the clinical intervention, the monitoring plan will provide the information to determine if change or adjustment is necessary to maintain or improve performance.

A variety of factors impact clinical interventions, including regulatory changes, economic burden, disease state advancement, technology, and innovation. Whether the change is pushed or pulled, monitoring performance over time allows you as the clinical coordinator and the stakeholder group to quickly respond or prepare for a change.

Share the Results

Communicating and sharing the results from the clinical intervention's evaluation and monitoring is a critical step in providing clinical services. We communicate results for many reasons including establishing buy-in and support, explaining additional resources, and gathering feedback. We may demonstrate a need for improvement and for allocation/reallocation of resources, establish a sense of urgency around a problem, or share successes.

Regarding opportunities for improvement, the closer you present the results to key decision makers, the better chance you have of engaging them and receiving useful input to achieve your target. Consider how your audience prefers to receive information as well as how to display the results to make the interpretation clear and efficient. Translating your results using a visual tool can help your audience deduce your message much more quickly than with an in-depth explanation. Based on your audience's perspectives, it may also be necessary to produce several renditions of the visual tool to align with the stakeholder's perspective. For example, front-line staff may want more detailed information around the process that immediately impacts them while executives may want to see only high-level summaries. It is important to clearly communicate results in a comprehensible way and show how the results align and impact the particular initiative's strategic priorities or goals.

PRACTICE TIPS

1. Remember that by completing the evaluation and monitoring, you can describe what is or is not working and gather evidence that your work is benefiting the patient.

2. The results that you track may not be what you expect. By tracking the process in addition to the outcome, you can continue to improve your process and evaluation to provide clarity around the clinical intervention's value. As you learn from failures, your skill set of how to capture the value of your clinical intervention will expand and enable you to identify the metrics that will clarify the value.

3. Establish a performance standard for what and how well the clinical intervention is completed. The standard will allow you a clear intervention to measure and monitor. The more variation that exists within your intervention the more difficult it is to show success. Setting clear expectations will allow a more direct path to what will be achieved by completing the clinical intervention.

4. Within your practice of evaluation and monitoring, make it an expectation that what you evaluate and monitor will be of high utility, practicality, feasibility, accuracy, and relevance. Each of these describes data that will make your role as a clinical coordinator much easier.

5. Maintain your data through the evaluation and monitoring process. Make it a habit to routinely update the data, report out your findings, and investigate any outliers. Continue to understand and be prepared to speak to the performance of the clinical intervention, and identify new ways to improve the clinical intervention.

6. Thoroughly understand and communicate the assumptions made in the data collection process. You may find that a variety of practices utilize similar data sets throughout the organization. When you communicate your results to stakeholders, they may have various interpretations of your data; it is your job to provide them with the background and assumptions to best understand the value you present. Initial assumptions may change over time due to an update in process or change in the source of your data, so it is critical to keep these up-to-date.

7. Keep your stakeholders (the key suppliers and customers impacted) engaged through constant communication about your project's status. Identify how often your key stakeholders need to hear about your interventions. Increase their knowledge of the process and value of the clinical interventions by sharing wins as well as key barriers that they potentially could help to overcome. Watch out for unintended consequences, such as positive or negative outcomes that may impact the valuation of your clinical intervention as well as unanticipated outcomes.

Summary

The advancement of pharmacy practice and expansion of pharmacy services requires you as a leader to monitor and evaluate the value provided to patients demonstrated through clinical interventions. By defining the purpose, clarifying a problem, and elucidating through measurements and analysis what your intervention will improve, you will be on your way to creating value for the patient. At times, tracking the performance of clinical metrics is complicated and or difficult; however, by completing the actions described in this chapter to understand, describe, and communicate performance, you will simplify your process and eliminate waste from patient care. These tools will help you utilize a technique to break down the hard work already done in caring for patients and identify easy ways to track its impact. The activities described will provide the tools to monitor and evaluate your clinical intervention and to share your results with stakeholders. Remember that practice makes perfect and what gets measured matters. The time that you spend learning your process through evaluation and monitoring will enrich your knowledge about what it takes to achieve the results needed to improve patient care.

References

1. The definition of clinical pharmacy. *Pharmacotherapy.* 2008;28(6):816-817.

2. Bond CA, Raehl CL. 2006 National clinical pharmacy services survey: clinical pharmacy services, collaborative drug management, medication errors and pharmacy technology. *Pharmacotherapy.* 2008;28(1):1-13

3. Google dictionary website. http://www.google.com/defition. Accessed May 13, 2015.

4. iSix Sigma Dictionary website. http://www.isixsigma.com/dictionary/cycle-time/. Accessed May 13, 2015.

5. 5W2H tools. http://healthit.ahrq.gov/health-it-tools-and-resources/workflow-assessment-health-it-toolkit/all-workflow-tools/5w2h. 2013. Accessed May 13, 2015.

6. SIPOC tools. http://asq.org/service/body-of-knowledge/tools-sipoc. Accessed May 13, 2015.

7. SIPOC diagram. http://www.isixsigma.com/tools-templates/sipoc-copis/sipoc-diagram/. Accessed on May 13, 2015.

8. Business dictionary website. http://www.businessdictionary.com/. Accessed May 13, 2015.

9. Doran GT. There's a S.M.A.R.T. way to write management's goals and objectives. Management review. 1981;70(11):35-36.

10. ASQ: pareto chart. http://asq.org/learn-about-quality/cause-analysis-tools/overview/pareto.html. Accessed May 13, 2015.

11. ASQ: histogram analysis. http://asq.org/learn-about-quality/data-collection-analysis-tools/overview/histogram.html. Accessed May 13, 2015.

12. ASQ: control chart. http://asq.org/learn-about-quality/data-collection-analysis-tools/overview/control-chart.html. Accessed May 13, 2015.

13. Kaplan RS, Norton DP. Using the balanced scorecard as a strategic management system. *Harv Bus Rev.* 1996;74(1):75-85.

14. Rough SS, McDaniel M, Rinehart JR. Effective use of workload and productivity monitoring tools in health-system pharmacy, part 1. *Am J Health-Syst Pharm.* 2010;67(4):300-311.

15. Rough SS, McDaniel M, Rinehart JR. Effective use of workload and productivity monitoring tools in health-system pharmacy, part 2. *Am J Health-Syst Pharm.* 2010;67(5):380-388.

Suggested Reading

Abu-Ramaileh AM, Shane R, Churchill W, et al. Evaluating and classifying pharmacists' quality interventions in the emergency department. *Am J Health-Syst Pharm.* 2011;68(23):2271-2275.

Bhavnani SM. Benchmarking in health system pharmacy: current research and practical applications. *Am J Health-Syst Pharm.* 2000;57(suppl 2):S13-S20.

George ML, Rowlands D, Price M, et al. *The Lean Six Sigma Pocket Toolbook.* Chicago, IL: McGraw-Hill Books; 2005.

Goetzel RZ, Guindon AM, Turshen IJ, et al. Health and productivity management: establishing key performance measures, benchmarks, and best practices. *J Occup Envir Med.* 2001;43(1):493-504.

Ling JM, Mike LA, Rubin J, et al. Documentation of pharmacist interventions in the emergency department. *Am J Health-Syst Pharm.* 2005;62(17):1793-1797.

Murphy JE. Using benchmarking data to evaluate and support pharmacy programs in health systems. *Am J Health-Syst Pharm.* 2000; 57(suppl 2):S28-S31.

Rough SS, McDaniel M, Rinehart JR. Effective use of workload and productivity monitoring tools in health-system pharmacy, part 1. *Am J Health-Syst Pharm.* 2010;67(4):300-311.

Rough SS, McDaniel M, Rinehart JR. Effective use of workload and productivity monitoring tools in health-system pharmacy, part 2. *Am J Health-Syst Pharm.* 2010;67(5):380-388.

Touchette DR, Doloresco FD, Suda KJ, et al. Economic evaluations of clinical pharmacy services: 2006–2010. *Pharmacotherapy.* 2014;34(8):771-793.

Leadership from the Clinical Coordinator's Perspective

David Hager

KEY TERMS

Change Management—The application of a structured process to lead people to a desired future state.

DiSC Assessment—A behavior-based assessment tool that centers on four different personality traits: **d**ominance, **i**nfluence, **s**teadiness, and **c**onscientiousness.

Time Management—The ability to use one's time effectively and productively.

Time Management Matrix—Stephen Covey's approach to separating tasks into four quadrants based on importance and urgency.

WIIFM—An acronym for "**w**hat's **i**n **i**t **f**or **m**e?" This term is used to describe identifying what is important to your audience so they will act on a new idea.

The true measure of leadership is influence—nothing more, nothing less.

—John C. Maxwell

Introduction

One of an effective clinical coordinator's greatest pitfalls is the belief that you are not a leader within the organization and your position does not require you to become one. Although you may not feel a part of your former team of peers as a front-line pharmacist, you may also not feel part of the management or leadership team. The differences between titles (e.g., clinical pharmacist, coordinator, manager, and director) are both miniscule and profound. Your title has likely afforded you more responsibility, accountability, and, hopefully, compensation for the expanded role that separates you from front-line staff. However, at the same time, you likely do not have the role power associated with the title of manager or director. This may feel like a large gap at first. It is essential that coordinators realize that role power or authority does not determine an individual's measure of leadership. In truth, this should be something pharmacists are uniquely comfortable with. There are very few interactions as part of a interprofessional team where pharmacists carry the role power to independently mandate change in the face of opposition. This is known as *leading from the middle*. It would benefit you to go back and reflect on those sources of influence that made you effective in your previous roles.

How one demonstrates leadership varies based on personal strengths and personality, but the fact remains that leadership is essential to a clinical coordinator's role. Peter Drucker defined an executive as "anyone who is responsible for actions and decisions, which are meant to contribute to the performance capacity of his organization."[1] That is exactly what a coordinator does. They make and are responsible for decisions such as standardizing care for a disease state to improve outcomes, positioning residents within our staffing model to maximize our ability to care for patients, or defining the role of a new ambulatory care pharmacist to reduce readmissions. Because you are accountable to the organization for those decisions and their outcomes, you are an executive (as are many knowledge workers). The first goal of any

executive should be effectiveness, which leads to influence and leadership.

Effectiveness is a result of a set of behaviors that can be learned. As Vince Lombardi once stated, "Leaders are made, they are not born. They are made by hard effort, which is the price which all of us must pay to achieve any goal that is worthwhile." Some of the technical expertise and approaches you relied on as front-line pharmacists may no longer apply to the clinical coordinator position. In many ways, you have moved out of the clinician role and into the role of executive. Along with this new role comes the difficult task of changing longstanding habits that were essential to your past success. You probably know individuals who have tried to take on new positions as coordinators or managers who did not succeed. So what behaviors do you need to learn, and how do you use them to be effective clinical coordinators and leaders?

Time Management

The first and most important behavior to develop is the ability to manage time. Actually, **time management** is a misnomer. Time cannot, in fact, be managed as it seems to move regardless of how much effort is put into trying to stop it. Everyone has had weeks during their careers where they say, "If only I had two solid days to actually get some things done—I'd get caught up;" however, no one has actually (ethically) found a way to accomplish that. In other words, as a coordinator it is extremely unlikely that at the end of any day all your projects will be completed or problems solved. Organizations are always trying to improve medication safety, reduce cost, or improve quality. This may be in contrast to your previous roles where you took care of patients and went home without much carryover to the next day. Because you cannot complete your list of tasks by the end of any given workday, you must choose, actively or passively, each day's priorities.

Given that time is the most important resource and prioritization is the only recourse, coordinators who effectively manage their priorities are the most successful. To be effective, you must first understand what your priorities are, and then put a majority of your time into achieving them. Having resources available to spend on what matters most will help ensure positive results. If you treat everything as a priority, then nothing will get accomplished. Most effective coordinators have one or two priorities. Anything beyond this is likely to be unsustainable as you will run out of time. A coordinator newly put in charge of antimicrobial stewardship might determine that the most important priority is to lower drug spending on a singular broad-spectrum antibiotic. This is selected because lowering use of that antibiotic will result in fewer resistant organisms, fewer cases of *Clostridium difficile*, and in developing systems to encourage de-escalation of anti-biotics in the organization. If the coordinator succeeds in achieving this priority, he or she will be judged as more effective than the coordinator who tries to simultaneously start a new infectious disease residency, develop new anti-biograms, and boost surgical care improvement project core measures (and only marginally achieves all of them). All of these are valuable priorities and may improve the organization, but the coordinator who focuses and completely achieves one priority is more effective.

To determine your priorities, the first step is to decide what you want to achieve. One process to determine priorities is outlined in **Table 14-1**. Next, you should write them down and make them prominently visible in your office or workspace as a reminder. Whenever new opportunities arise, you need to ask if it aligns with previously set priorities. The difficult part of setting priorities is that it is easy to determine what to work on and much more difficult to determine what to stop doing! As a coordinator, you are invited to many meetings that have bearing on your area of expertise, and it is tempting to decline these invitations or decline to serve on a committee that no longer matches your priorities. To continue to waste your time, however, also contains risks which should be weighed.

It is valuable to separate tasks into what is deadline-driven and feels urgent and then divide them into what is critical to achieving your priorities and what are time-wasters. This has been best described by Stephen Covey's four-quadrant **time management matrix**.[2] It is important to spend as much time as possible on tasks that are nonurgent and critical to success for your priorities as this is where you will be most effective and the area that is the most sustainable. For example, developing yourself and systems that prevent

crises or improve outcomes is time well spent. Coordinators who spend most of their time on tasks that are urgent and important will eventually burn out—this amount of stress is not sustainable. Typically, this leads to more time spent on time-wasting activities, such as those that are nonurgent and nonimportant. Anyone who has spent a day running from meeting to meeting, going home 2 hours later than usual, and feeling like nothing was accomplished does not spend the evening on self-development but instead spends time surfing the Internet/social media or watching television. The final group of tasks is a trap for many coordinators: urgent and nonimportant. It is easy to believe that because you operate "from the middle," that all email, meetings, and completing all other people's requests are equally important and urgent when in fact they are not. The overall goal is to be judicious with time by avoiding time-wasting activities, managing or delegating urgent and important tasks, prioritizing critical tasks that feel urgent but are not important, and then shifting as much time as possible to personal development.

There are some practical tools to regain and refocus your time to match your priorities. First, determine how and where you currently spend your time by setting up a work sampling time study. Although intimidating, this is a 3-day process to ensure your most important resource—time—is in alignment with your goals. To capture your time appropriately, create a recording form for your week's activities (**Figure 14-1**). Make each activity as specific as possible so you can drill down to the level of detail needed to reallocate your time based on the results of the analysis. Next, use a random time generator (https://www.random.org/clock-times/) to get a list of times during your work day to sample. To get an accurate picture, have a number of observations equal to every 10 minutes in your work day (e.g., 9-hour work day equals 54 observations). A 3-day to 5-day analysis should be sufficient to categorize your time depending on the amount of variation in your work week (more days for highly variable schedules). The next step is to program these times into a phone or pager so they silently remind you throughout the day to put a tally mark on the recording form for what you are doing at that moment. Once programmed, you can reacti-

Table 14-1. How to Determine Priorities

Audience	Questions	Purpose	Methods
Yourself	■ What are my strengths? ■ What can I leverage to improve the organization? ■ What measurable results will I demonstrate if I achieve this? ■ If I am honest with myself and I don't do this, what is the risk to patients or my career? ■ What I am currently doing does not help me achieve results, but is it because of obligation or outdated priorities?	■ Never focus on your weaknesses ■ Determine where you provide the most value and spend your time on those activities and measure your impact ■ There is risk in not doing tasks, but there is also risk in trying to do everything and accomplishing nothing	■ Complete a strengths assessment (Insights, StrengthsFinder, or Myers-Briggs Type Indicator) ■ At least quarterly, schedule time on your calendar to ask yourself these questions ■ Complete a time analysis to ensure you are spending your time on these priorities
Your supervisor	■ Why did you hire me for this position? ■ What are your priorities for the year? ■ What results will your supervisor hold you to? ■ How can I help you achieve your goals?	■ Your supervisor also has a supervisor who will judge his or her success based on the performance of the team ■ It is your professional obligation to help him or her achieve those goals	■ Meet with your supervisor and ask these questions ■ If there is a change in leadership or direction in the organization, re-ask these questions to determine if the priorities are the same
Your peers	■ What are your priorities for the year? ■ What results has our supervisor held you to in the past? What have you not been held accountable to, even when on your list of year-long goals? ■ What are we doing that overlaps and how can we partner to be more efficient?	■ Your peers have insights because of their different perspectives on the organization and your supervisor ■ You want as much information as possible to make sure you are headed in the right direction	■ Schedule regular peer meetings to build relationships with peers and ensure alignment

vate the alerts whenever a major change in your career or priorities occurs to reprioritize time as needed. Each tally mark represents 10 minutes spent on the activity. You can then convert this to the percentage of time you spend on activities of value that match your priorities, which will inform you what to eliminate or delegate.

Often, there are a few items that will surprise you when you complete this type of analysis. You may find that you attend standing meetings where you do not add unique value,

are not well run, or do not match your new priorities as a clinical coordinator. In these cases, you may decide to find a replacement to attend these meetings or ask the chair to allow you to step down. You might find that you spend more time than you thought on email or other distractions. This might cause you to turn off email notifications and schedule particular times to check email. You might find that you are not using your calendar effectively when you compare what is on your calendar against your time study. If you find major discrepancies, you

FIGURE 14-1. Time Study for Coordinators Form

Activity	Number of Observations
Project work—related to priorities	
Project work—unrelated to priorities	
Meeting attendance—status meetings with manager	
Meeting attendance—leadership team meetings	
Meeting attendance—related to priorities	
Meeting attendance—unrelated to priorities	
Meeting preparation (name of meeting _____)	
Meeting preparation (name of meeting _____)	
Chairing a meeting (name of meeting _____)	
Chairing a meeting (name of meeting _____)	
Student/resident precepting	
Student/resident evaluation (e.g., PharmAcademic, school of pharmacy forms)	
Clinical questions—providers	
Clinical questions—pharmacists	
Email	
Training or in-servicing others	
Personal learning (attending conference or in-service)	
Scholarship (e.g., manuscript creation, review, IRB application, presentation writing)	
Socializing	
Personal activities	
Travel	
IRB = institutional review board.	

will want to use your calendar not just to accept meetings, but also to block off time to work on your priorities or, when politically appropriate, to decline new meetings. As you schedule your time consider the following best practices:

- Spend a maximum of 90 minutes on any one project. If you spend more, you will not be as creative or productive.

- Schedule your priorities early in the day. Then, when new business comes up during the day, you will have already worked on your priorities.

- Do not let meetings take over more than 75% of any given day. As new work arrives you will not have the flexibility to respond.

- Dedicate time every week to review your calendar. Many find Sunday nights are a good time to spend 30 minutes reviewing your calendar and priorities for the next 2 weeks and make adjustments as needed. Consider putting this as a recurring appointment on your calendar.

- Do not try to multitask. Data continue to emerge that humans, while able to rapidly move focus, cannot actually multitask. Minimizing distractions and focusing on one task at a time is far more efficient.

Taken as a whole, these steps will help you identify and spend time on your priorities and minimize the chances to be distracted.

Work–Life Balance

All professionals struggle with how to balance their work life and personal life. Many feel pulled in two directions and feel that they never fully satisfy either set of obligations. This rapidly leads to job dissatisfaction, burnout, and, in extremes, loss of relationships or loss of employment. The term *work–life balance* implies that work and your life are equivalent and can be balanced through enough effort. This is a false assumption. Although work–life balance may be a myth, there are three steps to feeling more in control of your life.

1. Determine what success looks like for where you are in your career.
2. Commit yourself to focusing on the here and now.
3. Actively build support structures in your life by giving more than you take.

Your family and your relationships should be prioritized first. Your job and your supervisor may be amazing, but in the end your family and the relationships in your life will be with you no matter what happens. The same cannot be said of any career. Additionally, balance implies that through constant juggling of obligations you can succeed in keeping both happy. However, the resulting stress of this balancing act means that you do not engage meaningfully at work or at home. So balance cannot be the goal. We must determine how to effectively live in both worlds, focusing on each, so we can maximize our professional and personal satisfaction.

An important first step is to define what success is in your life. This is a highly personal assessment that will likely evolve over your career, which may last 30 to 40 years. With more dual-career couples, many careers expand early as responsibilities grow, wane when children arrive, and expand again when the children are raised and leave the house (**Figure 14-2**).[3] Remembering this is a typical course can remind you there are seasons in everyone's life, and definitions of success may change. Early in your career, you may consider success to be recognition from peers or physician colleagues, and later it might change to spending four nights a week at home with your family, and still later in your career, it could be recognition by professional organizations or the sense you are "making a difference." New practitioners often leave residency with a deep and diverse skill set and rapidly expand their role and influence. As you prioritize family or relationships in the "valley" of the M-shaped curve, it is important that you do not fall so far down as to lose the skills that allowed you to achieve early success. Taking time to define success for yourself is essential, so you can prioritize your time to match your definition of success for where you are on your career journey.[4]

To prioritize your time, first collaborate with your partner to commit to a time to be home every day. This might seem like an impossible or daunting task, so go slowly and commit 1 day a week, then expand to 2 days, and so on. What you might find is that the work you relegated to the end of the day either never really needed to be done at that time or, even if accomplished, was not done efficiently enough to have value. You will have to focus your time to get the necessary tasks completed because you no longer have the option of staying late. To be successful, you need to commit to be home at a specific time. There will always be high-priority projects that necessitate late hours, but if you keep your family informed, the occasional late days will not be a problem. Again, many find reviewing schedules for the next 2 weeks on Sunday nights and committing to times for returning home will help establish real work–life balance.

Using Technology for Scheduling Flexibility

Technology can be a significant barrier to focusing on work at work and home at home. Managing how you interact with email, text messages, voice mail, or social media is essential to feeling fully present at work or at home. Although it can make you feel important or

FIGURE 14-2. Evolution of Priorities Through a Career

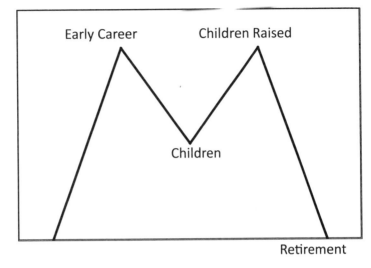

Source: Courtesy of Sara J. White, MS, FASHP.

valued by being available 24-hours-a-day, you may be propping up systems or people that are not sustainable. By sending more emails, you may actually be creating more work instead of focusing at home. Many times those communications would be more effective face to face. It will take discipline to turn your phone off or put it away when you are home. Alternatively, technology can provide flexibility by enabling you to leave earlier and then jump back into work later in the evening or early in the morning. Invest in technology at home and ask your organization for any required hardware or software to connect to your organization's networks. Use the technology to create flexibility in your schedule, without compromising your relationships, to create space for both work and home, without the work–life tradeoffs.

Building Support Networks

Finally, build support networks to support your busy life. Life and its emergencies require a network of extended family, neighbors, and friends to support you. Maintaining this personal network will give you the emotional support to endure and oftentimes can help you gain perspective on what is important. You might consider outsourcing some operational tasks such as grocery shopping, cooking, taxes,

yard work, and house cleaning so time at home can be spent more meaningfully. Alternatively, you could combine multiple needs in a single activity by working out with a friend or cooking meals for the week with your extended family. Your professional network of mentors and peers is also essential for your emotional and political support at work. One way to maintain these relationships is to schedule monthly lunches with peers and get to know them as individuals (who their spouse is, what their kid's names are, what they do outside of work, etc.). Because so much time is spent at work, it needs to be enjoyable, and developing these relationships will help make work and life more satisfying.

Change Management

The ability to create change within an organization is highly valued and an essential function of a coordinator. Hiring a coordinator is an organization's recognition that there are weaknesses to be corrected or opportunities for improvement to ensure long-term success. Most of these efforts cannot be accomplished alone and will require a team of people to change behaviors. When change is not managed, any new effort can be thwarted. Fortunately, there has been much written about how to manage change. When properly designed, change can be successfully implemented and sustained. John Kotter's *Leading Change* outlines an eight-step process to consider while engaging in any major **change management** process (**Table 14-2**).[5]

1. Establishing a Sense of Urgency

The current state is always most comfortable for everyone except for the leader. This means we have to make the current situation uncomfortable by connecting change with either collectively held values or by making *not* changing seem untenable. For example, although many organizations have pharmacist resources devoted to inpatient pharmacy services, there is increased recognition that more care and drug expense occurs in ambulatory settings. For example, you could use a few strategies to create a sense of urgency to convince pharmacists that it is essential to change the staffing model. You could have the pharmacists spend a day in the ambulatory clinic to identify the opportunities to improve care. A resident could do a pilot and measure the impact on reducing adverse drug events or

the number of interventions that are made. You could share stories from recent patient readmissions or adverse outcomes—even having the patient or their family members share their experiences. The modes of communication need to be highly relevant and personal; pep talks, presentations, and lectures are unlikely to create the sense of urgency required for large-scale changes. During this first step, you should have the end result in mind. If the improvement cannot be measured, it will not be possible to identify how close the organization is to success or if change has occurred. One organization struggling with a low-hand hygiene rate for years realized that repeating the data to the staff was not going to improve the situation.[6] The leadership team took the radical step to identify and asked patients to tell their stories about their experiences with nosocomial infections to each unit's staff members at team meetings. These very personal stories connected healthcare providers in real ways about the profound impact hand hygiene and prevention of nosocomial infection has on patients' well-being and their opinions of the medical community. Within 2 months, they had

Table 14-2. Kotter's Eight-Step Change Management Process

Eight Steps to Major Change Initiatives
1. Establishing a Sense of Urgency— Make the current state uncomfortable.
2. Creating a Coalition— Get the right mix of people with expertise, relationship, and role power to be a team.
3. Developing a Vision— Seeing the future state and developing a strategy to get there.
4. Communicating the Vision— Use all opportunities to discuss the new vision, empower the coalition to spread it.
5. Empowering Action from the Whole— Find the key new behavior(s) and remove barriers to accomplish them.
6. Generate Short-Term Wins— Plan for and share successes to leverage social pressure.
7. Never Let Up— Watch reward systems and make sure they are aligned with change, keep focused.
8. Incorporate New Approach into Culture— Ensure the environment reinforces the new approach, connect change to success.

Source: Adapted with permission from Kotter JP. Why transformation efforts fail. *Harvard Business Review.* 1995(March–April):61.

nearly 97% hand hygiene compliance across the organization.

2. Creating a Coalition

There must be a critical mass of support obtained for change to occur and be sustainable. Too often, a coalition of nonphysicians issue major policy changes that involve medical decision making or prescribing. These efforts are usually bound for failure. New ideas may begin with one or two people, but the coalition needs to grow to maintain momentum. Coordinators serving as coalition leaders must be present for change to occur, but they do not need to actively lead the change effort or be involved in the day-to-day tasks. However, they must support it by monitoring who is part of the coalition, who is already informed on the project, and who may need to be brought in. For example, when one organization tried to implement a risk evaluation and mitigation strategy alerting within the electronic health record, a physician champion was quickly identified along with administrative support from the drug information center. Identifying support and building a coalition that includes nursing, pharmacy, physician, administrative, laboratory, and informatics support is often required for large-scale change initiatives and should be planned for from the outset.

3. Developing a Vision

As the coalition grows and the need for change is increasingly accepted, a vision for the future needs to be clearly formulated. Everyone impacted by the change needs to not only understand but be able to visualize and describe succinctly what the new environment will look like. In one of the *Pharmacy Practice Model Initiative* spotlights, Spencer Hospital describes very clearly what implementing a new Tech-Check-Tech program and advanced technician position will mean to their ultimate goal of reprioritizing pharmacist time to provide clinical and cognitive services to their patients.[7] This two-paragraph description of their ideal state and a clearly defined vision overcame any hesitancy of existing technicians. They could see the value of their new roles in improving pharmacists' care for patients and what their new roles would entail. Kotter has a useful rule of thumb worth quoting, "If you can't communicate the vision to someone in five minutes or less and get a reaction that signifies both understanding and interest, you are not yet done."[5] Clearly, Spencer Hospital was able to do this.

4. Communicating the Vision

As the vision is clarified, the message of the new state needs to be communicated consistently and repeatedly. It is easy to forget the amount of communications someone might receive in a day, week, or month. If your change effort is one email out of 500 emails, agenda items, hallway discussions, and team huddle messages, your change effort is 0.002% of the communications available to those involved. This significantly increases the risk that people might not understand a change is underway or, when undercommunicated, they believe it is not really important or not a significant change. It is also essential to communicate in more than one medium. Email, although a powerful tool for quick communication, cannot be the extent of a communication plan. Unread emails, lack of comprehension, and possibility for subtle misunderstandings are all reasons to have a forum to discuss concerns to avoid outright resistance to change. Walk rounds, huddles, and town hall meetings are more likely to engage others in the change process. Continuing to hone and communicate the vision creates buy-in and increases momentum for change. Finally, ensure your actions are in alignment with the new vision. If you say an antimicrobial time-out is the correct strategy to control antibiotic use but do not lead by example, it will not take long for those who are not early adopters to create resistance to meaningful change.

5. Empowering Action from the Whole

Without having the tools available for change, no new behavior will take place. It is important to note that having the tools or processes in place becomes important at Step 5, not Step 1. All too often pharmacists are wired to think about the process before the vision and reason for change is communicated and becomes well established. Do not progress to Step 5 unless the others have already been accomplished. Just as best practices for patient education indicates not only convincing patients what to do, but also *why* they are doing it, the same needs to be true of your change efforts.

Focusing on the process is also important, and if barriers are present, all your motivation can lead to feelings of despair ("I know I have to change, but I don't have the skills for this new environment!"). These feelings will either cause entrenchment to the old way of doing things because the staff is comfortable or withdrawal from the change effort because they do not feel safe. When looking at the change, try to determine what the exact behaviors are that you will need for the new effort to be successful. Do not overestimate the abilities of those you work with, particularly interpersonal skills. For example, if you are going to implement a technician medication history and pharmacist medication reconciliation processes, you might identify the following pharmacist key behaviors: creating a complete medication list according to best practices, developing instant rapport with a patient, providing effective feedback to technicians, and making medication reconciliation recommendations to physicians. It would be easy to assume that pharmacists are already competent and confident in these areas. However, your change effort may fail if you find that the pharmacists do not give effective feedback, technicians obtain inaccurate medication histories, and a divide begins to appear between the two groups because the feedback is not delivered appropriately.

6. Generate Short-term Wins

To keep momentum up and continue to win over new people to support the cause for change, data demonstrating short-term wins need to be provided. In the absence of data, you should share stories of the project's initial successes with everyone involved in the change. Particularly for large change efforts, pilots or smaller tests of change that align with the overall goals should be completed and data collected to demonstrate the value of the new process. Without early successes people rarely sustain the initial momentum gained through visioning, and the change process will seem enormous in size and duration. Pilots make the change seem smaller, and the rewards seem more tangible. The data will also undermine those resisting the change and embolden stakeholders that they are on the right path. The pilot's short-term deadlines will sustain the sense of urgency. One example of a short-term win involved implementing a new

process for medication distribution with more frequent patient drawer exchanges so data were collected on the amount of time saved dealing with the large number of returns the old system produced. When technicians saw the work they were saving others by performing more work on the front end, the case for change was made. In fact, the original plan was to only increase the number of exchanges from daily to twice daily, but when the case for change was so strong and the data compelling, they settled on three-times-a-day cart exchanges and got technician buy-in for the new process with the smaller pilot data.

Celebrating success is also important. People need to feel that the level of excitement and urgency is high. Taking time to reward those visibly who are early adopters to the change will convince others that this change will become part of the organization's new expectations and will leverage social pressure to get others on board. The rewards can also offset the stress associated with these changes and help maintain overall morale.

7. Never Let Up

After early successes are demonstrated, you must be careful not to become a victim of your own short-term wins. Those who were early adopters can lose momentum if they feel their work is done. This lack of continued push combined with resisters who think the problem is completely solved, does not require continuing with the new ways, or was fixed so quickly it must not have been worth spending time on can lead to change efforts ceasing and allowing traditional practices to arise again.

Some practical ways of combating this regression is to continue to advance the change and align rewards with the change process. If your pilot succeeds in demonstrating a pharmacist's value in the oncology clinic reviewing oral chemotherapy orders for gynecology/oncology patients, continue to expand the role or scope of the pharmacist. Compounding the changes will send the message that you have not yet reached your vision of a pharmacist practicing as a provider in the clinic. Ask others to pilot new areas of practice or expanded roles and use the short-term wins to demonstrate to the clinic the need for continuing to adopt changes in workflows. Publicly display the results in clinic break rooms. Ensure reward systems are aligned with the change or your pilot might lead to downstream difficulties for early adopters. For example, if pharmacists are rewarded for publications in the organization's career ladder but now are expected to spend more time with patients in clinic, you might find regression to the old practices because awards are not properly aligned.

8. Incorporate New Approach into Culture

The new approach needs to become a part of the organization's mission and vision. If these new values do not become part of the employees' makeup and the urgency is lost, the gains will recede. You need to continually connect the way you do things to the organization's mission and vision. We must continue to focus on the *why*, such as "We have made investments in pharmacists in clinics because we know they improve care and lower cost" or "We continue to implement new technology to improve the safety of oncology drug preparation because we aim to be the safest hospital in the country to receive a dose of chemotherapy." These messages need to be part of the employees' work environment. Secondly, when hiring and terminating employees, as a coordinator you will often be part of interview teams and should specifically assess new hires for alignment with the key behaviors needed in the new environment. Additionally, you should use any means such as signs, bulletin boards, or meeting minutes to consistently reshare the mission, vision, and progress toward goals as these are excellent avenues to help instill the message into the department's culture.

Case Example

As part of an organization-wide initiative to lower readmission rates, all disciplines were required to train their staff members in direct, patient care roles on plain language and teach back patient education methods first studied at Boston University Medical Center as a part of Project RED (Re-Engineered Discharge). A coordinator was asked to lead this for the pharmacy department as part of their role in patient education and staff development. The Kotter change management technique was followed step-by-step as follows:

1. Sharing stories of patients who were readmitted due to poor understanding of their discharge medication instructions created a sense of urgency. Experienced pharmacists were asked to share their experiences with difficult discharge education sessions with patients where they were unsure the patient understood the instructions and how it felt when those patients were readmitted. Data on readmissions from our institution and reductions from other institutions adopting these methods were shared to create discomfort with the current state. Not only was the new technique taught, but expert faculty from the associated college of pharmacy was brought in to explain the adult education principles that underlay the techniques, so not only the "what" was taught, but the "why" as well.

2. A coalition was formed from the existing Pharmacy Patient Education Committee. This included representation from all areas of the department of those who were passionate about patient education and were seen as experts in this area by their peers. Department and senior leadership asked for the change, so they were constantly in the loop and visibly supported the effort.

3. A clear vision was provided for each patient to repeat back the vital instructions that would prevent them from being readmitted. The vision was not to complete the education as expeditiously as possible or to impress the patient with the amount of information the pharmacist knew. Monologues were discouraged, and many examples of how patients preferred to be engaged were provided.

4. This vision was shared at multiple department staff meetings, team meetings, email, a required computer-based training, pharmacy grand rounds, webinars, and training of residents and students in small groups early in the change process. As students and residents who had trained either at school or here on this new, more effective way to complete discharge education moved through the organization, they provided another voice. All patient education committee members were also asked to serve as champions of the change on each team and ensure that they personally trained each of their peers.

5. The new behaviors were clearly identified and put into a rubric. Student pharmacists

were asked to observe 10 pharmacist–patient education encounters and score them against the rubric. Barriers were identified via these observations and taken back to the patient education committee for assessment; re-education was provided as needed through one-on-one meetings or small group discussions.

6. The patient education committee gathered success stories, including testimonials from pharmacists who were early adopters about the new technique's impact on their satisfaction with the new process and their feedback from patients. Data demonstrating the rapid uptake of the new behaviors from the student pharmacist rubrics were shared, making everyone aware that other pharmacists were already engaging in these behaviors and, thereby, leveraging social pressure.

7. These stories were shared with department and organizational leadership. Data on the change's impact were presented at a state pharmacy society meeting and through the state's hospital association. Teams with the lowest readmission rates were recognized publicly.

8. The electronic medical record entries for documentation of patient education were altered to provide fewer options than use of the teach-back method. Verbal instruction was eliminated as an option sending the clear message of the organization's ongoing expectation. New alerts have been built to flag patients who failed to repeat back instructions so other resources can be found to prevent readmissions. All new hires in direct patient care roles (interns, residents, and pharmacists) are required to complete the same training undertaken at the project's outset. One continuing education presentation per year is dedicated to the topic with a new focus on barriers or challenging patients.

This project has led to significant gains for the organization and is an example of true practice change for experienced pharmacists. To ensure successful change management, it is essential to have a solid plan and follow it.

Leading from the Middle

A coordinator's first step toward better leadership is to understand that leaders are not determined by their place on the organizational chart. Although there are advantages and disadvantages as you move up an organization, believing that you become a leader once you have the title will lead to failure. As a coordinator, you are expected to lead from the middle and generate results for the organization. Managers and directors quickly learn that their titles and role power may change how interactions with their direct reports sound, but that true change in behavior or influence is not the result of that role power.[8] Role power is the weakest form of influence. Think about times you were told to do something because that is what your leader expected and how long you sustained or meaningfully engaged in that activity.

Three Sources of Influence

There are three important sources of influence within an organization: role power, expertise power, and relationship power. *Role power* is limited for coordinator with the notable exception of residents and students. Role power is merely the ability to rely on position within the organization to achieve a change in behavior. It is based on your area of accountability in your job description. Role power–facilitated changes are unlikely to be sustained and, if used too often, create dissatisfaction and burnout. This is especially true for knowledge workers like pharmacists who have far more freedom and independence in how they spend their time than other roles (e.g., production line workers) as they need to choose how much effort they put in to the new activity. Role power can be used when needed, for example, a resident who does not meet a project deadline or ignores clear directions; however, its use should be limited.

The second source of influence is *expertise power*, which relates to your mastery of a knowledge area, competency, or skill, such as being the only person in the department or organization that can run statistical tests, manipulate data, or is up-to-date in a given therapeutic area. The amount of influence is proportional to the value the organization places on that expertise. This information may help you decide what areas you want to oversee. If your organization values the legacy of their residency program, having expertise in the residency learning system or accreditation is a large source of influence. Alternatively, if the organization is trying to get into specialty pharmacy and you have mastery over rheumatoid arthritis therapy or relationships with those providers, you might also have a large source of influence. This is a powerful form of influence, particularly with peers and other clinicians. However, you must be careful not to rely too long on expertise power or it can become overbearing and demeaning to your coworkers who might feel that you are leveraging your knowledge or skills unfairly or selfishly. Additionally, expertise power can quickly evaporate if others develop those skills or if someone new is hired with those same knowledge sets. Laying a career foundation solely on expertise power can be risky.

Finally, *relationship power* is the strongest level of influence. At this level, people follow you because they want to. They understand you care about them as individuals and want them to succeed. They see the results you generate for the organization and respect you for it. They want to pay you back for the contributions you have made to their success or career. You should expand this sort of influence whenever possible.

To build relationship power takes time and attention. Human beings are not wired to have relationships with people who do not spend time with them, so maximizing the time you spend with the people you need to influence is essential. Many times coordinators believe that their projects or data are most important and therefore require the majority of their time. As much as possible, determine how you can work on those activities in ways that build relationships with others. For example, you could form a committee to look at the results of a medication-use evaluation instead of doing the analysis yourself or instead of sending an email to request information go and meet with that colleague. Take the time occasionally to have lunch or coffee with a peer. Additionally, whenever possible, give as much as you can. If someone is struggling with a project or a difficult issue, offer to assist with a last-minute interview, help review an article, or write part of a report. Internal networking is often more important early in one's career or position than traditional conceptions of networking with colleagues from across the country. Try to build relationships as broadly as possible. Focus first on building relationships with the individuals your supervisor relies on to make decisions or

the department's highest performers. Try to give as much as possible so when you need help, you will have a larger network to access. Have a mindset of helping others achieve.

There are more than enough opportunities for success and credit within an organization, and helping others succeed will not hinder your ability to get ahead. So, when you give, do not keep score or give for the purpose of getting in return; just give your time and talents to those who you need to build relationships with. Some find it valuable to schedule standing meetings with their peers to make sure they are maintaining these important relationships; just make sure it is more frequent than monthly or you will be creating another status report meeting where you will find yourself comparing notes with a colleague on projects but not building a relationship. Make sure you use your already scheduled meetings to touch base with your peers and build relationships; if you use the minutes between when people arrive and the meeting begins to frantically check email, you are missing the opportunity to grow important relationships. Also, build relationships by getting to know the other person as a whole, not just by who they are at work. This means learning about their family, interests, hobbies, pets, or whatever is important to them. You will also need to share these parts of your life as well. Connecting on this personal level provides a network of people who know you as a person and who you can rely on throughout your career.

There are some relationship-building behaviors to avoid as well. First, never sacrifice your department or your relationship with your supervisor in an attempt to further a new relationship or a project. You should accept blame if something goes wrong and never send the blame upward. Do not engage in conversations behind closed doors about how you would run the organization differently if you were in charge or how you wish your supervisor saw things as clearly as you. These are dangerous words that cannot be taken back. In the wrong hands, they can lead to disaster. Instead, if frustration arises, find a constructive way to disarm it either through spending time outside of work or filing these frustrations away for when you get promoted!

An internal network can serve as a way to influence the organization and can be a source of innovative ideas. As you meet with people and develop relationships, determine what has helped them be successful and if they have any pertinent ideas for your project. They may connect you with additional contacts outside or within other departments of your organization. You might find that there is, for example, a physician who also shares your concern about readmissions in geriatric patients who is looking for ways to combat the problem. These other innovators are those you want to identify and support. Building these relationships may help determine how to tackle the next change initiative. Another approach would be to identify individuals who helped your peers in their change efforts. These are the people you want to invest in relationally as they may be instrumental when you need support to make change happen. They can either play a role in your coalition for change or be part of the group that you make more visible by publicizing their early wins, but either way developing relationships with these smaller-scale leaders can make a huge impact on your level of influence within the organization.

The Value of Networking and the Politics of Decision Making

There will be times during your career where difficult decisions will have to be made between your recommendation and another's. These decisions can range from how to rank the resident applicants to what clinical services to cut. As coordinators, understanding the politics of these decisions can help determine what decision gets made. The first step is to understand your position. Many times an important decision will appear to be made based on the strength of data or story presented at a meeting. Sometimes seemingly large decisions will be made quickly and with little discussion, while small decisions will generate large debates. The cause for these different outcomes is less likely the skill of the person presenting the idea, but instead what took place prior to that meeting. What may actually have occurred is that the presenter met ahead of time with each of the decision makers in the room, determined the strengths and weakness of their position, adapted as needed to gather buy-in, and sealed the decision prior to the meeting. This means the actual presentation was, in essence, for show as the decision had

already been made through diligent work. This is how you want important decisions to go in your favor. To get there, it necessitates this sort of prewiring the meeting. Find informal ways to present your idea to colleagues who you know will support it and gather additional ideas for why this position is best. If everyone you go to does not like your idea, you have two options: reconsider your position or find a new way to reframe the issue. While you are determining how to prewire the meeting, consider who the decision maker is and how the decision will be made. Will it be a majority vote? Will the director or manager get to decide independently? Who does the director or manager look to when deciding the right course of action? In most of these intense situations, it will be a singular leader making the final decision, and he or she, in turn, will have two or three people to turn to for advice or take the lead. These are the people you should target prior to the meeting to explain your position and why you feel it has merit. To identify them, look for patterns when similar decisions were made as well as looking at your peers' patterns of influence. When you present your positions to the influential individuals and they do not see the issue the same way you do, try to understand what it would take for them to see it from your perspective. Getting buy-in with phrases like "if I could show you that we could implement this new service without expanding personnel budgets, would you support it?" can move the conversation past the conflict and into areas of agreement. Once you have the buy-in, the actual presentation usually is well executed because you are confident knowing the decision's outcome.

There may be times where you get outvoted, your proposal may be rejected, or another decision made. At these times, remember that your job as a professional is to accept that decision and move forward without hesitation or complaint. Compounding your loss with poor performance can lead to massive consequences, particularly if the new direction fails because of your poor performance and others remember you did not support the original idea. It is possible you could be painted as someone who attempted to sabotage the decision or were acting selfishly. This can cripple your relationships and eliminate the influence you had within the department. On the other hand, if you handle the situation with professionalism, the reverse will be true. People will remember that although you were originally against the idea, you put all your effort into the project and, yet, it still failed giving credence to your original idea and making you more credible the next time there is an important decision. Thus, a negative outcome turns into a relative win. However, there are times, for example, when the rest of the group entirely supports a proposal but there is little chance it can be stopped, so the better choice is to support the idea rather than risk being the lone dissenter. Unless the idea is unethical or you are willing to sacrifice your job for it, you should not fight moral victories when the outcome is predetermined. Because your main source of reliable influence is relationships, continuing to oppose an idea supported by those you want to maintain relationships with is detrimental and possibly harmful to your career. Making sure to monitor the political situations around us is a key skill worth developing.

Managing Up or How to Manage Your Supervisor

Managing up is commonly used to describe how someone would control the relationship between themselves and their direct superior. The problem with this concept is that you cannot actually manage your supervisor; he or she manages you. If you have ever had a resident ask you to drop everything and help them and you declined, then later your supervisor asked you to do the same and you complied, then you understand that you cannot manage up. However, you can tailor your approach to your relationship with your supervisor to maximize the chances that he or she sees you as an influential part of the team who generates positive results for the organization and wants you to continue to grow professionally.[8] Problems typically arise between supervisors and direct reports when they do not communicate effectively with each other. Communication breakdowns commonly occur when individuals do not perceive the world the same way. To become a better direct report, it would benefit you to understand your own tendencies as well as your supervisor's. Effective leaders demonstrate a high level of self-awareness and understand how their behavior affects others. They understand their reactions to other people, know how

to maximize what they do well, and know how to adapt their behavior to communicate effectively with their audience. Effective communication is the responsibility of the person sending the message.

DiSC Assessment Tool

One tool to understand our typical approach to work situations is the **DiSC** personality assessment.[10] This model has been thoroughly evaluated and found to be highly reliable and valid in multiple studies, correlating it with the 16 Personality Factor Questionnaire and the Myers-Briggs Type Indicator. The DiSC model supposes there are two dimensions that determine people's behavior. The first dimension is whether a person is typically focused on tasks or on people. The second is whether one perceives himself or herself as more powerful or less powerful than the work environment. This creates a four-sectioned model (**Figure 14-3**). There is no right or wrong DiSC profile to be a coordinator; it is simply the set of beliefs you operate from as a default. Additionally, all of us have parts of each of the four quadrants and demonstrate traits of each at any given time. Knowing how you are likely to think and how others perceive you makes this a powerful tool. Taking this or another validated assessment is recommended. In the DiSC model, it is simplified down to four primary profiles:

1. **Dominance**—You are task-focused and believe you are stronger than your environment. You are likely to be direct and decisive. You prefer to lead rather than to follow. Others perceive you as pushy, demanding, lacking empathy, blunt, and solitary. You direct others more than you ask for help, talk fast, get right to the issue, and sound authoritative. You want those around you to be direct, straightforward, and results focused. Think Donald Trump.

2. **Influence**—You are people-focused and believe you are stronger than your environment. You are likely to be animated, spontaneous, and warm. You prefer action to inaction and are excited about the next big idea. Others perceive you as attention-seeking, selfish, impulsive, disorganized, and lacking follow-through. You share stories or anecdotes frequently, talk about your emotions, are optimistic, have

FIGURE 14-3. DiSC Assessment Model

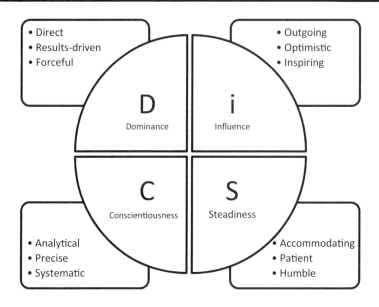

- Direct
- Results-driven
- Forceful

D Dominance

- Outgoing
- Optimistic
- Inspiring

i Influence

C Conscientiousness

S Steadiness

- Analytical
- Precise
- Systematic

- Accommodating
- Patient
- Humble

---

dynamic facial expression, laugh out loud frequently, and use humor in professional settings. You want those around you to be friendly, honest, and to recognize your contributions. Think Bill Clinton.

3. **Steadiness**—You are people-focused and believe you are weaker than your environment. You are likely to be supportive, tolerant, and collaborative. You prefer making sure everyone on the team is in harmony. Others perceive you as overly accommodating, resistant to change, and indecisive. You talk softly, make small talk frequently, listen more than you speak, are reserved with your opinions, and are embarrassed by public recognition. You want those around you to be relaxed, agreeable, cooperative, and show appreciation to each other. Think Mr. Rogers.

4. **Conscientiousness**—You are task-focused and believe you are weaker than your environment. You are likely to be ordered, meticulous, and focus on details. You prefer being right and having high standards. Others perceive you as overly critical, negative, having a tendency to overanalyze, and isolated. You are quiet, will not speak until you have all the information, are difficult to read, and have precise, detailed speech. You want those around you to minimize

socializing, give details, value accuracy, and have attention to detail. Think Bill Gates.

Once you understand your tendencies and place your supervisor in one of the four profiles, you can determine how to tailor communications with your supervisor to be most effective. For example, if your supervisor demonstrates mostly influence characteristics, he or she will respond better to interactions where you spend time on your relationship, generate new ideas (even those not vetted yet), express enthusiasm, use humor, and tell how you feel. This would make a supervisor who demonstrates mostly conscientiousness characteristics highly uncomfortable and may hurt his or her opinion of you. He or she would want a precise agenda that is not deviated from during meetings with them, plans for projects that are completely thought out, and a focus on deadlines and expectations. You have a one-in-four chance of having a supervisor that sees the world from the same perspective as you do, so leaving your effectiveness with them to chance by not adapting is dangerous. In my experience, pharmacists, whose training focuses on accuracy and precision, tend to be conscientiousness profiles. This may not be true of the management or leadership teams that might be filled with more influence and dominance types.

However, if you have ever been in a meeting full of pharmacists who are asked to brainstorm on a problem or spontaneously come up with new solutions and there is absolute silence, it is because you have a room of primarily conscientiousness-focused individuals; it is highly uncomfortable for them to come up with new ideas without all the information. They find it very difficult not to be negative about the ideas proposed by the influence types who love to speak up. You can see how using DiSC will help adapt our behavior and communications to match the default profile of your supervisor and increase your effectiveness.

Understanding Your Goals and Your Supervisor's Goals

Beyond the style of our supervisor, we need to understand our goals and our supervisor's goals. Your supervisor also probably has a supervisor who expects certain results. Prioritizing these items and delivering results will develop your relationship. You can accomplish this by asking early and often what the goals for the year are and what the supervisor sees as important. During meetings with your supervisor, watch for what he or she focuses time and attention on. You want to determine what the "what's in it for me" (**WIIFMs**) are and what motivates your supervisor to believe in your ideas. What does he or she highlight as recent successes in the department? Because there is usually much going on within an organization, what he or she highlights implies what is important. If you have the opportunity to see your supervisor at higher level meetings with other directors or members of the executive team, watch who he or she interacts with. Who are their allies? When your supervisor submits new ideas or requests to the executive team, who does he or she go to for support? Similarly, who does he or she avoid during meetings? Whose influence does he or she try to limit on the executive team? When you can identify your supervisor's allies and enemies, you can determine how to adjust your approach to these people in the future. You want to develop relationships with these allies and attempting to get on projects that align with these individuals may help you get ahead. You should let your supervisor know if you have been approached by one of the enemies to work on a project and ensure he or she agrees with your participation.

Meetings and Priorities

It is essential to know the standing meetings and reporting required of your supervisor. If your supervisor meets twice a month with his or her supervisor, you can expect that there might be changes in direction of projects based on those meetings. You should try to schedule your standing meetings after those meetings so you are not spending time on shifting priorities. Also, avoiding these same days for your meetings will likely mean fewer cancelled meetings and you will get more attention. If your supervisor has monthly reports due to their supervisor on a certain day, it will help you prioritize your time and communication. You will want to share success stories with your supervisor prior to your supervisor's reports going to their supervisor. Remember, it is your job as a direct report to make your supervisor look as good as possible and provide success stories that can be delivered up. Ensuring you have data or other measures of success is always helpful. As a success moves up an organization, it is simplified to be understandable outside of the specific discipline that created it. For example, a new pilot of pharmacist discharge medication reconciliation in the emergency department (ED) at a department level might include all the time studies of feasibility, measures of provider satisfaction with the process, all the workflow diagrams to determine how orders would be reviewed, and the details of overnight and weekend coverage. This might be simplified as a message to the organization to "using an existing full-time equivalent (FTE) ED pharmacist, a new pilot of discharge medication reconciliation reduced readmissions by 10%." Help preserve your relationship with your supervisor by never scheduling or allowing meetings to run longer than the allotted time on the days your supervisor is expected to send reports.

Never overestimate how well your supervisor understands what or how you spend your time or your relationship with him or her. As you move up an organization, your ability to keep a pulse on what everyone is doing decreases. Therefore, having a standing meeting to update progress and invest in the relationship is essential. When conducting this meeting, because it is labeled as "your time," you should expect to run the meeting. Do not show up waiting for your supervisor to provide the agenda. Of course, there will be times when he or she will decide the meeting's agenda. In those instances, to keep him or her from taking over the meeting's agenda, bring a hard copy of the meeting's agenda. Do not email the agenda prior to the meeting because your supervisor might focus more on computer tasks instead of the meeting. During your meeting with the supervisor, see what he or she pays attention to. Some people receive information most effectively in writing, so preparing a brief report might be the most productive. Others prefer verbal communication so questions can be asked in real-time. You will want to arrive on time or early for the meeting and, if possible, schedule it as early in the day as possible. Both of these signify the importance you place on your relationship and time. Early meetings, for example, allow the opportunity to replan your day to meet the new set of expectations.

Prioritizing Agenda Items and Relating Your Successes

When you create the meeting's agenda, prioritize the items. Provide updates on where you are on projects that relate to their priorities first. This is not an opportunity to impress your supervisor with a list of all the items you have worked on; this will instead make you look unfocused and busy without results. Also, share your small wins. Some consider this approach self-promotion, but when done correctly as selfless promotion, it will sell your supervisor on your accomplishments. John Maxwell's *The 360° Leader* clearly outlines the differences between self-promotion and selfless promotion (see **Table 14-3**), and you should approach sharing these successes considering these distinctions.[8]

Additionally, this is your time to ask for assistance. Good supervisors want to know how they can help their direct reports move initiatives ahead and want to know where barriers have been encountered proactively than have a long string of missed deadlines and excuses later. They might have the contacts you need to overcome resistance more efficiently than you can on your own. You should also ask how you can help them. In our desire to focus on relationships and giving as much as possible, ending conversations with "What else can I do to help you?" clearly sends the message that you are always available to them. Most times your supervisor will not take you up on this offer, but continually extending it also allows you to detect if something larger is going on. If you ask the same question at the end of the meeting every time and detect a hesitation or difference in the response tone, this can be an opportunity to probe further and see if there are new pressures, challenges, or opportunities

Table 14-3. Distinguishing Self-Promotion from Selfless Promotion

Self-Promotion	Selfless Promotion
Me first—"Here is what I accomplished."	**Others first**—"Here is what we accomplished."
Move up—"Here is how I feel I should be rewarded."	**Build up**—"Here is what I've learned from this."
Guard information—"I'll keep this to myself for the future."	**Share information**—"Here is what I learned about nursing's position on this issue."
Take credit—"Just so you know I worked on that too."	**Give credit**—"The resident did most of this; I helped on the politics side."
Hog the ball—"I'll be the project lead on that."	**Pass the ball**—"I'm happy to assist if you need me."
Dodge the ball—"That wasn't my project, the resident did that on their own."	**Share the ball**—"I know I could have done better assisting that project as well."
Manipulate others—"Here is what I would do in your situation."	**Motivate others**—Let's work together on this to get the results we are both looking for."

Source: Chart adapted from Maxwell JC, Emery S, Thompson M. *The 360° Leader.* Osprey, FL: Nelson Business; 2005. Used by permission of Thomas Nelson. www.thomasnelson.com. All rights reserved.

facing your supervisor. Knowing about these changes contemporaneously will assist you in refocusing your efforts when needed.

Finally, ask for feedback. Feedback is the key to improved performance, and good supervisors should give it consistently. This may not always be one of your supervisor's strengths or he or she may not interact with you in a way to provide feedback frequently. It is your responsibility then to pursue feedback. Recognizing that there is always room for improvement and asking for feedback opens up space in the relationship for honesty. Asking for feedback usually puts you in a more comfortable position to accept the feedback rather than receiving it unexpectedly. So, if you give a presentation to the staff and your supervisor is there, ask for feedback after the meeting; or if you present a report at your next status meeting, ask if there is anything that could make it more effective. All feedback, even delivered poorly, is valuable. It gives you insight into what your supervisor thinks about your skills and progress to date. It is always better to know what your supervisor thinks than to wait to be surprised later. Just because you do not know his or her opinion does not protect you from it later at performance appraisals or when new opportunities arise. Your only chance to adapt and to overcome these opinions is to ask for them and know them in advance.

Using Meetings to Develop Relationships

Spend time developing your relationship with your supervisor during these meetings and in day-to-day interactions. If you do not like your supervisor or if you do not respect him or her, this can be very difficult. Everyone gets to their positions in an organization because of some legitimate reason. No one is born into a management position. It is not always based on merit or accomplishments (it could be the result of great relationships!), but this does not excuse you from not finding and supporting your supervisor's strengths. Again, it is your job as a direct report to not try to "fix" your supervisor, but to maximize his or her strengths and help meet his or her goals. If your supervisor is successful, you are likely to be successful. When you focus on your supervisor's strengths instead of the weaknesses, it will help you develop the right mindset to have a successful relationship.

Another way to preserve your relationship is to ensure there are never any surprises. Getting your supervisor blindsided in a meeting or with an unexpected call of bad news or an important missed deadline can harm the trust in your relationship. Without trust, all behaviors can be interpreted in unfavorable ways. Use status meetings and other daily encounters to keep your supervisor up-to-date on projects and potential issues on the horizon. Burying bad news and hoping it will not come to light is risky. You need to be honest with your supervisor about concerns and avoid becoming a "yes man." These messages need to be delivered carefully (you should also consider the DiSC profile), but leaders need you to be honest with them about the situation's realities. It is almost always better to deliver these messages in person so tone and body language can make it clear why you are sharing this opinion. Additionally, try to bring potential solutions or options to address the concern to the in-person meeting; you want to inform and be a source of bad news with potential solutions.

As a coordinator, you must rely on relationships as our primary source of influence. The most important relationship is the one between you and your supervisor. It is your responsibility to adapt your messages to be effective and spend time engaged in meaningful discussions. You need to see your supervisor's strengths and maximize them. Be honest about problems on the horizon, be prepared to offer solutions that take those problems and turn them into opportunities, and deliver results in a way that can be easily shared up the organization.

Leading Through Difficult Times

Coordinators may be called on to lead in difficult times. There are many pressures facing healthcare, and not all organizations will adapt in time to be successful. Organizations may go through periods of difficult times such as budget cuts, layoffs, or significant reorganizations. If led appropriately, organizations can become stronger coming out of these periods of transition. To accomplish this, it will take both those in formal leadership positions as well as informal leaders, like coordinators, to work together and make the difficult decisions of how to adapt.

Understand and Define the Current State

The first step is to understand and define the current state. This is not the time to go back and try to rewrite history or to pretend no problem exists. The goal is to get everyone on the leadership team to understand the root causes of what got you to the current state and agree about where you are. A focus on short-term fixes will ultimately either lead to bad decision making or set the organization up to repeat the past failures. To truly understand the current state means encouraging dissent, getting multiple opinions on the root cause, including searching for the broadest underlying principle that led to the failure. For example, a pharmacy department forced to cut employees because of higher-than-budgeted drug costs might attribute it due to an increase in a specific, high-cost patient population (e.g., bone marrow transplant or hemophilia) and then later decide it was an exception and thus does not require a general solution. This would be an easy conclusion because it defers accountability. When a healthy leadership team digs deeper and encourages dissent, they may find that no one in the department was accountable for these costs, there were no physician relationships developed to influence prescribing, and there was a lack of financial trending or strategic planning done to anticipate and proactively deal with these changes. Once the full scope of the problem is defined, true solutions can be found.

Anticipate Possible Worse-Case Scenarios

The second step is to anticipate it will get worse. Do not try to sell a story to the staff that some quick short-term fixes will get the organization back on course. Although it is tempting to reassure employees, undershooting the amount of change needed and not capitalizing on the urgency these situations create can lead to far worse morale if a second wave of dramatic changes occurs. Crisis can create the burning platform needed for large-scale change that a department or organization might need to survive. The goal here is to make changes that, in the absence of complete information about the future, are conservative instead of trying to minimize the short-term change.

If the organization, for example, requests a 6% reduction in FTEs across all departments, leaders should prepare for more than 6% cuts in case further cuts are requested. Letting staff know you are preparing for more and are proactive about possible future changes will be more reassuring than trying to minimize the impact with small changes.

Get Staff Involved in Solutions

The next step is to get more people involved in the solutions and define the specifications of how to solve them. In crisis, it is easy for you to accept the entire burden and go into isolation. This reduces creativity and input that may be the key to better solutions. Regardless, you will need to manage the change and having a ready-made coalition to implement the changes is just as important as deciding what to do. Clearly, a crisis situation is not the time to poorly manage change. When you are meeting with this larger group to plan the change, clearly define the conditions for an acceptable solution. Clarity—viewing the broad scope of the situation—is essential when discussing how to solve the problem so the group can find meaningful solutions. For example, faced with cutting FTEs due to being over budget, the right conditions may not be simply cutting FTEs but also redeploying the remaining FTEs to prevent future budget overruns. Employing only one solution (cutting or redeploying) will not meet the conditions and will likely lead to failure.

Lead by Example

Others will look at how you react to determine what their response should be, so you need to lead by example through the crisis. If you are trying to find short-term solutions or trying to find ways to avoid the real problems facing the organization, others will likely do the same. If it is going to require large changes in responsibility and being flexible through change, show others your willingness by stepping up first to embrace new opportunities. If the organization is looking for someone willing to address the difficulties with oncology providers, for example, and you have spent your career in anticoagulation, this might be the time to use the skills you have learned as an effective coordinator to take on this new role. Your responsibility also includes remaining in emotional control. Stress will be high at work, and you will need to rely on your support network more than ever. Be clear with those around you about what you are going through and maintain professionalism at all times. Professionalism here should include keeping a positive attitude, being visible, avoiding fatalism, not taking your failures personally, and accepting responsibility for your past mistakes. You help set the tone for the organization as a respected leader, and your response to crisis may help determine the outcome.

Summary

The pharmacy coordinator is a position of leadership within a pharmacy department. Developing the leadership skills necessary to be effective will take effort and practice. This is a learned skill. Coordinators who recognize their position, manage their priorities, lead change, develop meaningful relationships, and lead by example through crisis will ultimately be successful in their current position and set themselves up for future promotions, if desired. Managers and directors utilize the skill set of a coordinator and add the human resource skills (and the role power associated with it) to further impact the organization. The skills you hone as an effective coordinator will develop and become the core of an effective executive skill set.

PRACTICE TIPS

1. Leadership is an ongoing process of improvement, and you will need to find experienced leaders to learn from. Find a mentor who can help guide you along the way. Mentors must be willing to provide feedback, advice, and strategic thinking.

2. Executive presence, which is functionally nonverbal communication tied with strong, clear verbal communication, may be more important than previously thought. This is an area to ask for feedback.

3. Become involved in professional organizations and advocacy efforts. This work will help you see the bigger picture of what is occurring in the profession and in healthcare. It will prepare you for the changes ahead and make you more flexible to change.

4. Pursue additional leadership training. Identify areas of opportunity in your leadership skill set. ASHP, state pharmacy societies, and many universities offer training in leadership specific to pharmacy or to healthcare.

5. Develop leadership and management skills jointly. Effective management skills (writing business proposals, running effective meetings, providing effective feedback) lay the groundwork for being an effective coordinator.

6. Do not neglect understanding budgets and financial spreadsheets. Knowing how your organization makes money, how payers think, and where money is spent will increase your value and help you find the right way to sell new ideas.

References

1. Drucker PF. *The Effective Executive: The Definitive Guide to Getting the Right Things Done.* 5th ed. New York, NY: HarperCollins; 2006:5.

2. Covey SA, Merrill R, Merrill RR. *First Things First: To Live, to Love, to Learn to Leave a Legacy.* New York, NY: Simon and Schuster; 1994.

3. White SJ. Integrating your personal life and career. *Am J Health-Syst Pharm.* 2007;64(4):358-360.

4. Groysberg B, Abrahams R. Manage your work, manage your life. *Harvard Bus Rev.* March 2014.

5. Kotter JP. *Leading Change.* Boston, MA: Harvard Business School Press; 1996.

6. Maxfield D, Grenny J, Lavendero R, et al. The silent treatment: why safety tools and checklists aren't enough to save lives. http://www.silenttreatment-study.com/media/Silent%20Treatment%20FAQ.pdf. Accessed April 20, 2015.

7. Mayer G. Practice spotlight: Spencer Hospital. http://www.ashpmedia.org/ppmi/docs/spotlight-Spencer_Hospital.pdf. Accessed April 20, 2015.

8. Maxwell JC, Emery S, Thompson M. *The 360° Leader.* Osprey, FL: Nelson Business; 2005.

9. Pastor J, White SJ. Managing your relationship with your boss. *Am J Health-Syst Pharm.* 2014; 71(5):369-371.

10. Cole P, Tuzinski K. *The DiSC Indra Research Report.* Hoboken, NJ: Inscape; 2003.

Suggested Reading

Allen D. *Getting Things Done: The Art of Stress-Free Productivity.* New York, NY: Penguin Books; 2002.

Auzenne M, Horstman M. Manager tools. https://www.manager-tools.com/all-podcasts?field_content_domain_tid=4. Accessed April 20, 2015.

Carnegie D. *How to Win Friends and Influence People.* New York, NY: Simon & Schuster; 2009.

Covey SR, Merrill AR, Merrill RR. *First Things First.* New York, NY: Simon & Schuster; 1994.

DePree M. *Leadership Is an Art.* New York, NY: Crown Business; 2004.

Drucker P. *The Effective Executive: The Definitive Guide to Getting the Right Things Done.* 5th ed. New York, NY: HarperBusiness Essentials; 2006.

Kotter JP. *Leading Change.* Boston, MA: Harvard Business Review Press; 2012.

Patterson K. *Influencer: The Power to Change Anything.* New York, NY: McGraw-Hill; 2007.

CHAPTER 15

Incorporating Students and Residents into It All

Antonia Zapantis

KEY TERMS

APPE—Advanced pharmacy practice experience.

Block Scheduling—The scheduling of two or more experiences at the same facility, which may or may not be consecutive.

Educational Coordinator—A person who is responsible for coordinating the training efforts of the department.

Flipped Classroom—The pharmacy students and/or residents read and prepare the materials prior to coming to the session.

Gap Rotation—A period of time where students complete a nontraditional rotation incrementally during a school break.

Instructional Objectives—Objectives that describe what the learner will be able to do after completing the activity.

IPPE—Introductory pharmacy practice experience.

Layered Learning—A team approach to patient care where the pharmacist oversees the pharmacy residents (PGY1 and PGY2), pharmacy students (APPE and IPPE), and pharmacy technicians.

Learner— A pharmacy student, pharmacy resident, or pharmacy fellow.

Learning Objectives—Objectives that incorporate the knowledge and skills the learner is expected to develop.

PGY1—Postgraduate year 1.

PGY2—Postgraduate year 2.

Introduction

With all of the stressors and demands placed on clinical coordinators, more needs to be done with fewer resources. One strategy to accomplish this goal is maximizing student and residency experiences. Accreditation Council of Pharmacy Education (ACPE) standards require pharmacy students to be practice-ready on graduation.[1] Schools of pharmacy rely on pharmacy practice experiences to provide students with real-world experiences to cement their education and prepare them for a pharmacy career. At the same time, the profession depends on postgraduate training experiences to enhance general competencies in managing medication-use systems and supporting optimal medication-therapy outcomes.[2] If the right approach is taken, this can be a symbiotic relationship between the clinical coordinator and the **learner**. This chapter focuses on using learners as a resource to meet the demands of contemporary pharmacy practice.

Why Include Learners into The Mix?

Below are recommendations from the ASHP Pharmacy Practice Model Summit:

- All patients should receive care from a pharmacist.
- Pharmacists must be responsible for patients' medication-related outcomes.
- Pharmacy departments should reallocate resources to devote more time toward medication management services.[3]

In the ASHP position statement, ASHP stresses the importance of student and resident roles in new pharmacy practice models. There is a myriad of evidence in the pharmacy literature of using pharmacy extenders to provide patient care services, especially in heavy workload, protocol-driven areas.[4-7] Pharmacy departments can leverage this training to augment, expand, and start many pharmacy services. Opportunities include transitions of care, medication history-taking, medication reconciliation, discharge instruction preparation, and discharge counseling. The first step, however, is to perform a needs assessment of your depart-

ment to see which services you can expand or develop with the use of learners as resources (see Chapter 11: Implementing New Clinical Pharmacy Programs—Step-by-Step for more discussion of needs assessment). Ensuring that there is pharmacy and organizational support is another important consideration, as these learning activities will take resources and time from your other responsibilities. **Table 15-1** lists the type of programs that can be implemented, and **Table 15-2** lists some of the benefits that can be achieved from the added services learners can provide your organization.

Getting Started

Logistics

In most organizations, the clinical coordinator, or **educational coordinator**, is responsible for managing the training efforts of the department. Once the decision has been made to use learners for assistance in providing pharmacy services, a few logistical issues will need to be addressed. Once the *why* has been addressed, attention needs to be given to *how* students will be incorporated and *who* will oversee the training, and, therefore, the pharmacy extenders. Like all new services, there will be early adopters and some pharmacists who will need encouragement to participate (see Chapter 14: Leadership from the Clinical Coordinator's Perspective). To ease this transition, your pharmacists need to know what is expected of them as preceptors. You, as the clinical coordinator, must make sure they understand your expectations, the residency

---

Table 15-1. Types of Services

Examples of Types of Services
■ Parenteral to oral (IV to PO)
■ Renal dose adjustment
■ Antimicrobial stewardship
■ Pharmacy consults
■ Anticoagulation
■ Pharmacokinetic
■ Direct patient care
■ Admission histories
■ Targeted disease state education
■ Discharge counseling
■ Bedside discharge delivery

Table 15-2. Byproducts of Pharmacy Extenders

Preceptors	Learners
▪ Expanding current pharmacy services ▪ Piloting new services ▪ Data collection ▪ Strengthens lifelong-learning skills ▪ Availability of student funds for preceptor development opportunities (e.g., conference fees, travel)	▪ Preparing for real-world pharmacy ▪ Preliminary training of potential new hires ▪ Providing opportunity to test drive career options

director's expectations (if different), the college of pharmacy's expectations, and ultimately, the learners' expectations. Additionally, pharmacist preceptors must have training and preceptor development to ensure that they have adequate skills to oversee the learner, as well as the tools to formally and informally assess learners for the purpose of providing feedback for improvement. The *Pharmacist Letter* has a webinar preceptor development series, and the *American Journal of Health-System Pharmacy* has a journal series that would greatly benefit your preceptors in their development. Additionally, *Hospital Pharmacy* has a journal club series to assist preceptors in guiding students through article reviews, and the ASHP website has resources to assist pharmacists that formally or informally precept students. You can schedule monthly seminars for your staff to view the webinars or have a journal club on the articles.

You will need to decide the optimal number of total learners (i.e., students and residents) on site for a given period of time (e.g., month, rotation, block, or year), taking into consideration the number of prepared preceptors, work space for learners, and your technology resources.[8] In addition, when scheduling students you should take into consideration your preceptors' availability, which could fluctuate during the holidays and school breaks. If there is a new service you are developing that would be sustained by pharmacy students, you may need to work closely with your school of pharmacy to ensure that you have a student every month of the year to ensure that the service impacting patient care continues without a lapse. Creating a master schedule incorporating the learner's level, the preceptors, the experiences, blocks, and availabilities (openings) offered will help you manage your

capacity. You also must determine if you will take students from one pharmacy school or multiple schools. Lastly, consideration must be made regarding acceptable ratios. Many states offer limits to the number of student interns per pharmacist, and the 2016 ACPE standards suggest no more than a two-to-one ratio.[1] **Appendix 15-1** has an example schedule coordinating introductory pharmacy practice experience (**IPPE**) students, advanced pharmacy practice experience (**APPE**) students, and residents. Once a schedule has been developed, you should review it and determine contingency plans for any holes in the calendar. How will the expanded patient care activities be completed if learners have scheduled time off from the practice site? One program addresses this challenge by developing a **gap rotation**, where students complete a nontraditional rotation incrementally during school breaks.[8] Another program utilizes evening and weekend hours for coverage.[5]

As each organization has specific requirements for orienting employees and nonemployees—in this case, residents and students—you should develop a plan for onboarding where the learners will be introduced to their new environments and responsibilities (see Chapter 8: Staff Development: 10 Factors to Guide Performance for a discussion on orientation). Orientation activities are also required per various accreditation bodies (e.g., ACPE, ASHP, and The Joint Commission). The duration of orientation activities will vary based on the duration of the experience and degree of previous experiences. For instance, a resident starting a new residency may have an extensive orientation that covers the facilities, computer systems, and expectations, while a resident starting their fourth rotation may just need to be oriented to the new responsibilities of the service. It is important to remember learners will have to comply with the employee or nonemployee orientation parameters as appropriate. **Table 15-3** reviews topics generally covered during orientation. Some of these requirements may be completed prior to learners starting the experience.

Managing Expectations

It is a good idea to review each stakeholder's expectations early in the experience, such as during orientation, to avoid disappointments. This is an opportune time for preceptors to define exemplary, passing, and deficient performance levels and behaviors, as well

Table 15-3. Topics to Cover During Orientation[a]

Orientation	Topics to Cover	Examples
Environment	Introductions	Key personnel including roles
	Introduction to practice	Tour, workspace, parking, restrooms, cafeteria, emergency exits
	Health and immunization requirements	Influenza vaccination policy
	Dress code	Badges, lab coat
	License and certification documentation	Intern license, basic life support (BLS) card
	Technology	Computer and documentation training
	Policies and procedures	Hospital, pharmacy, and nursing
	Dos and don'ts	
Experience	Overview of experience	Syllabus
	Preceptor expectations	Formal and informal assessment parameters
	Calendar	Typical hours and days for experience Due dates Absence procedure
	Baseline assessment	Career plans Previous experiences
	Learning activities	Daily responsibilities
	Evaluation process	Mechanisms and frequency of formal and informal evaluations
	Targeted training	Medication history, reconciliation processes, targeted disease-state education, and discharge education
	Dos and don'ts	

[a]For more information, see https://www.ashp.org/DocLibrary/MemberCenter/InpatientCare/APPEOrientationChecklist.aspx.

as reviewing patient care activities and the importance to the institution. A review of the individual learning and precepting styles should be incorporated into this discussion. Learners should have a good understanding as to why they will be asked to perform patient care activities and how success will be measured (i.e., number and type of interventions, HCAHPS [Hospital Consumer Assessment of Healthcare Providers and Systems] scores, etc.). This helps to ensure that learners understand their patient care responsibilities. Preceptors can use the orientation period to better understand the learners' expectations of the experience. This is the time to appreciate what skills and knowledge learners would like to obtain or how they can leverage this experience in developing their career plans. It is also an opportunity to review a preliminary calendar, as learners usually come into each experience anxious about the unknown. **Appendix 15-2** has an example of an APPE calendar. Program expectations are defined by the experience objectives set by the experiential or residency program director; **instructional objectives** describe what the learner will be able to do after completing the activity; and **learning objectives** incorporate the knowledge and skills the learner is expected to develop. Program expectations should be utilized in the assessment of the learner. Further clarification can be obtained by the program director. Students expect preceptors to have the following core values: professionalism, a desire to educate and share their knowledge, willingness to mentor, time committed for precepting, respect for others, and a willingness to work with a diverse student population.[9]

Team Approach

Using a team approach to provide orientation as a group can ensure all learners will have the same baseline guidance and similar expectations and maximize preceptor efficiency. Preceptors can rotate the orientation responsibilities, or a few preceptors can be designated to provide orientation at the beginning of each experience. Individual preceptors may still need to supplement the group orientation to cover rotation-specific matters and preceptor expectations. Ideally, the learners would have the same start date to help facilitate group orientation. Other opportunities for instilling team

spirit include collaborative patient and topic discussions. Learners can obtain perspectives from varied practitioners, in addition to allowing preceptors to divide time devoted to teaching thereby lessening their time commitment, which is often cited as a barrier to precepting. A conference room should be reserved for the same time each day with a schedule noting the topic and patient case discussions. You can also involve the department's pharmacists to divide up these sessions. This allows for more staff participation, ownership, and professionalism with the student development. You should have a master calendar with the appointments sent electronically to the students, and the staff member facilitating the session can attach prereading materials or worksheets to it. Some organizations repeat the topics every month to ensure all students who rotate through the site have the opportunity to focus on the topic. Organizations with a core group of students who are only at their site usually provide each topic once a year.

It is also important to consider the methods used for team teaching. It can be either a didactic lecture or a **flipped classroom** where the pharmacy students and/or residents prepare the materials and reading prior to coming to the session. The entire topic discussion is case-based active learning for a better application of the material rather than lectures that result in little subject matter retention. It is important to remember that the preceptor is ultimately responsible for the learner—especially students who practice under the preceptor's license. Pharmacy practice laws vary from state to state regarding student and resident training, so you should check with your state boards.

Opportunities for Layering

Organizations have used the layered learner model to provide pharmacy services. **Layered learning** involves the pharmacist overseeing the pharmacy residents (postgraduate year 1 and 2 [**PGY1** and **PGY2**]), pharmacy students (APPE and IPPE), and pharmacy technicians.[10] This approach is similar to that of the medical training model. The level of independence should be based on the learners' educational and clinical experiences (**Figure 15-1**). However, even using a team approach, each layer can exhibit precepting characteristics:

FIGURE 15-1. Layers of Learning with Respective Goals

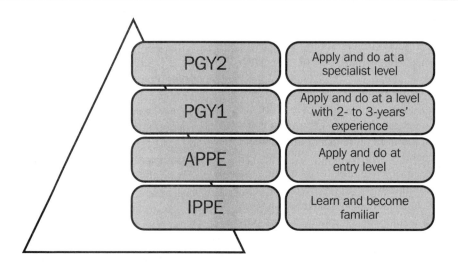

APPE = advanced pharmacy practice experience; IPPE = introductory pharmacy practice experience; PGY1 = postgraduate year 1; PGY2 = postgraduate year 2.

direct instruction, modeling, coaching, and facilitating.[2] In this method, each layer above the learner can help the learner with targeted skills and concepts with the preceptor having ultimate responsibility.

Block Scheduling for APPE Students

Block scheduling is when a student completes two or more APPEs at the same practice site. The pharmacy school and the practice site may require specific types and/or number of experiences to be completed and will determine whether the experiences will be consecutive or contingent on a successful application for competitive block scheduling.[8] The pharmacy department and the experiential program must discuss and agree on these requirements. Additionally, block programs can be incorporated into track programs to promote postgraduate training.[11] Advantages of block scheduling:

- Minimizing logistics
- Extending pharmacy services
- Increasing efficiency use of teaching resources
- Enhancing communication across experiences and preceptors

- Strengthening educational experiences continuity
- Developing opportunities to engage in longitudinal projects and patient care
- Building professional relationships and networks
- Preparing for practice and postgraduate training

Drawbacks of block scheduling include limiting practice site experiences and complacency regarding the learners' educational experience (i.e., perceptions of learners as cheap labor).[8] Block scheduling also affords both parties the opportunity for long-term, relationship building.

Keeping within the Boundaries of Accreditation Standards

Both ACPE and ASHP set accreditation standards for pharmacy school education and residency training, respectively. These standards are in place to ensure a minimum educational standard is met. Each accrediting body develops these standards based on the changing practice environments, feedback from stakeholders, and experience during accreditation visits. You must know the requirements for your practice site to ensure quality training is provided.

Precepting Tips

Assessment

The preceptor needs to provide assessment of the learner both formally and informally. At a minimum, feedback is conducted at the midpoint and end of the experience. Ongoing and midpoint evaluations typically are formative, where the learner has the opportunity to improve behaviors and optimize activities. A final evaluation is a summary of the learner's abilities during the stated experience. These evaluations are perfect opportunities for learners to apply your feedback to future experiences. If you completed evaluations on the first of a 4-month block, you are optimizing the learners' value to your institution for the next 3 months.

Learners should know exactly where and when the evaluations would be done, as well as which goals and objectives are tied to which activities. An example of mapping learning activities to goals can be found in **Table 15-4**.

Motivating Unmotivated Learners

In an ideal world, all learners would be motivated to provide the best patient care possible and secure all possible learning opportunities available at your practice site. However, that is not always the case. Even though each learner has made sacrifices to be at your site, not all learners are 100% committed. Learners have financial, personal, and educational competing factors. Residents could be behind on their research projects or be preparing for a pending presentation. Students could be juggling work with rotations or not interested in your practice setting. It is sometimes difficult to motivate learners to focus on the task at hand. Beginning with a proper orientation and training period will help empower learners to their patient care responsibilities. Also, frank discussions about the impact their rotational activities have on patient care can help with motivation, as will accountability for the results.

Summary

Providing educational opportunities for student and resident learners can be mutually beneficial for all parties. Learners will gain insight and practice experience, while preceptors can build their clinical competence and the organization can leverage existing resources to expand current clinical activities and patient care. Your organization's willingness to expand, capacity, learner scheduling, and any regulatory issues regarding experiential training must be considered. Expanding and augmenting pharmacy services have the potential to increase your department's visibility to patients and other healthcare providers.

Table 15-4. Mapping Goals to Learning Activities

Activity/Assignment	Specifications	Due Date	Goal
Accurately gathers, organizes, and analyzes patient information	Prior to team rounds	Ongoing	R2.4
Actively participates in internal medicine rounds	See calendar for team assignments and call schedule	Daily	R1.2 R2.4 R2.8
Provides therapeutic interventions during rounds and thereafter	Incorporating patient-specific and formulary considerations	Ongoing	R1.2 R2.2 R2.4 R2.6 R2.7 R2.8 R2.13

PRACTICE TIPS

1. Incorporating students and residents into your department can help to expand services, bring new ideas, and ensure up-to-date practices. It can help to expand services if hiring additional full-time employees is not an option.

2. Preparation before the students and residents arrive goes a long way for a successful learning experience. The coordinator's careful thought and consideration to orientation and team teaching will ensure that staff, residents, and students feel welcomed and part of the department and, in turn, they can be successful in their learning experiences.

3. At the beginning of the experience, the preceptor and the learner must set goals and expectations to ensure there is no miscommunication regarding the outcomes of the rotation.

4. Remember what it was like to be a student or resident. The experience will be enjoyable for all if you keep this in mind.

References

1. Accreditation Council of Pharmacy Education. Accreditation Council for Pharmacy Education draft standards 2016. 2014. https://www.acpe-accredit.org/pdf/Standards2016DRAFTv60FIRSTRELEASE VERSION.pdf. Accessed December 1, 2014.

2. ASHP. ASHP accreditation standard for postgraduate year one (PGY1). 2012:1-23. http://www.ashp.org/DocLibrary/Accreditation/ASD-PGY1-Standard.aspx. Accessed December 1, 2014.

3. ASHP. Pharmacy practice model summit: executive summary. *Am J Health-Syst Pharm.* 2011;68:1079-1085.

4. Bock LM, Duong MT, Williams JS. Enhancing clinical services by using pharmacy students during advanced experiential rotations. *Am J Health-Syst Pharm.* 2008;65(6):566-569.

5. Delgado O, Kernan WP, Knoer SJ. Advancing the pharmacy practice model in a community teaching hospital by expanding student rotations. *Am J Health-Syst Pharm.* 2014;71(21):1871-1876.

6. Wilhelm SM, Petrovitch E. Implementation of an inpatient anticoagulation teaching service: expanding the role of pharmacy students and residents in patient education. *Am J Health-Syst Pharm.* 2011;68(21):2086-2093.

7. Dalal K, Mccall KL, Fike DS, et al. Pharmacy students provide care comparable to pharmacists in an outpatient anticoagulation setting. *Am J Pharm Educ.* 2010;74(8):1-4. http://www.ajpe.org/doi/pdf/10.5688/aj7408139.

8. Hatton RC, Weitzel KW. Complete-block scheduling for advanced pharmacy practice experiences. *Am J Health-Syst Pharm.* 2013;70(23):2144-2151.

9. American Society of Health-System Pharmacists. Core values for preceptors. 2014. http://www.ashp.org/menu/MemberCenter/SectionsForums/NPF/DevelopmentalResources/CoreValuesforPreceptors.aspx. Accessed on December 15, 2014.

10. Pinelli NR. The layered learning practice model: toward a consistent model of pharmacy practice. 2013;(3). http://www.ashpfoundation.org/Pinelli Abstract. Accessed December 1, 2014.

11. New J, Garner S, Ragucci K, et al. An advanced clinical track within a doctor of pharmacy program. *Am J Pharm Educ.* 2012;76(3):43. http://www.ajpe.org/doi/pdf/10.5688/ajpe76343.

Suggested Reading

ASHP Preceptor Skills Resource Center. http://www.ashp.org/preceptorskillsASHP Preceptor Toolkit. http://www.ashp.org/menu/MemberCenter/SectionsForums/SICP/Resources/ASHPPreceptorsToolKit.aspx.

Local College or School of Pharmacy, Experiential Department. Pharmacy school locator: http://www.aacp.org/resources/student/pages/schoollocator.aspx.

National Association of Boards of Pharmacy. http://www.nabp.net/boards-of-pharmacy.

National Pharmacy Preceptor Conference. http://www.ashp.org/menu/events/conferences#nrpc.

Pharmacist's Letter. http://pharmacistsletter.therapeutic research.com/ptrn.

Appendix 15-1

Sample Yearly Schedule

Preceptor	IPPE	APPE	Resident Experience	May	Jun	Jul	Aug	Sept	Oct	Nov	Dec	Jan	Feb	Mar	Apr
P1	IPPE1		Orientation			R1 R2		I1, I2, I3, I4							
	IPPE2											I1, I2, I3, I4			
P2		IM	IM	A1			A3 R1	A5		A7		A9		A11	
P3		IM	IM			A2	A4 R2		A8		A6		A10		A12
P4		GenClin		A4		A2		A6		A8		A10		A12	
P5		Anticoag			A1	A3			A7		A5		A9		A11
P6		ED	ED	A3		A1	A2	A7 R1	A5 R2			A11		A9	
P7		TOC	TOC		A4			A8 R2	A6 R1				A12		A10
P8		CritCare	CritCare	A2		A4				A5 R1		A12 R2			
P9		Nutrition	Nutrition				A1			A7			A11 R1	A10 R2	
P10		ID	ID		A3					A8			R2		A9 R1
P11		Peds	Peds						A6						
P12		Admin	Admin							R1 R2					
P13		Elective								R2		R1		R1	R2

Admin = administration; Anticoag = anticoagulation; APPE = advanced pharmacy practice experience; CritCare = critical care; ED = emergency department; GenClin = general clinician; ID = infectious disease; IM = internal medicine; IPPE = introductory pharmacy practice experience; Peds = pediatrics; TOC = transitions of care.

Appendix 15-2

Sample APPE Calendar

Monday	Tuesday	Wednesday	Thursday	Friday	Student Assignments Due
26 Team A On Call	**27**	**28 Team B On Call**	**29**	**30 Team A On Call**	■ Pt monitoring (goal = 4) ■ 1 ADR/error ■ 1 intervention ■ 1 pt education ■ 3 pt discharge documenta-tions
■ 7:30 a.m.— Meet in hospital lobby ■ 8 a.m.— Morning report ■ 9:30 a.m.— Orientation/ syllabus review ■ 10:30 a.m.— Tour ■ 12 p.m.— Lunch ■ 1 p.m.— Computer orientation ■ 2 p.m.—Pt discharge training	■ 8 a.m.— Morning report ■ 9 a.m.— Rounds ■ 12 p.m.— Lunch ■ ~2 p.m.—Pt discharges ■ 4 p.m.—Pt presentation	■ 8 a.m.— Morning report ■ 9 a.m.— Rounds ■ 12 p.m.— Lunch ■ ~1 p.m.— Singer ABX rounds ■ ~2 p.m.—Pt discharges ■ 4 p.m.—Team B reports to ED	■ 8 a.m.— Morning report ■ 9 a.m.— Rounds ■ 12 p.m.— Lunch ■ ~2 p.m.—Pt discharges ■ 4 p.m.—Pt presentation	■ 8 a.m.— Morning report ■ 9 a.m.— Rounds ■ 12 p.m.— Lunch ■ ~2 p.m.—Pt discharges ■ 4 p.m.—Team A reports to ED	
2	**3 Team A On Call**	**4**	**5 Team B On Call**	**6**	■ Pt Monitoring (goal = 5) ■ Rough draft in-service ■ 1 ADR/error ■ 2 interventions ■ 2 pt education ■ Journal club ■ 5 pt discharge documenta-tions
■ 8 a.m.— Morning report ■ 9 a.m.— Rounds ■ 12 p.m.— Lunch ■ ~2 p.m.—Pt discharges ■ 4 p.m.— Pneumonia discussion	■ 8 a.m.— Morning report ■ 9 a.m.— Rounds ■ 12 p.m.— Lunch ■ ~2 p.m.—Pt discharges ■ 4 p.m.—Team A reports to ED	■ 8 a.m.— Morning report ■ 9 a.m.— Rounds ■ 12 p.m.— Lunch ■ ~1 p.m.— Singer ABX rounds ■ ~2 p.m.—Pt discharges ■ 4 p.m.— Acute MI discussion	■ 8 a.m.— Morning report ■ 9 a.m.— Rounds ■ 12 p.m.— Grand rounds ■ ~2 p.m.—Pt discharges ■ 4 p.m.—Team B reports to ED	■ 8 a.m.— Morning report ■ 9 a.m.— Rounds ■ 12 p.m.— Lunch ■ ~2 p.m.—Pt discharges ■ 4 p.m.— Journal club and midpoint evaluation	

Monday	Tuesday	Wednesday	Thursday	Friday	Student Assignments Due
9 Team B On Call	*10*	*11 Team A On Call*	*12*	*13 Team B On Call*	▪ Pt monitoring (goal = 5) ▪ Final in-service ▪ 1 ADR/error ▪ 2 Interventions ▪ 2 pt education ▪ 7 pt discharge documenta-tions
▪ 8 a.m.—Morning report ▪ 9 a.m.—Rounds ▪ 12 p.m.—Lunch ▪ ~2 p.m.—Pt discharges ▪ 4 p.m.—Team B reports to ED	▪ 8 a.m.—Morning report ▪ 9 a.m.—Rounds ▪ 12 p.m.—Lunch ▪ ~2 p.m.—Pt discharges ▪ 4 p.m.—VTE discussion	▪ 8 a.m.—Morning report ▪ 9 a.m.—Rounds ▪ 12 p.m.—Lunch ▪ ~1 p.m.—Singer ABX rounds ▪ ~2 p.m.—Pt discharges ▪ 4 p.m.—Team A reports to ED	▪ 8 a.m.—Morning report ▪ 9 a.m.—Rounds ▪ 12 p.m.—In-Service ▪ ~2 p.m.—Pt discharges ▪ 4 p.m.—Pt presentation	▪ 8 a.m.—Morning report ▪ 9 a.m.—Rounds ▪ 12 p.m.—Lunch ▪ ~2 p.m.—Pt discharges ▪ 4 p.m.—Team B reports to ED	
16	*17 Team B On Call*	*18*	*19 Team A On Call*	*20*	▪ Pt (goal = 5) ▪ 1 ADR/error ▪ 2 interventions ▪ 2 pt education ▪ 7 pt discharge documenta-tions ▪ Final case ▪ Final exam
▪ 8 a.m.—Morning report ▪ 9 a.m.—Rounds ▪ 12 p.m.—Lunch ▪ ~2 p.m.—Pt discharges ▪ 4 p.m.—Pt presentations	▪ 8 a.m.—Morning report ▪ 9 a.m.—Rounds ▪ 12 p.m.—Lunch ▪ ~2 p.m.—Pt discharges ▪ 4 p.m.—Team B reports to ED	▪ 8 a.m.—Morning report ▪ 9 a.m.—Rounds ▪ 12 p.m.—Lunch ▪ ~1 p.m.—Singer ABX rounds ▪ ~2 p.m.—Pt discharges ▪ 4 p.m.—Prepare for final presentation and exam	▪ 8 a.m.—Morning report ▪ 9 a.m.—Rounds ▪ 12 p.m.—Lunch ▪ ~1 p.m.—Singer ABX rounds ▪ ~2 p.m.—Pt discharges ▪ 4 p.m.—Team A reports to ED	▪ 8 a.m.—Morning report ▪ 9 a.m.—Rounds ▪ 12 p.m.—Lunch ▪ ~1 p.m.—Pt discharges ▪ 3 p.m.—Final case presentation and exam ▪ 4 p.m.—Final evaluation	
28	29	30			
Team A: Debbie and Andy			Team B: Jennifer and Georgia		

ABX = antibiotics; ADR = adverse drug reaction; ED = emergency department; MI = myocardial infarction; pt = patient; VTE = venous thromboembolism.

CHAPTER 16

Putting It All Together: The Effective Clinical Coordinator

Lynn Eschenbacher

Introduction

Being a clinical coordinator is an excellent opportunity to see if you enjoy the management aspect of pharmacy. It is a great first step from only participating in direct patient care activities. The blend between developing a clinical practice and maintaining the management/leadership side of pharmacy will help you determine opportunities for your future. Some pharmacists find they really enjoy a blend of both and remain clinical coordinators their entire career. Some pharmacists find they really miss the day-to-day direct patient care activities and return to being clinical pharmacists. Finally, some pharmacists find they enjoy management and leadership and pursue leadership roles. The wealth of available opportunities is why it's great to be a pharmacist.

Clinical Practice, Staff Development, Competency, and Trust

Keeping up your clinical practice can be challenging. You must stay on top of the recent evidence-based medicine by reading journals and critically evaluating the information, as well as subscribing to Listservs to see what your peers are considering in their practices. Using this information to determine areas of advancement for the pharmacy department is critical to expand and develop existing services. You and your staff can make a positive impact on patient care by having and using a clear strategic plan to guide your involvement in the organization and provide a strong infrastructure. Hardwiring your department with a long-term strategic plan that will be nimble and adjusting with acute trends will ensure your staff and senior leaders are confident in your leadership abilities. In addition, you must keep your staff members up-to-date by using active-learning techniques, such as the flipped classroom and small groups. Assessing their competency so you know they are retaining and applying what you have taught them is essential. Having the best ideas and new services to start are not enough to ensure success if your team is not ready or is not making the correct patient care recommendations. You need to invest in your staff on a continual basis and reassess that knowledge as well. It is important to be an authentic leader who is clear and transparent with your staff. The more your staff trusts you, the more effective you will be in implementing new ideas or services. Above all, you must do your best not to violate that trust. Sometimes you will have to make decisions that will be difficult, and sometimes you may not be able to share all information, but if your staff members know that you have their best interest in mind, you will succeed. Always think about how you would want to hear the message and what you would want to know.

Key Relationships and Project Management

Developing trust with those outside of your department will help ensure your success as a clinical coordinator. You will be collaborating with many departments, including patient safety, risk management, finance, materials management, nursing, and medical staff. Developing the foundation and infrastructure for these relationships far in advance of needing them is key to your effectiveness. It is much easier to work with people you already know rather than cold-calling them when you need a favor, their opinion, or assistance in critical times. Within your department, clinical and operations staff work extremely close together and need to be aware of what each other is doing. As a clinical coordinator, your responsibilities extend beyond clinical areas to include a strong operations component. For example, in pediatrics the best practice would be pulling up individual oral syringes for each patient rather than having bulk bottles for the nurses to pull up their own doses. The clinical aspect could be helping to determine the medications and dosing, and the operations aspect would be where to perform pulling up the oral syringes, which oral syringes to use, and how to build this in the informatics systems.

You should be involved in all aspects of an initiative to ensure safe and effective implementation for the patients and the staff. Your guidance and feedback to each team working on the initiative will ensure its success. When the initiative is ready for implementation, you should clearly communicate to your staff members the new expectations and hold them

accountable. If an initiative is initially followed, but within 6 months it is no longer used, then you must determine if there is a better way to do it, if staff members need a refresher on the process, and if they need a reminder about your expectations and their accountability for adhering to the plan. You will gain respect if you clearly set expectations and hold employees accountable. Helping staff members understand why an initiative is being implemented increases better adoption and incorporation into their daily routine.

Clinical Expertise—Formulary and Cost-Savings Ideas

As the department's clinical expert, it is imperative that you keep up with evidence-based medicine to ensure you implement and provide the best patient care. Reviewing order-sets and computerized prescriber order-entry programming on the front end, as well as analyzing the outcome data for prescribing patterns and patient outcomes on the back end, will ensure procedures are making a positive difference. In your clinical coordinator role, you will make recommendations and work with expert decision teams to review new formulary medications and utilization of current medications to ensure optimal patient outcomes. You will also need to determine if there are therapeutically equivalent outcomes or opportunities to restrict based on providing more cost-effective use of the medications. You should subscribe and use Listservs, collaborate with your network of clinical coordinators, and read available literature. Coming up with ideas for cost savings based on improving patient outcomes might seem difficult at first. If you begin with a report of the highest in dollars and highest in volume, you can start at the top and brainstorm opportunities. Ideas could include alternative medications, different presentations (a vial and bag rather than a premixed product), restrictions based on indications, or using a generic drug instead of a brand name drug. You should conduct medication-use evaluations (MUEs) on a monthly basis to ensure the policies, guidelines, and restrictions you recommended to the pharmacy and therapeutics (P&T) committee are still in place and followed. You can use students, residents, pharmacy technicians, and pharmacists to help with the MUEs. Keep a list of all the suggested

MUEs available for students who might need to complete a project.

Finance

It may seem strange as a clinical coordinator to need to know so much about finance, but in today's healthcare environment, you must be well versed in the terminology, monitor weekly and monthly reports, and be proactive with budgets. In the area of full-time equivalent (FTE) management, you need to understand how many employees you can hire based on the staffing model that you want to deploy. If you want to have pharmacists on all the patient care units, you must determine which units, which times of the day, and what other services to offer. Do you need just one pharmacist to do anticoagulation monitoring or antimicrobial stewardship? If so, that would require two or more dedicated FTEs. However, if you educate your staff members and have assessed their competence, then you can build that into their daily workflow; the result would be more expansive coverage of the patient care areas rather than one person dedicated to each service. Also, remember to count in nonproductive time. When staff members are on vacation, taking a sick day, or at a conference, this counts into each month's final FTE budget numbers. You also need to assist with developing the annual drug budget as well as maintaining the monthly adherence to the budget. If your department is grossly over the budget, you will need to assist with analyzing the data to determine, for example, which medication(s) went over budget. Then you can determine if there is a future strategy. If it was a nonformulary medication, you should work with the prescribers and the pharmacists to decide if the medication could be administered in an outpatient setting.

Medication Safety and Accreditation

If there is no medication safety officer or accreditation manager assigned to your department, then, as the coordinator, it is your responsibility. If there are pharmacists working in these other roles, the coordinator is responsible for working closely with staff members to ensure they are knowledgeable and incorporating these processes into the daily workflow. The coordinator should also review the medication safety information to determine if there are trends or opportunities to modify practices and make them safer. The coordinator might be a part of a root cause analysis or failure mode and effects analysis and should be well educated on all aspects of the process. If an error occurred, it is important to ascertain the facts rather than assume what happened. The coordinator will often need to talk with the front-line employee involved in the incident. Remember to be caring, listen, and ask questions. You want to be careful not to lead the employee to answer the way you think he or she should answer. It might be a difficult conversation with the employee, so it is imperative that you find a private place to talk. If the employee is upset by the discussion, he or she may need to take time away from patient care to calm down and not make another error. You need to determine if the error was a system breakdown or if the employee violated a safety practice. Based on the answer, you will need to either help fix the system or address the issue with the employee and human resources if there was a violation.

For accreditation, you must ensure you know all the rules and regulations. For example, if you are being surveyed by The Joint Commission, you need to know the Medication Management Standards and the National Patient Safety Goals. It is necessary to proactively inspect your areas and ensure your staff knows the information and is prepared for a survey visit. There are many checklists and fun ways to keep your staff informed and involved, such as morning huddles, bulletin boards, or electronic postings.

Human Resources—Building and Managing the Team

Staff involvement, buy-in, and team work are very important to your success and, ultimately, directly contribute to the best patient care. You need to invest in your team members through individualized time to know more about them and their career plans, their skill sets, and their competency. Working with them individually will help them grow and develop. As a team, foster collaboration and teamwork to benefit patient care. If your staff members work in silos, they will not know if another area desperately needs help. Working as a team will enable you to achieve more. Develop staff satisfaction by knowing what is important to them. Listen to how they want to be rewarded and recognized for a good job. Rewards and recognition do not have to always cost money. Some creative ways to recognize staff include handwritten notes, a simple trophy or award that is passed around based on certain performance practices or scheduling benefits. The schedule will probably be a big part of what you do unless you have a dedicated scheduler. You must have a clear staffing model and know if you want to have 8-hour, 10-hour, or 12-hour shifts, or a combination. Do you allow only full-time staff, or do you have part-time and supplemental staff? Once you decide how you want to staff your department, you can build a schedule based on requested days off and preferences. The earlier you can create the holiday schedule, the more satisfied your staff members will be so they can make plans accordingly.

Onboarding and orientation are critical to set the clear expectations from the first day so that staff members will know what they need to do to be successful. Your orientation program should cover all aspects of their jobs. Checklists to ensure all areas are covered are important (e.g., for general orientation, sterile compounding, order entry, automated dispensing cabinets, anticoagulation, pharmacokinetics, controlled substances, progress notes, pediatrics, chemotherapy, and antimicrobial stewardship). Setting expectations is essential so that you can hold your staff accountable. Staff members need to know that if they do not meet expectations, there will be repercussions. You should reset the expectations at least annually with the new strategic plan as well as review these at each staff meeting. You should also share with the staff your progress toward achieving the strategic plan. Expectations should be reviewed annually and individually as needed. If someone is not meeting expectations, it is essential to have that crucial conversation as soon as possible.

Be real and authentic in your conversation. They are never easy, but over time, you will become more comfortable having these conversations. Your human resources department can help with wording conversations. Take notes when talking with the human resources representatives so that you have those talking points for your discussion with the employee. Always document your conversations and keep a record in your files.

You should also mentor your staff members or help them find mentors. Encourage them to get involved in state and national pharmacy organizations as well as doing posters and presentations. Your staff can also get involved by precepting students and residents or facilitating topic discussions. There are many opportunities to invest in your staff, and the more you do the more successful you and your department will be.

Vision

You will set the clinical tone for the department. Do you have a vision for what the pharmacists should be doing? What services should they be providing? What does the practice model look like? Are the pharmacists on the patient care areas? You will develop the plan and then prepare the staff to fulfill that plan every day. Share your vision with the staff, your leadership, and the hospital leadership. As pharmacists we need to do a better job of making sure the chief executive officer, chief operating officer, and the chief nursing officer, etc., knows what value pharmacy can bring to the organization and why we need to be involved in the direct patient care. You need to demonstrate what pharmacists can do and share those stories of "great catches" and how we made a difference. As a coordinator, you are the champion and cheerleader for pharmacy involvement and all that we can do.

Monitoring to ensure that your vision is actually making a positive impact is important. You may want to add something new, but that may mean it is necessary to stop doing something that they are currently doing. How do you decide what adds the most value? You need to routinely follow metrics and measures to determine the value added by the pharmacists and technicians. There are many different metrics that you can monitor. For medication safety, voluntary reports should not be trended to measure a safety improvement because these are reliant on the staff taking the time to report and knowing what to report. Voluntary reports are a good measure of the culture of safety and triggers; systematic surveillance is a good measure of improvement in safety.

Benchmarking and productivity measures can be difficult and are not always an accurate reflection of what is truly being done. There are many ways to measure, and you need to know what your organization uses as well as its pros and cons so that you can speak to the variances when asked and advocate for other methods if the current one does not accurately reflect your team's work.

You are the leader of your team. Surround yourself with individuals that you believe will lead to a successful team. Invest in your team and develop them. If you set high expectations and hold them accountable, you and your team will achieve great things. Try not to micromanage your team, but give them guidance and support where needed. Treat your team how you would want to be treated, and you and your team will be successful.

Clinical Services

Often you may want to expand services but may not have the FTEs that you can hire. Here are two suggestions that do not require hiring additional FTEs. First, you can collaborate with the schools of pharmacy for pharmacy student rotations. Ask if they can provide a student every month so that you can provide the service consistently. You would not want to stop the service in July and December because there are no students in those months. This is an excellent opportunity to have a progressive, hands-on rotation for students to apply their learning. A second option is to develop your staff members' competency so they can incorporate the service into their daily workflow. Services that could be decentralized include antimicrobial stewardship, anticoagulation dosing and monitoring, pharmacokinetic dosing and monitoring, code response, and transitions of care.

To further develop clinical services, you can help the staff identify clinical opportunities for interventions. Use alerts to signal when a specific criterion is met or if a specific action is required. The action that the pharmacist takes could either be automatic based on a P&T protocol, or the pharmacist could contact the physician. Metrics can be documented on the number and types of interventions made. In addition, you can help improve overall patient care by modifying an order set or updating a process.

Leading from the Middle

As a clinical coordinator, you are often in the middle—between the front-line staff and the senior management. You try to represent the staff, learn about politics, and effectively run a department to provide value to the organization. The middle can be a difficult place. Staff members may think you do not understand or represent them, and the department's leadership may wonder why you do not address certain decisions. Remember to do your best and, if you use all the advice and guidance from this handbook, you will be a successful pharmacy clinical coordinator.

Time Management

Sometimes it is difficult to balance all of your clinical practice duties, such as addressing human resource issues; developing other clinical practices and services; investigating clinical therapeutic and standardization opportunities that align with evidence-based medicine; being involved in professional organizations; precepting students and residents; investing in your staff members through education; and providing pertinent feedback to staff members so they can provide the best patient care. Scheduling time for each activity may be one strategy; however, acute issues may come up that need immediate attention. Being flexible is important, but also be careful because your time can be consumed with projects and requests. Time management is critical to ensure you meet deadlines and promptly address issues. It might take some time to figure out how to prioritize, so consult with your direct boss to see if you are correctly identifying priorities. It can be challenging as a coordinator to identify your top priority. Try to determine a process that shows the organization's global focus so that you can try to align your department's priorities. Patient care and human resource issues usually are top priority. Remember that addressing issues immediately is the best practice.

Your Development

Be thoughtful about your career development. Develop a network of clinical coordinators through your state organizations or national professional pharmacy organizations. Identify several mentors for feedback and coaching. Your mentors can help you grow and develop as well as act as a sounding board when you need advice. Make sure you keep in touch on a regular basis and do not just contact them when you need something. Take time to build the mentor relationship and nurture it. Get involved at the state or national levels. Join a committee or group working on a project. Work or collaborate on a research project, prepare a poster or a presentation, or submit a proposal to present at a meeting. Consider precepting students, participating on a panel for a class discussion, or presenting a topic for a class. The more involved you are, the more your career and overall satisfaction will benefit. Be a mentor to others. Introduce your mentee at professional organizations. Pharmacy is a small world, and you can really help to develop your relationships as well as those you mentor.

Words of Wisdom from Our Contributors

Carrie Berge: There will be many opportunities for a clinical coordinator to expand or improve clinical pharmacy services; do not become overwhelmed with all the choices. Pick one that you and your health system feel strongly could be improved or optimized. Take advantage of the tools this handbook provides, and reach out to your ASHP network.

Jennifer Burnette: Be team-oriented. Promote a primary focus on team achievements rather than individual success. As the formal team leader, set a team-centric tone by using *we* instead of *I*. When you or someone on your team wins, then the entire team wins.

Steve Carlisle: Cutting-edge, best practice clinical pharmacy programs must exist in concert and in support of state-of-the-art dispensing and operational excellence. All programs and all staff must work together to help create, maintain, and evolve departmental practices and policies. Patient care, morale, and overall success will suffer if operational and clinical services function in silos. Significant thought and effort must be dedicated to obtaining global pharmacy and institutional support for all clinical programs. Only by working together can all pharmacy team members ensure that the myriad of critical components of pharmacy services function as they should. With appropriate effort and coordination, clinical pharmacy programs will be a shining star within a successful and innovative pharmacy department.

Noelle Chapman: *"If you don't like something, change it. If you can't change it, change the way you think about it."* I love this quote adapted from Maya Angelou as I think it encompasses the power we all have as individuals to embrace various situations. It is easy to get caught in the weeds and lose sight of your goals or to get frustrated with perceived boundaries. However, I hope in those moments this centers you and reminds you that we always have the power to alter our own viewpoint to be more effective, accepting, understanding, and fearless.

Jean Douglas: The song by the Rolling Stones, "You Can't Always Get What You Want" says hard work and creative thinking are needed to achieve goals. Clinical coordinators never seem to have enough time, have the staff to do what is desired, complete all the training plans and protocols, or get in front of the key decision maker at the exact time needed. What a clinical coordinator *does* have is the opportunity to lead those who want to provide patient care services, prevent drug-related problems, precept future pharmacists, and make the most of the resources and talents available to drive patient pharmacotherapy outcomes. There is no one path to follow; decide what you want, and build on your needs with all of your gusto.

Robert Granko: Adapted in part from Richard St. John's *8 to Be Great: The 8-Traits That Lead to Great Success*, this is my take on the eight (plus my two add-ons) to be great! These secrets of success have helped guide me through my last decade of leadership and have served as an anchor for me personally and professionally as I continuously strive to self-improve. I share these with all learners in the hopes that they interpret and apply them in their own way.

1. *Purpose and Intent*—What do I want to achieve and what are my reason(s) for doing it? Your personal and professional purpose should answer that question. Your purpose will help you through the personal and professional obstacles that will be placed in your path.

2. *Work Hard*—Commit to working hard *and* smart while having fun; celebrate your wins no matter how small, and take time to reflect on what has made your particular initiative successful or not.

3. *Practice*—Practice makes you great and recognized as an expert in your field. You must hone your craft over and over, all the while learning and self-reflecting. It has been said that it takes 10,000 hours of investment in a particular area to be considered an expert.

4. *Focus*—Given the multitude of what we have to manage, having a focused and detailed plan in place may not ensure success, but it will certainly improve your odds. Work to actively prune nonvalue-added activities through a planned abandonment approach. If select daily activities do not add personal or professional value, work to shed them and repurpose saved time.

5. *Push*—You have to want to be successful. If you are struggling, reach out to those around you who re-energize you and fill/refill your reserves. Pay this forward *and* backward—repaying those who have filled your buckets and those that need their buckets filled.

6. *Network*—You must develop and cultivate a strong network. This is easy to accomplish by doing for, and investing in, those around you in a kind, thoughtful, and considerate way.

7. *Serve*—Strive to be a servant leader, genuinely enriching and inspiring those around you. This applies both to formal and informal leadership positions. If you have to ask, permission is granted!

8. *Share Ideas*—Share your many ideas, develop them, be courageous, build consensus and momentum around them, and deploy them. When your ideas don't work, try #5: Push (above). Help others with their ideas and problems; be inquisitive, watchful, and ask thoughtful and helpful questions

9. *Be Persistent*—You must ethically persist through doubts, through criticism, and through it all. Your core and emotional intelligence quotient can serve as your compass.

10. *Sustain Family Relationships*—You must not lose focus on having both personal *and* professional success. Your family unit is key to your sustained success, and as leaders we must remain cognizant that we continuously borrow from the ones we love. Be sure to replace what you take, and do your very best to leave it better than you found it.

David Hager: The coordinator position is an organization's recognition of a need for focus on an area of weakness or perceived lack of quality. This means tangible results are expected and required, oftentimes very rapidly, because patient outcomes or regulatory compliance is at risk. A great organization, however, will recognize that large-scale transformative change will require more than expertise and hard work. Nothing in healthcare can be fixed by one person; the field is much too interprofessional and collaborative (or political depending on your perspective) to allow for unilateral decision making. When you start your new position, ask that your organization provide 60 to 90 days to meet people from across the organization so that you can understand the current environment before results are required. Even if you have worked at the organization for years, ask for this time so you can look at the issues with a new perspective and view the department from the perspective of an outside consultant. Beginning without these relationships and understanding the environment in which you are operating could lead to unnecessary political entanglements and opposition to needed change. When you implement your first set of improvements, carefully measure the impact. This methodical process will have meaningful results at the end and will ensure you begin your new position in a position of strength, rather than desperation.

Jenna Huggins: Relationship building has the power to turn your ideas into reality. If someone seems like they may be a good contact for an aspect of healthcare where pharmacists could have an impact, foster that relationship. It almost always will prove useful in the future.

Scott Knoer: There are several universal truths to personal and leadership success. The first is that every day is a job interview. Your colleagues and staff will notice how you treat others and how you solve problems. Healthcare is a small world, and how you act today will impact how you are perceived tomorrow. It is also important to have a positive attitude and a bias for *yes*. Successful leaders can "smell" opportunity and capitalize on it to move initiatives forward. If you are viewed as a can-do team member who achieves results, you will be given more opportunity. Seizing opportunity creates success, and success breeds more success. Finally, it is critical to nurture relationships if you want to be effective. Very few people put their heart into accomplishing tasks because they have to. People achieve greatness when they are passionate about issues and because they want to serve patients. Creating a compelling vision and demonstrating your commitment to improving patient care will make people want to help you achieve it.

Laurimay Laroco: From my clinical coordinator experience, I have learned a tremendous amount about pharmacy management strategies. One of the most important aspects of my job is that I am able to incorporate staffing my clinical area of expertise into my coordinator schedule. This is the same area of practice where my employees directly staff in, as well as the area of practice where I can implement new pharmacy clinical services. By actively participating in this area, I gain respect and trust from my team members as well as directly experience their daily workflows. This experience gains me important insight when reviewing their performance, targeting the team's areas for improvement and strengths, identifying new ideas for clinical pharmacy services and its feasibility into the workflow, and understanding employees' areas of concern or issues. Lastly, through this opportunity, I work side by side with the physicians, nurses, and other healthcare professionals, which allows me to build important relationships to support my pharmacy team, assist in identifying new ideas where my team can support or manage, and create a sense of trust and teamwork that

facilitates implementation of new services or initiatives. Find ways to stay active into your team's daily workflows and to work with other healthcare professionals in your team's area of practice.

Bob Lobo and Mark Sullivan: Those of us who are entrusted to make policy decisions on behalf of patients should always keep in mind the purpose of the healthcare enterprise, which is to provide optimal patient outcomes. When it comes to medication-use policy decisions, the clinical coordinator must balance this purpose with the potential economic and operational challenges that are unique to each health system. When the clinical coordinator engages a broad array of pharmacy, nursing, and medical staff members and includes them in the process, the best medication-use policy decisions and, ultimately, the most optimal patient outcomes occur.

Trista Pfeiffenberger: Learn who the informal leaders are in your work group. Informal leaders influence the group's response to changes and new initiatives without having a position of authority. You want to know who these people are and learn how to work with them early in the process of a new initiative so that they are onboard and can assist with implementation instead of creating any resistance. If your work group's informal leaders generally go with the flow, then at a minimum you will want to notify them of new initiatives or changes shortly before implementation. If your informal leaders generally resist change, then you may need to engage them in any new initiative or change process very early on so that they have some degree of ownership in it.

Jennifer Schultz: It is so easy to get bogged down with your projects and emails. Remember that success begins with the relationships you develop with your staff members. Put them first and help them to develop. I used to try to "fix" whatever people wanted, and I ended up so overwhelmed with tasks that I was not proactive in building and maintaining work relationships. Now, I prioritize my projects and have developed staff councils that I can rely on to fix many of the issues that must be resolved. This system has nurtured ownership and accountability. Don't forget about yourself; continue to develop your own skills in leadership and clinical practice. Also, practice a work–life balance to prevent yourself from burnout. One of the most rewarding aspects of my professional career has been my active involvement in ASHP. I encourage you to get involved in a professional pharmacy organization as it will help keep you excited about the pharmacy profession and help you develop a large professional network. Lastly, love your job! You have the power to mold your position into one that brings meaning to your career and your organization. All the best to you!

Antonia Zapantis: It is essential to make contacts with individuals in similar positions at different organizations. You always hear networking is important, but you don't realize how important it is until you have a situation that you don't know how to best approach. These colleagues can share experiences and help you through your problem.

Rhonda Zillmer: Focus on building and maintaining strong relationships with those inside pharmacy as well as outside pharmacy, such as nursing, physicians, respiratory, etc. When you need their assistance and support, they will know who you are and understand your role. Maintain regular and open communication with your direct supervisor. Find out your manager's specific initiatives or tasks and identify ways your work supports their needs. Use your regularly scheduled one-on-one meetings with your manager to share your tasks or projects, discuss anticipated requests or needs, and inquire what your manager needs from you. It is important for your manager to be informed about what you are doing.

Do walking rounds. Spend time each week walking the floors and checking in with the frontline pharmacists. This is especially important if in your role as coordinator you are not staffing in these areas. These walking rounds allow you to get the pulse of their daily activities and observe where your staff members are succeeding, what challenges they are facing, and how you can support them.

Be sure to finish pilots. Often new ideas, assignments, or tasks start as pilot projects. We often must start a pilot project in one unit or during one time of the day. Work hard to implement pilots that are transferrable to a departmental or hospital-wide level. Otherwise, you may end up with a boutique or concierge-type service that is not sustainable or available to all who could benefit from it.

Connect with others outside of your department and hospital, and push yourself to build and maintain these relationships. They will help you to continue and grow yourself professionally. These may be local and national pharmacy organizations, universities, or a network of colleagues at other local hospitals. The key is to push yourself to stay open to other ideas and practice models that you could implement in your own practice setting.

Closing Thoughts

Being a clinical coordinator is a great opportunity to try something new. As pharmacists, we are lucky because there are so many opportunities. If you are just thinking about taking the job, have already taken the job, or have been in the job for years, the advice in this book should help you determine if this is the next step you want to take, how to start the new role, and how to enhance what you are already doing. You have a lot of opportunities to do your best and be as successful as you can to ultimately impact patients and their healthcare.

Index